Handbook of
Hypertension

This is book is dedicated to my loving and wonderful parents, R.R. Houston and Mary Ruth Houston, my incredible wife, Laurie, and all of my marvelous children, Helen Ruth, Marcus (Bo), John, and Kelly. Without them, and God, I could not have achieved my dreams, my goals, or received all of the blessings in my life. I am thankful and grateful.

Handbook of Hypertension

Mark C. Houston, MD, MS, FACP, FAHA

Associate Clinical Professor of Medicine
Vanderbilt University School of Medicine
Director, Hypertension Institute and Vascular Biology Section
Saint Thomas Hospital and Health Services
Nashville, Tennessee, USA

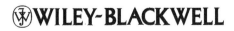

A John Wiley & Sons, Ltd., Publication

Library of Congress Cataloging-in-Publication Data
Houston, Mark C.
  Handbook of hypertension / Mark C. Houston.
      p. ; cm.
  Includes bibliographical references and index.
  ISBN 978-1-4051-8250-8
  1. Hypertension—Handbooks, manuals, etc. I. Title.
  [DNLM: 1. Hypertension—Handbooks.   2. Antihypertensive Agents—therapeutic use—Handbooks.
  3. Hypertension—drug therapy—Handbooks. WG 39 H843ha 2009]
    RC685.H8H653 2009
    616.1'32—dc22

                                                                          2008039512

ISBN: 978-1-4051-8250-8

A catalogue record for this book is available from the British Library.

Set in 7.75/10.5 pts, Frutiger light by Macmillan Publishing Solutions

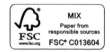

Contents

Part 5 The Clinical Trials of Hypertension

Part 6 Special Considerations in the Management of Hypertension Based on the Hypertension Clinical Trials

Part 7 The Antihypertensive Drugs

The author would like to kindly acknowledge Ralph Hawkins MD, LLM, FRCPC for his contribution on the "Kidney and Hypertension" section which was incorporated and revised from the previous handbook: Hypertension Handbook for Clinicians and Students, 2005, ANA Publishing in Birmingham, AL, USA.

Abbreviations

ACE	angiotensin-converting enzyme
Ang-II	angiotensin II
ARB	angiotensin II receptor blocker
AV	atrioventricular
BB	beta-blocker
BP	blood pressure
BUN	blood urea nitrogen
CHD	coronary heart disease
CHF	congestive heart failure
CO	cardiac output
CRF	chronic renal failure
CVA	cerebrovascular accident
D	diuretic
DBP	diastolic blood pressure
DHEAS	dehydroepiandrosterone sulfate
DHP	dihydropyridine
EPI	epinephrine
GFR	glomerular filtration rate
GITS	gastrointestinal therapeutic system
HCTZ	hydrochlorothiazide
HDL	high-density lipoprotein
HR	heart rate
HsCRP	high sensitivity CRP
IBW	ideal body weight
IGCP	intraglomerular capillary pressure
ISA	intrinsic sympathomimetic activity
IVP	intravenous pyelogram (pyelography)
LDL	low-density lipoprotein
Lp(a)	lipoprotein A
LVFP	left ventricular filling pressure
LVH	left ventricular hypertrophy
MAO	monoamine oxidase
MAP	mean arterial pressure
MI	myocardial infarction
MIBG	metaiodobenzylguanidine
MRI	magnetic resonance imaging
MSA	membrane-stabilizing activity
NE	norepinephrine
NPI	neuro-peptidase inhibitors
NSAIDs	nonsteroidal anti-inflammatory drugs
PET	positron emission tomography
PFTs	pulmonary function tests
PIH	pregnancy-induced hypertension
PRA	plasma renin activity
PWP	pulmonary wedge pressure
RAAS	renin–angiotensin–aldosterone system

RBC	red blood cell
RBF	renal blood flow
RI	renin inhibitor
RPF	renal plasma flow
RVR	renal vascular resistance
SARA	serum aldosterone receptor antagonist
SBP	systolic blood pressure
SNS	sympathetic nervous system
SV	stroke volume
SVR	systemic vascular resistance
TPA	tissue plasminogen activator
UTI	urinary tract infection
VLDL	very-low-density lipoprotein
VMA	vanillylmandelic acid

Part 1
General Introduction to Hypertension

Handbook of Hypertension. By M.C. Houston. Published 2009 by Blackwell Publishing, ISBN: 978-1-4051-8250-8

Hypertension Prevalence and Consequences

Hypertension is one of the major risk factors for coronary heart disease (CHD), myocardial infarction (MI), cerebrovascular accidents (CVA), chronic renal failure (CRF), and congestive heart failure (CHF) in the United States and in westernized or industrialized countries around the world. In industrialized countries, the risk of becoming hypertensive (blood pressure [BP] >140/90 mm Hg) over a lifetime is >90%. CHD is the leading cause of death in the United States, accounting for more than 800 000 deaths per year (more than one death per minute), and CVA is the fourth leading cause of death in the United States.

The annual expenditure for CHD is over 200 billion dollars [1–3]. Essential hypertension is defined as an increase in BP of unknown cause that increases the risk for cardiovascular (CV) diseases such as cerebral, cardiac, large artery, and renal events. However, subclinical vascular target organ damage (TOD) occurs very early in the course of hypertension and can be identified with noninvasive testing. These subtle CV findings include left ventricular hypertrophy (LVH), diastolic dysfunction, microalbuminuria, abnormal vascular compliance, and abnormal cognitive dysfunction or vascular dementia.

Hypertension Syndrome

Hypertension is a part of heterogeneous condition that is best described as an atherosclerotic syndrome or hypertension syndrome with genetic and acquired structural and metabolic disorders (Figure 1) including the following [4, 5, 147]:

1. Dyslipidemia or hyperlipidemia
2. Insulin resistance, impaired glucose tolerance, and diabetes mellitus (DM)
3. Central obesity (android or portal obesity)
4. Endocrine and neurohormonal changes (sympathetic nervous system [SNS], Renin-Angiotensin-Aldosterone System [RAAS])
5. Renal function abnormalities (sodium, water, uric acid, protein load excretion, and microalbuminuria)
6. Abnormalities of vascular and cardiac smooth muscle structure and function such as arterial compliance abnormalities with loss of arterial elasticity, diastolic dysfunction, and LVH.
7. Membranopathy and abnormal cellular cation transport (Ca^{++}, Mg^+, Na^+, and K^+)
8. Abnormalities of coagulation (prothrombotic)
9. Endothelial dysfunction
10. Vascular inflammation (high sensitivity C-reactive protein [HS-CRP])
11. Aging
12. Accelerated atherogenesis

**The Hypertension syndrome—
It's more than just blood pressure**

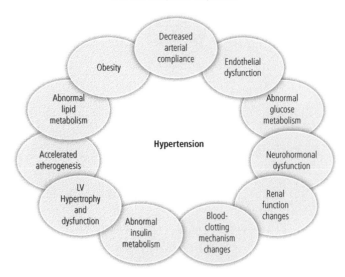

It is estimated that over 70% of patients with genetic hypertension have one or more of the coexisting metabolic or functional disorders that increase the risk of vascular damage, artherosclerosis, and target organ damage.

Figure 1 The Hypertension Syndrome.

Subsets of Hypertension Approach to Treatment

By definition, all antihypertensive drugs lower BP, which is clearly the most important determinant for the reduction of CV risk. However, differences exist among the various antihypertensive drug classes, as well as within the same class, with respect to target organ disease and prevention of major CV events. The majority of hypertensive patients will require two or more drugs to reach newer BP goals, and those hypertensive patients with high risk for CV disease will need concomitant statin use as well to maximize CV risk reduction. However, despite effective drug for hypertension, the majority of patients around the world remain uncontrolled, with the United States having the best overall BP control.

The clinician seeking optimal antihypertensive drug therapy must recognize a myriad of new challenges and concepts. Individualization of treatment is recommended on the basis of *the subsets of hypertension approach* [5]. An essential component of individualized treatment is a logical and tailored selection of drug therapies based on:

1. Pathophysiology and vascular biology
2. Renin and aldosterone profiling
3. Hemodynamics
4. Risk factor reduction and end-organ damage reduction
5. Concomitant medical diseases or problems
6. Demographics
7. Quality of life (QOL) and adverse effects of treatment
8. Compliance with therapy
9. Total health care cost

This will be discussed in detail in the following chapters.

Clinical Hypertension Trials: A Perspective

This first edition of *The Hypertension Handbook* includes many new concepts, changes in philosophy, clinical information, clinical trials, new antihypertensive drugs, and nonpharmacological treatment. Large-scale clinical trials comparing the older antihypertensive drug regimens with newer agents have been completed, and many others are in progress. The recently published studies include Antihypertensive Therapy and Lipid Lowering Heart Attack Prevention Trial (ALLHAT), Anglo-Scandinavian Cardiac Outcomes Trial (ASCOT), TROPHY, International Nifedipine GITS Study: Intervention as a Goal in Hypertension Trial (INSIGHT), Nordic Diltiazem Study (NORDIL), Losartan Intervention For Endpoint reduction in hypertension (LIFE), African American Study of Kidney Disease and Hypertension (AASK), Randomized Evaluation of NIDDM with the Ang-II antagonist Losartan (RENAAL), Irbesartan Diabetes Nephropathy Trial (IDNT), IRMA, Controlled Onset Verapamil Investigation of Cardiovascular Endpoints (CONVINCE), ANBP-2, Valsartan Antihypertensive Long-Term Use Evaluation (VALUE), JIKEI, and MOSES.

The Systolic Hypertension Trial in Europe (SYST-EUR), Shanghai Trial of Nifedipine in the Elderly (STONE), Systolic Hypertension in China (SYST-CHINA), Hypertension Optimal Treatment (HOT), and the Chen-Du Nifedipine Trial, INSIGHT, NORDIL, NIC-EH, CONVINCE, Prospective Randomized Evaluation of Vascular Effects of Norvasc Trial (PREVENT), Verapamil in Hypertension and Atherosclerosis Study (VHAS), Study Group on Long-term Antihypertensive Therapy (GLANT), Practitioners Trial on the Efficacy of Antihypertensive Treatment in the Elderly (PATE), Swedish Trial in Old Patients–2 (STOP-2), VALUE, ALLHAT, and ASCOT have documented significant reductions in CV and cerebrovascular morbidity and mortality with calcium channel blockers (CCBs), especially the dihydropyridine CCBs.

The Captopril Prevention Project (CAPPP) and ANBP-2 showed that angiotensin-converting enzyme inhibitors (ACEIs) reduce CV morbidity and mortality in hypertensive patients equal to or better than conventional diuretic and beta-blocker (BB) therapy. The Heart Outcomes Evaluation (HOPE) and EUROPA studies showed that ACEIs reduced CV death in a high-risk nonhypertensive population.

The treatment of the hypertensive patient with DM with proteinuria has now been shown in SYST-EUR, CAPPP, RENAAL, IDNT, IRMA, LIFE, VALUE, and ASCOT to be better with ACEIs, Angiotensin receptor blockers (ARBs), and CCBs than with conventional diuretic or BB therapy in reducing CV morbidity and mortality.

The STOP-2 showed that calcium blockers and ACEIs are equal to conventional therapy in reducing CV morbidity and mortality and superior in reducing CVA and equal BP levels. The PROGRESS trial, STOP-2, MICROHOPE, QUIET, SCAT, AASK, Appropriate Blood Pressure Control in Diabetes Trial (ABCD), ALLHAT, Fosinopril and Amlodipine Cardiac Events Trial (FACET), GLANT, ANBP-2, and PATE have proven significant reductions in CV morbidity and mortality with ACEIs.

New data on BBs, serum aldosterone receptor antagonists (SARAs), ACEIs, and ARBs in cardiac disease (CHF, MI, and post-MI as well as angina) are positive as well.

ARBs (Losartan) significantly reduced cerebrovascular and CV morbidity and mortality in the LIFE trial. Valsartan reduced CV morbidity and mortality in the VALUE trial. Eprosartan reduced CV morbidity and mortality in the MOSES trial. Prehypertension treatment reduced CV events in the TROPHY trial with candesartan.

ASCOT clearly demonstrated that in the high-risk hypertensive patient, the combination of a statin (atorvastatin) with antihypertensive agents significantly reduced all CV events compared with placebo. The combination of atorvastatin with amlodipine +/− perindopril was superior to the BB/diuretic combination in all CV events and in reducing the onset of type 2 DM.

No single antihypertensive drug can meet every need in all hypertensive patients. However, emerging clinical trials indicate that CCBs, ACEIs, ARBs, SARAs, and the newer alpha/beta-blockers have distinct advantages in reducing CV risk, type 2 diabetes, and renal disease compared with treatment with diuretics and the older BBs. The new vasodilating BBs and renin inhibitors (RIs) also have excellent BP control, metabolic, and vascular effects. Clinical trials are in progress with the drug classes. Combination antihypertensive therapy has gained foothold an initial treatment. Fortunately, the armamentarium is large and rapidly growing.

Vascular Biology and Hypertension

The goals in the treatment of hypertension are to reduce intra-arterial pressure, improve vascular biology, vascular health, treat the hypertension syndrome optimally, and reduce TOD (Figure 2). Ideally, the optimal treatment should maximize reduction in all end-organ damage, including CHF, CHD, MI, CVA, CRF, LVH, large arterial disease, as well as total mortality.

Recent advances in our understanding of the physiology and pathophysiology of the blood vessel show that endothelial function, inflammation, oxidative stress, autoimmune vascular dysfunction, and abnormal arterial compliance play an important role in end-organ damage. Attention must be directed at promoting *vascular health* in order to achieve optimal reduction for end-organ damage. The accurate assessment of global CV risk is required in each patient in order to select the optimal antihypertensive regimen as well as appropriate concomitant therapy for dyslipidemia, DM, renal disease, or other CV diseases and risk factors.

The blood vessel is an organ. In fact, it is the largest organ in the body, about five times the heart in mass and six times as tennis court in area. The vascular system regulates vascular health and tone through a chronic active balance between vasoconstrictors, inflammatory/autoimmune mediators, oxidative stress mediators, procoagulants, and growth promoters vs. vasodilators, anti-inflammatory/autoimmune mediators, antioxidants, anticoagulants, and growth inhibitors (Figures 3 and 4).

Figures 5 and 6 illustrate the complexity of the processes mediated by the endothelium in carrying out its various regulatory functions. The vasorelaxant substances nitric oxide (NO), prostacyclin, and endothelium-derived hyperpolarizing

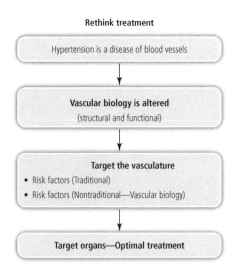

Rethink treatment

Hypertension is a disease of blood vessels

↓

Vascular biology is altered
(structural and functional)

↓

Target the vasculature
• Risk factors (Traditional)
• Risk factors (Nontraditional—Vascular biology)

↓

Target organs—Optimal treatment

Figure 2 New Approach to Hypertension Treatment.

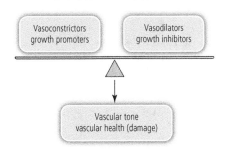

Figure 3 The Balance for Vascular Tone.

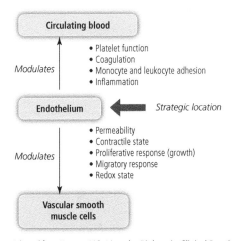

Adapted from Houston MC. *Vascular Biology in Clinical Practice* 2000.

Figure 4 The Vascular Endothelium: Strategic Location and Modulation Factors in Blood and VSM.

factor (EDHF) released by the endothelium promote vasodilation and inhibit growth of vascular smooth muscle cells (SMCs). Ang-II and endothelin are potent vasoconstrictors and growth-promoting factors released from the endothelium. Bradykinin, through a receptor-mediated mechanism, stimulates release of NO. Increased expression of angiotensin-converting enzymes (ACE) in the endothelium escalates production of Ang-II and degradation of bradykinin, leading to decreased synthesis/release of NO from the endothelium. NO prevents platelet adhesion/ aggregation and mediates synthesis of tissue plasminogen activator (t-PA), whereas Ang-II promotes platelet aggregation and formation of plasminogen activator inhibitor-1 (PAI-1).

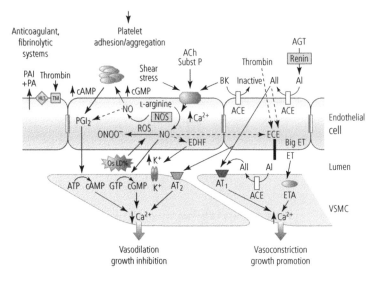

Figure 5 Functional Endothelium.

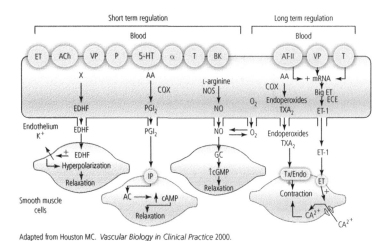

Adapted from Houston MC. *Vascular Biology in Clinical Practice* 2000.

Figure 6 Endothelium-Dependent Responses (Not Present in All Blood Vessels).

Blood Vessel Structure

The walls of the artery consist of the intima, media, and adventitia (Figure 7). The intima, the smooth inner lining of the vessel, comprises the endothelium and underlying connective tissue. Metabolically active endothelial cells line the lumen.

The middle layer, the media or muscularis, comprises SMCs that are surrounded by an extracellular protein matrix containing collagen, elastin fibers, fibroblasts, and an internal elastic lamina. Small arteries contain greater proportions of smooth muscles than large arteries. The media of large arteries (e.g., the aorta) has a relatively large amount of elastic tissue.

The adventitia, or outer layer of the arterial wall, comprises connective tissue that acts to maintain the shape of the vessel and limit distention. The structural heterogeneity in large vs. intermediate vs. small vessels is potentially important in terms of disease processes and therapeutic responsiveness.

The Blood Vessel Structure

■ Serosa   ■ Muscularis   ■ Endothelium

Structural and functional changes may cause dysfunction leading to vascular damage and target organ damage

The Arterial Wall

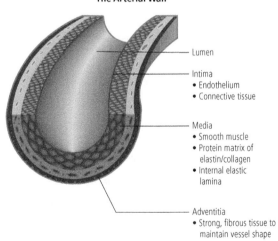

- Lumen
- Intima
  - Endothelium
  - Connective tissue
- Media
  - Smooth muscle
  - Protein matrix of elastin/collagen
  - Internal elastic lamina
- Adventitia
  - Strong, fibrous tissue to maintain vessel shape

Modified from Ross R. Atherosclerosis—An Inflammatory Disease. *N Engl J Med* 1999; 340:115–126; Mulvany MJ, Aalkjaer C. Structure and function of small arteries. *Physiol Rev* 1990; 70: 921–961.

Figure 7 Blood Vessel Structure.

Endothelial Function and Dysfunction

The endothelial function and dysfunction is shown in Figure 8.

Normal vascular functions of endothelium

Maintain tone (vasodilation and vasoconstriction) and structure
Regulate cell growth and migration
Regulate thrombotic and fibrinolytic properties
Mediate inflammatory, oxidative st ress, and immune mechanisms
Regulate leukocyte and platelet adhesion to surface of endothelium
Modulate oxidation (metabolic activity)
Regulate permeability

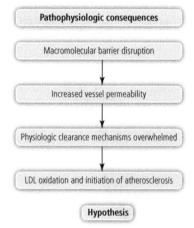

Definition

■ Injury or activation of the endothelial cell leads to altered endothelial function that may promote disease

■ The dysfunctional state may be characterized by numerous features such as an imbalance between endothelium-derived relaxing and contracting factors or growth-promoting factors

Pathophysiologic consequences

Macromolecular barrier disruption

↓

Increased vessel permeability

↓

Physiologic clearance mechanisms overwhelmed

↓

LDL oxidation and initiation of atherosclerosis

Hypothesis

■ Normal endothelium maintains balance between relaxant and constrictive factors

■ Endothelial dysfunction promotes vasoactive substance imbalance
↓ NO (nitric oxide)
↑ tissue ACE
↑ Ang-II

From Lüscher TF. *J Myocard Ischemia 1995;* 7(Suppl. 1): 15–20.
ACE = angiotensin-converting enzyme; Ang-II = angiotensin-II; LDL = low-density lipoprotein.

Figure 8 Endothelial Dysfunction.

Endothelial dysfunction

Physiological dysfunction
1. Vasospasm (vasoconstriction vs. vasodilation)
2. Thrombosis (procoagulant vs. anticoagulant)
3. Atherosclerosis (proinflammatory, oxidative stress, autoimmune vs. anti-inflammatory, antioxidative stress, and antiautoimmune)
4. Restenosis (growth promotion vs. inhibition)

Structural dysfunction
1. Vascular hypertrophy
2. Vascular hyperplasia
3. Vascular polyploidy

The process of endothelial dysfunction
Injury or activation of the endothelial cell leads to altered endothelial function that may promote disease (Figure 8). The dysfunctional state may be characterized by numerous features such as an imbalance between endothelium-derived relaxing and contracting factors or growth-promoting factors.

Pathophysiologic consequences include
Macromolecular barrier disruption
Increased vessel permeability
Physiologic clearance mechanisms overwhelmed
Low-density lipoprotein (LDL) oxidation and initiation of atherosclerosis
From Lüscher TF. *J Myocard Ischemia* 1995; 7 (Suppl. 1): 15–20.

New Treatment Approach to Hypertension Based on Concepts of Endothelial Dysfunction and Vascular Biology

Hypertension is a disease of the blood vessel in which the vascular biology is altered. A myriad of emerging, nontraditional and traditional CV risk factors lead to oxidative stress, inflammation, and autoimmune dysfunction of the vasculature (Figures 9 and 10). The endothelial and vascular wall dysfunction leads to atherosclerosis and TOD. It is imperative that new treatment approaches be directed at both the abnormal vascular biology and the hypertension in order to achieve optimal vascular health and reduce CV events (Figures 8 and 9). New treatment concepts and clinical hypertension trials suggest that the best drugs for CV risk reduction include CCBs, ACEIs, and ARBs. The SARAs, RIs, and third generation alpha/beta and vasodilating BBs show promising early data as well. However, the use of diuretics and first- and second-generation BBs (nonselective, cardioselective, and those with intrinsic sympathomimetic activity [ISA]) should be discouraged as

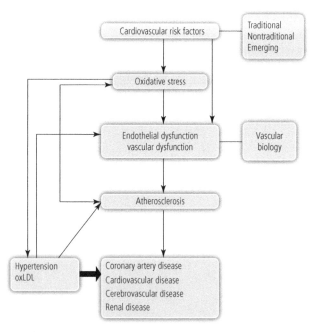

Oxidative stress to the blood vessels plays a major role in directly inducing endothelial dysfunction, vascular smooth muscle dysfunction, and atherosclerosis. Thus, oxidative stress is the mediator between cardiovascular risk factors and target organ damage.

oxLDL = oxidized low-density lipoprotein.

Figure 9 Key Concepts in Endothelial Dysfunction, Atherosclerosis, CV Disease, and CHD [155A].

first or event second-line therapy due to adverse effects on glucose, DM, other metabolic disturbances, and possibly renal dysfunction with long-term use.

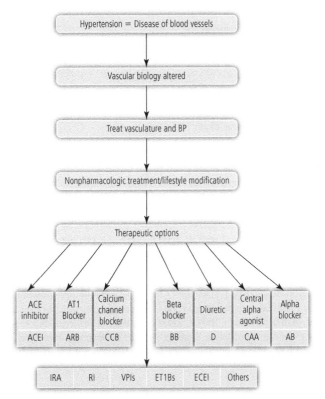

ECEI = endothelin-converting enzyme inhibitor; ETIB = endothelin receptor blocker type B; IRA = imidazolindine receptor antagonist; RI = renin inhibitor; VPI = vasopeptidase inhibitor.

Figure 10 New Treatment Approach.

Treatment of Impaired Endothelial Function: A Global CV Approach

- Cholesterol lowering (statins, fibrates, niacin, resin binders, small intestinal cholesterol inhibitors, nutraceuticals, nutrition, weight reduction, exercise, lifestyle changes, etc.)
- Antioxidant, vitamins, and minerals
- Weight reduction and improve body composition
- ACEIs
- ARBs
  RIs
  SARAs
- CCBs
- Omega-3 fatty acid supplementation
- Exercise training (aerobic and resistance)
- Improve insulin resistance (diet, weight reduction, metformin, thiazolidinediones, sitagliptin, and glucose intestinal uptake inhibitors, etc.)
- Low-dose aspirin (81 mg); optimal nutrition and other lifestyle modifications
- Lower homocysteine with vitamin B6, B12, and folate
- Discontinue all tobacco products

Hypertension is a disease of the blood vessel, which is characterized by endothelial dysfunction and abnormalities of vascular smooth muscle that precede clinical CV events by decades. Essential hypertension is a syndrome consisting of a constellation of metabolic, functional, and structural abnormalities that increase global CV risk and must be considered when selecting the best antihypertensive agents. Emerging clinical data suggest that CCBs, ACEIs, and ARBs have beneficial effects on CV events beyond their BP lowering effect and are preferred therapy in most patients with hypertension. The RIs, vasodilating BB, and alpha/beta-blockers also have excellent early clinical data. Diuretics, with the exception of indapamide, and the first- and second-generation BBs have taken a secondary or tertiary role in the treatment of hypertension.

Part 2
What is Hypertension

Handbook of Hypertension. By M.C. Houston. Published 2009 by Blackwell Publishing,
ISBN: 978-1-4051-8250-8

Hypothesis: Essential Hypertension and End-Organ Damage

The primary goal in the treatment of essential hypertension is to prevent and reduce all end-organ damage by reducing BP, improving various components of the hypertension syndrome, and promoting optimal vascular health or vascular biology (endothelial function and vascular smooth muscle function and structure). Hypertension is associated with an increased risk of cerebrovascular, CV, and renal morbidity and mortality. Pharmacologic therapy with some antihypertensive drug classes has partially reduced some, but not all, of these complications [5]. To achieve optimal decreases in morbidity and mortality in hypertension-related diseases, the overall impact of antihypertensive drug therapy on vascular risk factors, risk markers, vascular biology, and the pathogenesis of damage to each end organ must be considered.

Although a higher percentage of deaths occurs in patients with diastolic blood pressure (DBP) > 105 mm Hg, patients with DBP < 105 mm Hg account for more deaths [5]. The majority of patients with hypertension have the mild form [5]. The risks of therapy vs. the benefits of therapy are particularly critical in this group. Pharmacologic therapy of mild to moderate hypertension (DBP < 110 mm Hg) has reduced the complications of most pressure-related (arteriolar) damage such as CVA, CHF, and some cases of CRF, but the atherosclerotic complications (CHD, angina, MI, and sudden death) have not been reduced to the extent predicted by the degree of BP reduction in those prospective clinical trials in which diuretics and BB were the primary antihypertensive drugs used [5]. The only exception, to date, for this statement is the Antihypertensive and Lipid-Lowering Treatment to Prevent Heart Attack Trial (ALLHAT), in which the fatal and nonfatal CHD primary endpoint was equivalent among the chlorthalidone, amlodipine, and lisinopril treated subjects [150]. It should be noted, however, that this was a high-risk elderly population (average age of 67 years) prospective clinical trial with numerous methodological flaws when left open to question many of the ALLHAT investigators conclusions about the role of diuretics in the treatment of hypertension [150].

Systolic hypertension has emerged as an equal or more sensitive predictor of CV risk in most age groups (especially after age 50) than diastolic pressure [5, 213, 238]. The selection of initial and combination antihypertensive drug therapy is a complex decision based on numerous factors such as goal BP, concomitant risk factors, renal function, age, gender, race, metabolic and hemodynamic parameters, pathophysiology, vascular biology, adverse effects, compliance, economics, and finally, clinically proven ability to reduce TOD. The role of BB monotherapy in reducing CHD in the elderly has been questioned [130]. Recent studies indicate that BBs are no longer recognized as appropriate therapy in any patient with essential hypertension due to inferior reduction in central aortic pressure and all clinical CV events including CHD, MI, CVA, and total mortality [130, 222–227]. In addition, the indiscriminate use of some diuretics (hydrochlorothiazide [HCTZ], chlorthalidone, and thiazide-like diuretics, but not indapamide) in hypertensive patients may be associated with a higher incidence of insulin resistance, glucose intolerance, new onset of type 2 DM, renal cell carcinoma, and progressive renal insufficiency [90, 148, 222, 228–232, 234–237].

There is even a suggestion in many clinical trials of superiority of some antihypertensive drugs in reducing specific TOD (i.e., CCB for CVA; ACEI, ARB for CRI; ACEI, ARB, or diuretic for CHF; CCB, ACEI, ARB for CHD and MI) [5, 226, 238, 239].

A more sophisticated pharmacologic approach based on pathophysiology and our knowledge of vascular biology, endothelial dysfunction (ED), and the complex interplay of the components of the hypertension/atherosclerotic syndrome is reviewed in this *Handbook of Hypertension*.

Hypertension Classification and Guidelines Worldwide

Hypertension in the United States and Classification and JNC 7 [213]

1. Approximately 50–60 million people in the United States have hypertension with a BP reading >140/90 mm Hg [6]. Only 27% of this population has their hypertension under control according to National Health and Nutritional Examination Survey III (NHANES III) (Figures 11 and 12) and only 31% have it under control according to NHANES IV (Table 1).

2. *Joint National Committee 7 (JNC 7) Guidelines*: Classification and management of BP for adults aged 18 years or older [213] (Table 2).

3. Prevalence rates: highest in African Americans, men, and the elderly. African Americans have the greatest morbidity and mortality [5, 238].

4. Hypertension occurs in approximately 60% of non-Hispanic whites, 70% of non-Hispanic blacks, and 61% of Mexican Americans aged 60 years or older [6] (Figure 13).

5. A large proportion (60%) of the excess mortality, disability, and morbidity attributable to hypertension occurs among those with stage I hypertension [6].

6. Hypertension is the most common medical problem seen by the US physicians, accounting for more office visits and prescriptions than any other disease [5, 238]. The annual cost is over 10 billion dollars.

7. In the United States and other industrialized societies, BP increases with age, especially systolic blood pressure (SBP) [5, 238].

8. SBP and wide pulse pressure (PP) correlate with TOD better than DBP in most age groups except younger patients (<50 years of age). The higher the BP the greater is the TOD with a linear increase in CV events per 1 mmHg of BP [5, 213, 238, 240].

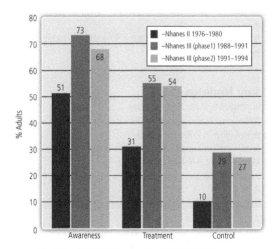

Adapted from Burt et al. *Hypertension* 1995; 25: 305–313.
NHANES = National Health and Nutritional Examination Survey.

Figure 11 NHANES III: High Blood Pressure in US Adults (1976–1994).

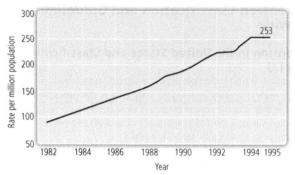

Adapted from Burt et al. *Hypertension* 1995; 25: 305–313.

Figure 12 NHANES III: Cardiovascular Disease Trends (End Stage Renal Disease).

Table 1 Trends in the Prevalence, Awareness, Treatment, and Control of High BP in Adults in the United States (1976–1994)*

Percent	NHANES II	NHANES II (Phase 1)	NHANES III (Phase 2)	NHANES IV (Phase 3)
	1976–1980	1988–1991	1991–1994	1994–2000
Awareness	51	73	68	68.9
Treated	31	55	53	58.4
Controlled	10	29	27	31

Adapted from Ref. [217].
DBP = diastolic blood pressure; NHANES = National Health and Nutritional Examination Survey; SBP = systolic blood pressure.
*Adults with hypertension (SBP > 140 mm Hg or DBP > 90 mm Hg) or taking antihypertensive medication. Age 18–74 years.

NHANES IV: key findings [217]

NHANES IV: key findings are illustrated in Tables 3–5.
- Hypertension prevalence in the United States increased from 25% in 1988 to 28.7% of the population in 2000 (p = 0.5).
- Hypertension awareness remained unchanged in 2000 compared to 1988 (68.9% in 2000 vs. 69.2% in 1988) (p = 0.58).
- Hypertension treatment has increased since 1988 from 52.4 to 58.4% (p = 0.007).
- Hypertension control overall has increased from 24.6% in 1988 to 31% in 2000 (p = 0.05).
- BP control among hypertensive diabetics has not improved since 1988 (28.5% achieving contemporary target in 1988, 25.4% achieving target BP in 2000) (p = 0.70).

Conclusion: Hypertension prevalence in the United States is increasing, and control rates are unacceptably low.

Table 2 Joint National Committee 7 (JNC 7). Classification and Management of BP for Adults Aged 18 Years or Older

BP classification	Systolic blood pressure (mm Hg)*		Diastolic blood pressure (mm Hg)*	Management*		
				Lifestyle modification	Initial drug therapy	
					Without compelling indications	With compelling indications
Normal	<120	and	<80	Encourage		
Prehypertension	120–139	or	80–89	Yes	No antihypertensive drug indicated	Drug(s) for the compelling indications[†]
Stage I hypertension	140–159	or	90–99	Yes	Thiazide-type diuretics for most; may consider ACEI, ARB, BB, CCB, or combination	Drug(s) for the compelling indications[†] Other antihypertensive drugs (diuretics, ACEI, ARB, BB, CCB) as needed
Stage II hypertension	≥160	or	≥100	Yes	Two-drug combination for most (usually thiazide-type diuretics and ACEI or ARB or BB or CCB)[‡]	Drug(s) for the compelling indications Other antihypertensive drugs (diuretics, ACEI, ARB, BB, CCB) as needed

Adapted from *JAMA*, May 21, 2003; 289 (19).

ACEI = Angiotensin-converting enzyme inhibitor; ARB = angiotensin receptor blocker; BB = beta-blocker; BP = blood pressure; CCB = calcium channel blocker.

*Treatment determined by highest BP category.

[†]Treat patients with chronic kidney disease or diabetes to BP goal of <130/80 mm Hg.

[‡]Initial combined therapy should be used cautiously in those at risk for orthostatic hypotension.

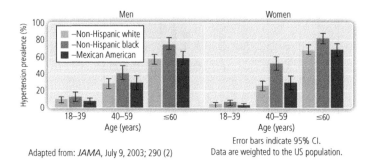

Error bars indicate 95% CI.
Adapted from: *JAMA*, July 9, 2003; 290 (2)   Data are weighted to the US population.

Figure 13 Hypertension Prevalence by Age and Race/Ethnicity in Men and Women.

Hypertension Guidelines

JNC 7 key recommendations [213]
1. In people >50, SBP is a more important risk factor for CVD than DBP.
2. CVD risk doubles with each 20/10 mm Hg BP increment above 115/75 mm Hg.
3. People with SBP 120–139 or DBP 80–89 mm Hg should be considered prehypertensive and require lifestyle modifications to prevent CVD.
4. Thiazide-type diuretics should be used either alone or in combination for most patients with uncomplicated hypertension. (*Note:* Most authorities and worldwide hypertension guidelines do not agree with this recommendation or its validity, nor do I.) Certain high-risk conditions are compelling indications for use of other agents as first-line therapy (ACEI, ARB, CCB, BBs).
5. Most patients require two or more drugs to achieve goal BP (<140/90 or <130/80 mm Hg especially for patients with diabetes or chronic kidney disease).
6. If BP is >20/10 mm Hg above target level, consider initiating therapy with two agents one of which should be a thiazide-type diuretic. (*Note:* Most authorities and worldwide hypertension guidelines do not agree with this recommendation to use thiazide diuretics as initial or second drug therapy in most patients, nor do I.)
7. Clinician empathy builds trust and motivates patients to comply with therapy.

Canadian Hypertension Society [214, 247]
Canadian Hypertension Education Program (CHEP) Recommendations [214, 247]:
    "Based on ALLHAT, is it fair to conclude that diuretics should be recommended as sole 'first line' therapy in the management of hypertension in patients without other compelling indications?" Considering the evidence to date, the answer would have to be "No." (Quoted from CHEP 2003 Recommendation Summary.) Please refer to Table 6 for specific guideline recommendations for drug therapy. These are updated in 2007 [247] and are very similar to JNC 7.

European Societies of Hypertension and Cardiology Guidelines (ESH–ESC) [215, 241, 242, 243]
"Emphasis on identifying the first class of drugs to be used is probably outdated by the need to use two or more drugs in combination in order to achieve goal BP" [215].
    These guidelines have been updated in 2007 [241–243].

Table 3 Age-Specific and Age-Adjusted Prevalence of Hypertension by Sex and Race/Ethnicity [217]. In the US Population, 1988–2000[a]

Characteristics	Prevalence, % (SE)			Change, 1988–2000	
	1988–1991	1991–1994	1999–2000	% (95% CI)	p-Value
Age-specific data					
Age, years					
18–39	5.1 (0.6)*	6.1 (0.6)*	7.2 (1.1)*	2.1 (−0.3 to 4.5)	0.05
40–59	27.0 (1.4)*	24.3 (2.2)*	30.1 (1.8)*	3.1 (−1.4 to 7.6)	0.09
>60	57.9 (2.0)	60.1 (1.1)	65.4 (1.6)	7.5 (2.4 to 12.5)	0.002
Age-adjusted (to 2000 US population) data					
Overall	25.0 (1.5)	25.0 (1.7)	28.7 (1.8)	3.7 (0 to 8.3)	0.02
Sex					
Men	24.9 (2.1)	23.9 (2.6)	27.1 (2.7)	2.2 (−4.5 to 8.9)	0.26
Women	24.5 (1.7)	26.0 (1.8)	30.1 (2.4)	5.6 (0 to 11.4)	0.03
Race/ethnicity					
Non-Hispanic white	25.9 (1.8)	25.6 (2.1)	28.9 (2.3)	3.1 (−2.7 to 8.7)	0.14
Non-Hispanic black	28.9 (2.2)	32.5 (2.1)**	33.5 (3.2)**	4.6 (−3 to 12.2)	0.12
Mexican American	17.2 (1.6)*	17.8 (2.0)*	20.7 (2.7)*	3.5 (−2.7 to 9.7)	0.13
Sex and race/ethnicity					
Men					
Non-Hispanic white	26.7 (2.7)	24.4 (2.4)	27.7 (3.4)	1.0 (−7.5 to 9.6)	0.41
Non-Hispanic black	29.1 (3.3)	29.5 (2.9)	30.9 (4.9)b	1.8 (−9.8 to 13.4)	NA
Mexican American	17.9 (2.6)	17.8 (1.8)	20.6 (3.9)b	2.7 (−6.5 to 11.9)	NA
Women					
Non-Hispanic white	25.1 (2.1)	26.8 (2.3)	30.2 (3.1)	5.1 (−2.2 to 12.4)	0.09
Non-Hispanic black	28.6 (2.7)	35.0 (2.7)	35.8 (4.2)b	7.2 (−2.6 to 17.0)	NA
Mexican American	16.5 (2.2)b	17.9 (2.1)b	20.7 (3.4)	4.2 (−3.8 to 12.2)	NA

Adapted from Ref. [217].
NA = Not Applicable due to unreliable data.
[a]Data are weighted to the US population.
[b]Estimates are unreliable because of National Health and Nutrition Examination Survey minimum sample size criteria or coefficient of variation of at least 0.30.
**p < 0.01 for the difference among racial/ethnic groups, with non-Hispanic whites as referent, or for the difference among three age groups, with >60 years as referent.
*p < 0.001 for the difference among racial/ethnic groups, with non-Hispanic whites as referent, or for the difference among three age groups, with >60 years as referent.

Table 4 Multiple Regression Analysis [217]. Association Between Hypertension Prevalence, Demographic Factors and BMI

Factors	Regression Coefficient (SE)		
	1988–1991	1991–1994	1999–2000
Age (per 1-year increase)	1.2 (0.04)*	1.2 (0.03)*	1.3 (0.04)*
Sex (referent: women)	3.5 (1.3)	0.03 (0.7)	1.4 (1.5)
Race/ethnicity (referent Mexican American)			
Non-Hispanic white	−1.1 (0.9)	−0.2 (1)	0.6 (1.4)
Non-Hispanic black	7.0 (1.4)*	10 (0.1)*	8.2 (1.7)*
BMI (per 1 unit of increase)[a]	1.3 (0.07)*	1.3 (0.1)*	1.2 (0.1)*
R^2	0.30	0.30	0.31

Adapted from *JAMA*, July 9, 2003; 290 (2): 203.
[a] Body mass index (BMI) was calculated as weight in kilograms divided by the square of height in meters.
* $p < 0.001$ for the independent association between hypertension prevalence and each factor after adjusting for the remaining factors.

Table 5 Awareness, Treatment, and Control Among Participants with Hypertension [217]. US Population, 1988–2000

Characteristics	Prevalence, % (SE)			Change, 1988–2000	
	1988–1991 ($n = 3045$)	1991–1994 ($n = 3045$)	1999–2000 ($n = 1565$)	% (95% CI)	p-Value
Awareness	69.2 (1.3)	67.8 (l.8)	68.9 (1.5)	−0.3 (−4.2 to 3.6)	0.58
Treatment	52.4 (1.4)	52.0 (1.0)	58.4 (2.0)	6.0 (1.2–10.8)	0.007
Control					
Among those treated	46.9 (2.2)	43.6 (1.7)	53.1 (2.4)	6.2 (0–12.6)	0.03
Among all with hypertension	24.6 (1.4)	22.7 (1.1)	31.0 (2.0)	6.4 (1.6–11.2)	0.004
<140/90 mm Hg (among treated hypertensive diabetic individuals)	53.1 (4.5)	41.6 (5.8)*	46.9 (4.7)	−6.2 (−19.0 to 6.6)	0.83
<130/85 mm Hg (among treated hypertensive diabetic individuals)	28.5 (4.2)	17.2 (4.2)*	25.4 (4.0)	−3.1 (−14.5 to 8.3)	0.70

Adapted from *JAMA*, July 9, 2003; 290 (2): 203.
Data are weighted to the US population.
*Estimates are unreliable because of National Health and Nutrition Examination Survey minimum sample size criteria or coefficient of variation of at least 0.30.

Table 6 Canadian Hypertension Society [214]. Considerations in the Individualization of Antihypertensive Therapy

	Initial therapy	Second-line therapy	Notes and/or cautions
Hypertension without other compelling indications	Thiazide diuretics, BBs, ACEI, ARBs, or long-acting dihydropyridine CCBs	Combinations of first-line drugs	ABs are not recommended as initial therapy. BBs are not recommended as initial therapy in those over 60 years of age. Hypokalemia should be avoided by using potassium-sparing agents in those who are prescribed diuretics. ACEIs are not recommended in blacks.
Isolated systolic hypertension without other compelling indications	Thiazide diuretics, ARBs, or long-acting dihydropyridine CCBs	Combinations of first-line drugs	Hypokalemia should be avoided by using potassium-sparing agents in people who are prescribed diuretics.
DM with nephropathy	ACEIs or ARBs	Addition of one or more of thiazide diuretics, cardioselective BBs, long-acting CCBs, or an ARB/ACEI combination	N/A
DM without nephropathy	ACEIs, ARBs, or thiazide diuretics	Combination of first-line drugs or addition of cardioselective BBs and/or long-acting CCBs	If the serum creatinine level is > 150 μmol, loop diuretic should be used as a replacement for low-dose thiazide diuretics if volume is required.
Angina	BBs (consider adding ACEIs)	Long-acting CCBs	Avoid short-acting nifedipine
Prior MI	BBs and/or ACEIs	Combinations of additional agents	N/A
Heart failure	ACEIs (thiazide or loop diuretics, BBs, spironolactone as additive therapy)	ARBs or hydralazine/isosorbide dinitrate	Avoid nondihydropyridine CCBs (diltiazem, verapamil)
Past CVA or transient ischemic attack (TIA)	ACEI/diuretic combinations	N/A	BP reduction reduces recurring cerebrovascular events
Renal disease	ACEIs (diuretics as additive therapy)	Combinations of additional agents	Avoid ACEIs if bilateral renal artery stenosis
LVH	ACEIs, ARBs, dihydropyridine CCBs, diuretics (BBs for patients under 55 years)	N/A	Avoid hydralazine and minoxidil
PAD	Does not affect initial treatment recommendations	Does not affect initial treatment recommendations	Avoid BBs with severe disease
Dyslipidemia	Does not affect initial treatment recommendations	Does not affect initial treatment recommendations	N/A

AB = Alpha-blocker; ACEI = angiotensin-converting enzyme inhibitor; ARB = angiotensin receptor blockers; BB = beta-blocker; BP = blood pressure; CCB = calcium channel blocker; CVA = cerebrovascular accident; DM = diabetes mellitus; MI = myocardial infarction; LVH = left ventricular hypertrophy; PAD = peripheral arterial disease; TIA = transient ischemic attack.

WHAT IS HYPERTENSION

Summary of recommendations

1. The guideline's role is educational and not prescriptive or coercive for the management of individual subjects who may differ widely in their personal, medical, and cultural characteristics.

2. BP has a unimodal distribution in the population as well as a continuous relationship with CV risk.

3. The real threshold for defining hypertension must be considered as flexible, being high or low based on the total CV risk of each individual (Figure 14).

4. The classification of patients is based on relation to the grades of hypertension and the total CV risk resulting from the coexistence of different risk factors, organ damage, and disease (Figure 14). This represents the 10-year risk of a fatal or nonfatal CV event.

5. Treatment strategies are dependent on the initial level of CV risk.

6. CV risk is categorized as low, moderate, high, and very high with "added risk" referring to the risk additional to the average one.

7. Relative and absolute risk are calculated, but in younger patients relative risk is a better indicator of risk in the presence of other risk factors since age may bias the actual risk category to a lower level.

8. Utilization of rigid cutoffs of absolute risk over 10 years is not recommended.

9. Clinical variable should be used to stratify the total CV risk (Table 7).

10. Office, home, and 24-hour ambulatory BP are recommended depending on the clinical situation.

11. Drug therapy should be decided on by two criteria: The level of SBP and DBP and the level of total CV risk.

12. Drug therapy should be initiated promptly in grade 3 hypertension as well as in grades 1 and 2 when the total CV risk is high or very high (Figure 15).

13. In grade 1 or 2 hypertensive patients with moderate total CV risk, drug treatment may be delayed for several weeks and in grade 1 hypertensive patients without any other risk factor for several months. However, even in those patients, lack of BP control after a suitable period should lead to initiation of drug treatment.

14. When the BP is in the high normal range, the decision on drug intervention heavily depends on the level of risk. In the case of diabetes, history of CVA, CHD, or peripheral arterial disease (PAD), the recommendation to start BP-lowering drugs is justified by the results of controlled trials.

15. The primary goals of treatment are to achieve maximum reduction in long-term total and CV risk by treating hypertension and associated reversible risk factors, lower BP to at least 140/90 mm Hg or lower levels as tolerated and to 130/80 mm Hg in patients with diabetes or high or very high risk such as those with stroke, MI, renal dysfunction, or proteinuria. Early treatment is recommended before significant CV damage occurs.

16. Treatment with lifestyle changes should be instituted initially with or without drugs depending on level of risk and BP levels.

17. The choice of antihypertensive drugs are based on concomitant conditions present in the patients, effects on CV risk factors and the CV risk of the patient, subclinical or clinical CV disease, renal disease or diabetes, drug interactions, adverse effects contraindications, duration of action, BP-lowering effect and cost (Tables 8 and 9). However, diuretics and BBs are not recommended for patients with metabolic syndrome or high risk for DM.

18. Combination therapy is appropriate for initial treatment and is usually required to achieve BP goals. Fixed-dose combinations improve compliance and simplify treatment. Some combinations are preferred (Figures 16 and 17).

Blood pressure (mm Hg)					
Other risk factors, OD, or disease	Normal SBP 120–129 or DBP 80–84	High normal SBP 130–139 or DBP 85–89	Grade 1 HT SBP 140–159 or DBP 90–99	Grade 2 HT SBP 160–179 or DBP 100–109	Grade 3 HT SBP ≥ 180 or DBP ≥ 110
No other risk factors	Average risk	Average risk	Low added risk	Moderate added risk	High added risk
1–2 risk factors	Low added risk	Low added risk	Moderate added risk	Moderate added risk	Very high added risk
3 or more risk factors MS, OD, or diabetes	Moderate added risk	High added risk	High added risk	High added risk	Very high added risk
Established CV or renal disease	Very high added risk	Very high added risk	Very high added risk	Very high added risk	Very high added risk

Stratification of CV risk in four categories of added risk.
CV = Cardiovascular; DBP = diastolic blood pressure; HT = hypertension;
MS = metabolic syndrome; OD = subclinical organ damage; SBP = systolic blood pressure.

Figure 14 Stratification of Cardiovascular Risk and Blood Pressure.

Table 7 Factors Influencing Prognosis

Risk factors

- Systolic and diastolic BP levels
- Levels of PP (in the elderly)
- Age (M > 55 years; W > 65 years)
- Smoking
- Dyslipidemia
  - TC > 5.0 mmol/L (190 mg/dL)
  or:
  - LDL cholesterol > 3.0 mmol/L (115 mg/dL)
  or:
  - HDL cholesterol: M < 1.0 mmol/L (40 mg/dL)
  W < 1.2 mmol/L (46 mg/dL)
  or:
  - TG > 1.7 mmol/L (150 mg/dL)
- Fasting plasma glucose 5.6–6.9 mmol/L (102–125 mg/dL)
- Abnormal glucose tolerance test
- Abdominal obesity (waist circumference >102 cm (M), >88 cm (W))
- Family history of premature CV disease (M at age <55 years; W at age <65 years)

Subclinical organ damage

- Electrocardiographic LVH (Sokolow-Lyon > 38 mm; Cornell > 2440 mm/ms) or:
- Echocardiographic LVH• (LVMI M ≥ 125 g/m^2, W ≥ 110 g/m^2)
- Carotid wall thickening (IMT > 0.9 mm) or plaque
- Carotid–femoral PWV >12 m/sec
- Ankle/Brachial BP index < 0.9
- Slight increase in plasma creatinine: M: 115–133 mmol/L (1.3–1.5 mg/dL) W: 107–124 mmol/L (1.2–1.4 mg/dL)
- Low estimated glomerular filtration rate•• (<60 mL/min/1.73 m^2) or creatinine clearance••• (<60 mL/min)
- Microalbuminuria 30–300 mg/24 hour or albumin–creatinine ratio: ≥22 (M); or ≥31 (W) mg/g creatinine

(Continued)

Table 7 (Continued)

Diabetes Mellitus	Established CV or Renal Disease
• Fasting plasma glucose ≥7.0 mmol/L (126 mg/dL) on repeated measurement or: • Postload plasma glucose > 11.0 mmol/L (198 mg/dL)	• Cerebrovascular disease: ischemic stroke; cerebral hemorrhage; transient ischemic attack • Heart disease: MI; angina; coronary revascularization; heart failure • Renal disease: diabetic nephropathy; renal impairment (serum creatinine M > 133; W > 124 mmol/L); proteinuria (>300 mg/24 hour) • Peripheral artery disease • Advanced retinopathy: hemorrhages or exudates, papilledema

Note: The cluster of three out of five risk factors among abdominal, obesity, altered tasting plasma glucose, BP ≥130/85 mm Hg, low HDL cholesterol, and high TG (as defined above) indicates the presence of metabolic syndrome.

BP = Blood pressure; C = cholesterol; CV = cardiovascular; HDL = high density lipoprotein; IMT = intima–media thickness; LDL = low density lipoprotein; LVH = left ventricular hypertrophy; LVMI = left ventricular mass index; M = men; MI = myocardial infarction; PP = pulse pressure; PWV = pulse wave velocity; TC = total cholesterol; TG = triglycerides; W = women. • = risk maximal for concentric (wall thickness/radius ratio ≥ 0.42); •• = MDRD formula; ••• = Cockroft Gault formula.

International Society of Hypertension in Blacks (ISHIB) [216]

Recommendations for African-American patients to initiate monotherapy for newly diagnosed patients with one of these medications (Figure 18) are diuretic, BB, CCB, ACEI, and ARB.

American Heart Association Council for High Blood Pressure Research (AHA) and the Councils on Clinical Cardiology and Epidemiology and Prevention: Treatment of Hypertension in the Prevention and Management of Ischemic Heart Disease [244]

The primary treatment options for the hypertensive patient with ischemic heart disease and CHF is summarized in Tables 10 and 11.

BHS/NICE/NCC-CC: British Hypertension Society and the National Institute for Health and Clinical Excellence and the Royal College of Physicians [245, 246] (Table 12 and Figure 19)

The primary treatment options for the hypertensive patient recommended by the BHS are quite different from JNC 7 and ESH/ESC. These are summarized in Table 11 and Figure 19.

JBS 2: Joint British Societies' Guidelines on Prevention of Cardiovascular Disease in Clinical Practice [223]

Joint British Societies' Guidelines on Prevention of Cardiovascular Disease in Clinical Practice are shown in Figures 20–22.

Blood pressure (mm Hg)					
Other risk factors, OD, or disease	Normal SBP 120–129 or DBP 80–84	High normal SBP 130–139 or DBP 85–89	Grade 1 HT SBP 140–159 or DBP 90–99	Grade 2 HT SBP 160–179 or DBP 100–109	Grade 3 HT SBP ≥ 180 or DBP ≥ 110
No other risk factors	No BP intervention	No BP intervention	Lifestyle changes for several months then drug treatment if BP uncontrolled	Lifestyle changes for several months then drug treatment if BP uncontrolled	Lifestyle changes + immediate drug treatment
1–2 risk factors	Lifestyle changes	Lifestyle changes	Lifestyle changes for several months then drug treatment if BP uncontrolled	Lifestyle changes for several months then drug treatment if BP uncontrolled	Lifestyle changes + immediate drug treatment
≥3 risk factors, MS, or OD	Lifestyle changes	Lifestyle changes and consider drug treatment	Lifestyle changes + drug treatment	Lifestyle changes + drug treatment	Lifestyle changes + immediate drug treatment
Diabetes	Lifestyle changes	Lifestyle changes + drug treatment	Lifestyle changes + drug treatment	Lifestyle changes + drug treatment	Lifestyle changes + immediate drug treatment
Established CV or renal disease	Lifestyle changes + immediate drug treatment	Lifestyle changes + immediate drug treatment	Lifestyle changes + immediate drug treatment	Lifestyle changes + immediate drug treatment	Lifestyle changes + immediate drug treatment

BP = Blood pressure; CV = cardiovascular; MS = metabolic syndrome; OD = subclinical organ damage; SBP = systolic BP.

Figure 15 Selection of Treatment Based on Blood Pressure, Risk Factors and CoMorbid Conditions.

Table 8 Conditions Favoring the Use of Some Antihypertensive Drugs vs. Other

Subclinical organ damage	
LVH	ACEI, CA, ARB
Asymptomatic atherosclerosis	CA, ACEI
Microalbuminuria	ACEI, ARB
Renal dysfunction	ACEI, ARB
Clinical event	
Previous stroke	Any BP-lowering agent
Previous MI	BB, ACEI, ARB
Angina pectoris	BB, CA
Heart failure	Diuretics, BB, ACEI, ARB, antialdosterone agents
Atrial fibrillation	
Recurrent	ARB, ACEI
Permanent	BB, nondihydropyridine CA *(Continued)*

Table 8 (*Continued*)

Tachyarrhythmias	BB
ESRD/proteinuria	ACEI, ARB, loop diuretics
Peripheral artery disease	CA
LV dysfunction	ACEI
Condition	
ISH (elderly)	Diuretics, CA
Metabolic syndrome	ACEI, ARB, CA
DM	ACEI, ARB
Pregnancy	CA, methyldopa, BB
Black people	Diuretics, CA
Glaucoma	BB
ACEI induced cough	ARB

ACEI = Angiotensin-converting enzyme inhibitors; ARB = angiotensin receptor blocker; BB = beta-blocker; CA = calcium antagonist; ESRD = end-stage renal disease; ISH = isolated systolic hypertension; LVH = left ventricular hypertrophy; LV = left ventricular; MI = myocardial infarction.

Table 9 Contraindications to Use Certain Antihypertensive Drugs

	Compelling contraindications	Possible contraindications
Thiazide diuretics	Gout	Metabolic syndrome
		Glucose intolerance
		Pregnancy
BBs	Asthma A-V block (grade 2 or 3)	Peripheral artery disease
		Metabolic syndrome
		Glucose intolerance
		Athletes and physically active patients
		Chronic obstructive pulmonary disease
Calcium antagonists (dihydropyridines)		Tachyarrhythmiast
		Heart failure
Calcium antagonists (verapamil, diltiazem)	A-V block (grade 2 or 3)	
	Heart failure	
	Pregnancy	
ACEIs	Angioneurotic edema	
	Hyperkalemia	
	Bilateral renal artery stenosis	
	Pregnancy	
ARB	Hyperkalemia	
	Bilateral renal artery stenosis	
Diuretics (antialdosterone)	Renal failure	
	Hyperkalemia	

ACEI = Angiotensin-converting enzyme inhibitors; ARB = angiotensin receptor blocker.

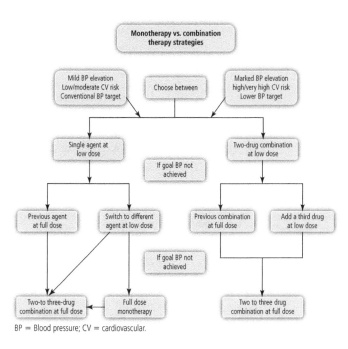

BP = Blood pressure; CV = cardiovascular.

Figure 16 Selection of Therapy: Monotherapy or Combination.

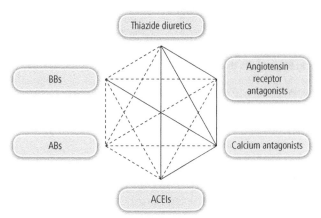

The preferred combinations in the general hypertensive population are represented as thick lines.
The frames indicate classes of agents proven to be beneficial in controlled intervention trials.
ABs = Alpha-blockers; BBs = beta-blockers;
ACEIs = angiotensin-converting enzyme inhibitors.

Figure 17 Preferred Combinations of Drugs for Hypertension.

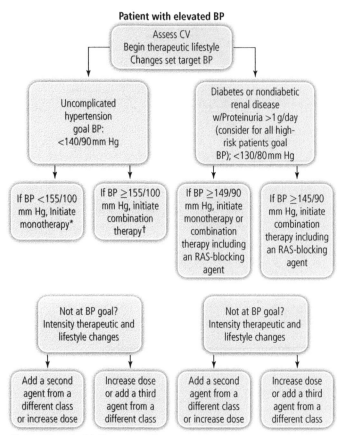

Patient with elevated BP

Assess CV
Begin therapeutic lifestyle
Changes set target BP

Uncomplicated
hypertension
goal BP:
<140/90mm Hg

Diabetes or nondiabetic
renal disease
w/Proteinuria >1g/day
(consider for all high-
risk patients goal
BP); <130/80mm Hg

If BP <155/100
mm Hg, Initiate
monotherapy*

If BP ≥155/100
mm Hg, initiate
combination
therapy†

If BP ≥149/90
mm Hg, initiate
monotherapy or
combination
therapy including
an RAS-blocking
agent

If BP ≥145/90
mm Hg, initiate
combination
therapy including
an RAS-blocking
agent

Not at BP goal?
Intensity therapeutic and
lifestyle changes

Not at BP goal?
Intensity therapeutic and
lifestyle changes

Add a second
agent from a
different class
or increase dose

Increase dose
or add a third
agent from a
different class

Add a second
agent from a
different class
or increase dose

Increase dose
or add a third
agent from a
different class

Not at BP goal with three agents?
• Consider factors that may decrease compliance or efficacy with current regimen
• Consider referral to BP specialist

Adapted from *Arch Intern Med* 2003; 163: 525–541.
ACEI = angiotensin-converting enzyme inhibitor; ARB = angiotensin
receptor blocker; BB = beta-blocker; BP = blood pressure;
CCB = calcium channel blocker.

RAS indicates renin-angiotensin system.
To initiate monotherapy at the recommended starting dose with an agent from any
of the following classes: diuretics, BBs, CCBs, ACEIs, or ARBs. To initiate low-dose
combination therapy with any of the following combinations: BBS, ACEI diuretic,
ACEIs/CCB, or ARB/diuretic.

Figure 18 Clinical Algorithm for Achieving Target BP in African-American Patients with High BP.

Table 10 Summary of Main Recommendations

Area of concern	BP target (mm Hg)	Lifestyle modification[†]	Specific drug indications	Comments
General CAD prevention	<140/90	Yes	Any effective antihypertensive drug or combination[‡]	If SBP ≥160 mm Hg or DBP ≥100 mm Hg, then start with two drugs
High CAD risk*	<130/80	Yes	ACEI or ARB or CCB or thiazide diuretic or combination	If SBP ≥160 mm Hg or DBP ≥100 mm Hg, then start with two drugs
Stable angina	<130/80	Yes	BB and ACEI or ARB	If BB contraindicated, or if side effects occur, can substitute diltiazem or verapamil (but not if bradycardia or LVD is present) Can add dihydropyridine CCB (not diltiazem or verapamil) to BB A thiazide diuretic can be added for BP control
UA/NSTEMI	<130/80	Yes	BB (if patient is hemodynamically stable) and ACEI or ARB[§]	If BB contraindicated, or if side effects occur, can substitute diltiazem or verapamil (but not if bradycardia or LVD is present) Can add dihydropyridine CCB (not diltiazem or verapamil) to BB A thiazide diuretic can be added for BP control
STEMI	<130/80	Yes	BB (if patient is hemodynamically stable) and ACEI or ARB[§]	If BB contraindicated, or if side effects occur, can substitute diltiazem or verapamil (but not if bradycardia or LVD is present) Can add dihydropyridine CCB (not diltiazem or verapamil) to BB A thiazide diuretic can be added for BP control
LVD	<120/80	Yes	ACEI or ARB and BB and aldosterone antagonist[¶] and thiazide or loop diuretic and hydralazine/isosorbide dinitrate (blacks)	Contraindicated: verapamil, diltiazem, clonidine, moxonidine, ABs

(Continued)

Table 10 (*Continued*)

ACEI = Angiotensin-converting enzyme inhibitors; ARB = angiotensin receptor blocker; BB = beta-blocker; BP = blood pressure; CCB = calcium channel blocker; DBP = diastolic BP; DM = diabetes mellitus; HF = heart failure; LVD = left ventricular dysfunction; LVEF = left ventricular ejection fraction; MI = myocardial infarction; NSTEMI = nonsegment elevation myocardial infarction; PAD = peripheral arterial disease; SBP = systolic BP; STEMI = segment elevation myocardial infarction; UA = unstable angina.

Before making any management decisions, you are strongly urged to read the full text of the relevant section of the scientific statement.

*DM, chronic kidney disease, known CAD or CAD equivalent (carotid artery disease, PAD, abdominal aortic aneurysm), or 10-year Framingham risk score ⩾10%.

†Weight loss if appropriate, healthy diet (including sodium restriction), exercise, smoking cessation, and alcohol moderation.

‡Evidence supports ACEI (or ARB), CCB, or thiazide diuretic as first-line therapy.

§If anterior MI is present, if hypertension persists, if LV dysfunction or HF is present, or if the patient has DM.

¶If severe HF is present (New York Heart Association class III or IV, or LVEF <40% and clinical HF). See text.

Table 11 Recommendations

1. The treatment of hypertension in patients with HF should include behavioral modification such as sodium restriction, and a closely monitored exercise program (*Class I; Level of Evidence C*). Other nonpharmacological approaches are the same as for patients without HF.

2. Drugs that have been shown to improve outcomes for patients with HF generally also lower BP. Patients should be treated with diuretics, ACEIs (or ARBs), BB, and aldosterone receptor antagonists (*Class I; Level of Evidence A*).

3. Thiazide diuretics should be used for BP control and to reverse volume overload and associated symptoms. In severe HF, or in patients with severe renal impairment, loop diuretics should be used for volume control, but these are less effective than thiazide diuretics in lowering BP. Diuretics should be used together with an ACEI or ARB and a BB (*Class I; Level of Evidence C*).

4. Studies have shown equivalence of the benefit of ACEIs and ARBs, candesartan or valsartan, in HF. Either class of agents is effective in lowering BP. Drugs from each class can be used together, provided that the patient is hemodynamically stable and not in the immediate post-MI period (*Class I; Level of Evidence A*).

5. Among the BBs, carvedilol, metoprolol succinate, and bisoprolol have been shown to improve outcomes in HF and are effective in lowering BP (*Class I; Level of Evidence A*).

6. The aldosterone receptor antagonists spironolactone and eplerenone have been shown to be beneficial in HF and should be included in the regimen if there is severe HF (New York Heart Association class III or IV or LVEF <40% and clinical HF). One or the other may be substituted for a thiazide diuretic in patients requiring a potassium-sparing agent. If an aldosterone receptor antagonist is administered with an ACEI or an ARB or in the presence of renal insufficiency, the serum potassium should be monitored frequently. These drugs should not be used, however, if the serum creatinine level is ⩾2.5 mg/dL in men or ⩾2.0 mg/dL in women, or if the serum potassium level is ⩾5.0 mEq/L. Spironolactone or eplerenone may be used together with a thiazide diuretic, particularly in patients with refractory hypertension (*Class I; Level of Evidence A*).

Table 11 (*Continued*)

7. Consider the addition of hydralazine/isosorbide dinitrate to the regimen of diuretic, ACEI or ARB, and BB in black patients with NYHA class III or IV heart failure (*Class I; Level of Evidence B*). Others may benefit similarly, but this has not yet been tested.

8. Drugs to avoid in patients with HF and hypertension are nondihydropyridine CCBs (such as verapamil and diltiazem), clonidine, and moxonidine (*Class III; Level of Evidence B*). Alpha-adrenergic blockers such as doxazosin should be used only if other drugs for the management of hypertension and HF are inadequate to achieve BP control at maximum tolerated doses (*Class IIa; Level of Evidence B*).

9. The target BP is <130/80 mm Hg, but consideration should be given to lower the BP even further to <120/80 mm Hg. In patients with an elevated DBP who have CAD and HF with evidence of myocardial ischemia, the BP should be lowered slowly, and caution is advised in inducing falls of DBP below 60 mm Hg if the patient has DM or is over the age of 60 years. In older hypertensive individuals with wide PP, lowering SBP may cause very low DBP values (<60 mm Hg). This should alert the clinician to assess carefully any untoward signs or symptoms, especially those due to myocardial ischemia and worsening HF (*Class IIa; Level of Evidence B*)

ACEI = Angiotensin-converting enzyme inhibitor; ARB = angiotensin receptor blocker; BB = beta-blocker; BP = blood pressure; CAD = coronary artery disease; DBP = diastolic BP; DM = diabetes mellitus; HF = heart failure; MI = myocardial infarction; NYHA = New York Heart Association; PP = pulse pressure; SBP = systolic BP.

Table 12 Recommendations That Are Not Changing

The GDG is not proposing to change the following recommendations from section 1.4 of the original NICE clinical guideline on hypertension in primary care (CG 18). These recommendations will still apply after publication of the updated guideline, and are not part of the consultation.

1.4.1	Drug therapy reduces the risk of CVD and death. Offer drug therapy to: • patients with persistent high BP of 160/100 mm Hg or more; • patients at raised CV risk (10-year risk of CVD ≥20% or existing CVD or TOD) with persistent BP of more than 140/90 mm Hg.	A
1.4.2	Provide appropriate guidance and materials about the benefits of drugs and the unwanted side effects sometimes experienced in order to help patients make informed choices.	D
1.4.3	Offer drug therapy, adding different drugs if necessary, to achieve a target of 140/90 mm Hg, or until further treatment is inappropriate or declined. Titrate drug doses as described in the British National Formulary noting any cautions and contraindications.	A
1.4.10	Offer patients with isolated systolic hypertension (SBP >160 mm Hg) the same treatment as patients with both raised systolic and diastolic BP.	A
1.4.11	Offer patients over 80 years of age the same treatment as other patients over 55 years, taking account of any comorbidity and their existing burden of drug use.	A
1.4.12	Where possible, recommend treatment with drugs taken only once a day.	A
1.4.13	Prescribe nonproprietary drugs where these are appropriate and minimize cost.	B

NICE clinical guideline 18 was developed by the Newcastle Guideline Development and Research Unit. It is available from www.nice.org.uk/CG018

BP = Blood pressure; CV = cardiovascular; CVD = cardiovascular disease; GDG = generation data group; NICE = National Institute for Health and Clinical Excellence; SBP = systolic BP TOD = target organ damage.

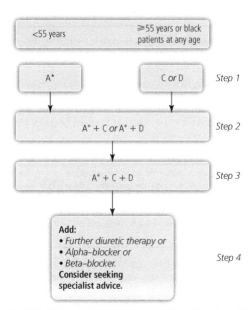

<55 years	≥55 years or black patients at any age
A*	C or D	Step 1

A* + C or A* + D   Step 2

A* + C + D   Step 3

Add:
• *Further diuretic therapy or*
• *Alpha–blocker or*
• *Beta–blocker.*
Consider seeking specialist advice.   Step 4

A = ACE inhibitor (* or ARB if ACEI-intolerant); C = calcium channel blocker; D = thiazide-type diuretic. Beta-blockers are not a preferred initial therapy for hypertension but are an alternative to A in patients <55 years in whom A is not tolerated, or contraindicated (includes women of child-bearing potential). Black patients are only those of African of Caribbean descent. In the absence of evidence, all other patients should be treated according to the algorithm as non-black.

Figure 19 Algorithm: Treatment of Newly Diagnosed Hypertension.

Major recommendations regarding BP

1. CVD risk should be assessed with all major CV risk factors including smoking, BP, lipids, and diabetes using risk calculation tables (Figure 20) which are stratified by age and then refined with additional historical clinical and test results to make an overall clinical judgment about the person's total CVD risk and need for drug treatment. A total CVD risk over 20% in 10 years is considered sufficiently high to justify the use of antihypertensive and other therapies.

2. Antihypertensive drug therapy is summarized in Figures 21 and 22. The combined use of diuretics and BBs is discouraged due to the increased incidence of type 1 diabetes. In general, the BBs are reserved for specific indications but not for primary use in hypertension. The diuretics are not recommended for patients under the age of 55.

3. The ABCD system is now replaced with the ACD system of drug selection (Figure 22).

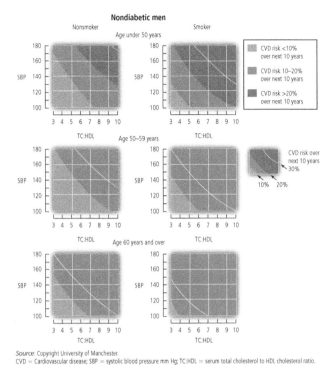

Source: Copyright University of Manchester.
CVD = Cardiovascular disease; SBP = systolic blood pressure mm Hg; TC:HDL = serum total cholesterol to HDL cholesterol ratio.

Figure 20 JBS CVD Risk Prediction Chart: Nondiabetic Men.

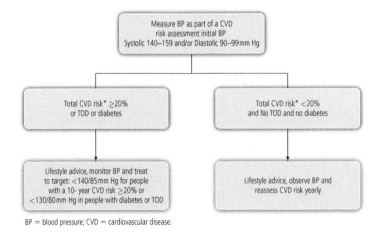

BP = blood pressure; CVD = cardiovascular disease.

*Assessed with CVD Risk Chart.

Figure 21 Risk Thresholds and Targets for BP in Asymptomatic People without CVD.

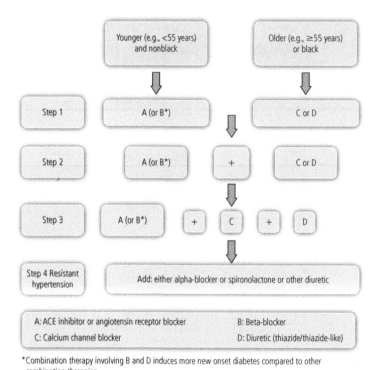

| Step 1 | A (or B*) | | C or D |

| Step 2 | A (or B*) | + | C or D |

| Step 3 | A (or B*) | + C + D |

| Step 4 Resistant hypertension | Add: either alpha-blocker or spironolactone or other diuretic |

| A: ACE inhibitor or angiotensin receptor blocker | B: Beta-blocker |
| C: Calcium channel blocker | D: Diuretic (thiazide/thiazide-like) |

*Combination therapy involving B and D induces more new onset diabetes compared to other combination therapies

Figure 22 Recommendations for Combining BP Drugs/ABCD Rule.

Global CV Risk Calculation [248–252]

Numerous CV calculators have been proposed to determine global CV risk including *Framingham* [250], *BHS*, *SCORE* [251], *INTERHEART* [252], and *COSEHC* [248, 249] (Tables 13–16). The most complete and updated CV risk calculator is that of *COSEHC* and it is the one recommended at this time [248, 249]. Tables for men and women are shown in both US and metric units to allow for easy conversion.

Absolute scores over 40 or relative risks over 60% are high risk for CV death and require aggressive therapy. The absolute scores represent the risk of CV death within 5 years.

Absolute score between 30 and 40 represents moderately high risk, absolute score of 20–30 is moderate risk and below 20 is low risk.

Table 13 COSEHC CV Risk Score for Women

Merged PROCAM and INDANA data

Risk factor	Addition to risk score											Risk score
Age (years)	35–39 0	40–44 +5	45–49 +9	50–54 +14	55–59 +18	60–64 +23	65–69 +27	70–74 +32				
Extra for cigarette smoking	+13	+12	+11	+10	+10	+9	+9	+8				
SBP (mm Hg)	110–119 0	120–129 +1	130–139 +2	140–149 +3	150–159 +4	160–169 +5	170–179 +6	180–189 +8	190–199 +9	200–209 +10	≥210 +11	
Total cholesterol concentration (mg/dL)	≤193 0	194–231 0	232–269 +1	270–308 +1	309–347 +2	≥348 +2						
Height (inches)	<57 +6	57–<61 +4	61–<65 +3	65–<69 +2	≥69 0							
Creatinine concentration (mg/dL)	<0.6 0	0.6 +1	0.7 +1	0.8 +2	0.9 +2	1.0 +2	1.1 +3	1.2 +3	>1.2 +4			
Homocysteine (µmol/L)	≤5 −4	5–5.9 −3	6–6.9 −2	7–7.9 −1	8–9.9 0	10–10.9 +1	11–11.9 +2	12–12.9 +3	13–13.9 +4	14–14.9 +5	15–15.9 +6	≥16 +7
Uric acid	<6.0 add 0		>6.0 add +3									
Microalbuminuria	Absent add 0		Present add +3									
Prior MI	No 0		Yes +8									
Prior stroke	No 0		Yes +8									
LVH	No 0		Yes +3									
Diabetes	No 0		Yes +9		If not diabetic see below							

Nondiabetic, FBS (mg/dL)	≤71	72–77	78–84	85–95	96–101	102–107	108–113	114–119	120–125	≥126	Diabetic (above)
	−1.5	**−1**	**−0.5**	**0**	**+0.5**	**+1**	**+1.5**	**+2**	**+2.5**		Total risk score=

Scores exceeding 40 are HIGH ABSOLUTE RISK category; 60th percentile RELATIVE RISK SCORES by age-range are **18** for age 35–39; **21** for age 40–44; **27** for age 45–49; **31** for age 50–54; **36** for age 55–59; **41** for age 60–64.

Absolute risk score	% dying from CVD in 5 years
0	0.04
5	0.07
10	0.11
15	0.19
20	0.31
25	0.51
30	0.84
35	1.4
40	2.3
45	3.7
50	6.1
55	9.8
60	15.6
65	24.5
70	37.0

CVD = Cardiovascular disease; FBS = fasting blood sugar; LVH = left ventricular hypertrophy; MI = myocardial infarction; SBP = systolic BP.

Table 14 COSEHC CV Risk Score for Men

Merged PROCAM and INDANA data tables

Risk factor	Addition to risk score												Risk Score
Being male	Add 12 points												**+12**
Age (years)	35–39	40–44	45–49	50–54	55–59	60–64	65–69	70–74					
	0	**+4**	**+7**	**+11**	**+14**	**+18**	**+22**	**+25**					
Extra for cigarette smoking	**+9**	**+7**	**+7**	**+6**	**+6**	**+5**	**+4**	**+4**					
SBP (mm Hg)	110–119	120–129	130–139	140–149	150–159	160–169	170–179	180–189	190–199	200–209	≥210		
	0	**+1**	**+2**	**+3**	**+4**	**+5**	**+6**	**+8**	**+9**	**+10**	**+11**		
Total cholesterol concentration (mg/dL)	≤193	194–231	232–269	270–308	309–347	≥348	*Only if total ≤193 see below*						
	0	**+2**	**+4**	**+5**	**+7**	**+9**							
LDL cholesterol (mg/dL)	*If total cholesterol ≤193; LDL:*			*<100*	*100–129*	*130–159*	*160–189*						
				0	**+1**	**+3**	**+4**						
HDL cholesterol (mg/dL)	*If total cholesterol ≤ 193; HDL:*			*<35*	*35–44*	*45–54*	*≥55*						
				+4	**+2**	**+1**	**0**						
Triglyceride (mg/dL)	*If total cholesterol ≤193; TG:*			*<100*	*100–149*	*150–199*	*≥ 200*						
				0	**+0**	**+1**	**+1**						
Height (inches)	<63	63–<67	67–<71	71–<75	≥75								
	+6	**+4**	**+3**	**+2**	**0**								
Creatinine concentration (mg/cL)	≤0.8	0.9	1.0	1.1	1.2	1.3	1.4	>1.4					
	0	**+1**	**+1**	**+2**	**+2**	**+3**	**+3**	**+4**					
Homocysteine (μmol/L)	≤5	5–5.9	6–6.9	7–7.9	8–8.9	9–9.9	10–11.8	11.9–12.9	13–13.9	14–14.9	15–15.9	≥16	
	−6	**−5**	**−4**	**−3**	**−2**	**−1**	**0**	**+1**	**+2**	**+4**	**+5**	**+6**	

Uric acid	<7.0 add 0	>7.0 add +2	
Microalbuminuria	Absent add 0	Present add +3	

	No	Yes
Prior MI	0	+8
Family history of MI pre-60	0	+1
Prior stroke	0	+8
LVH	0	+3
Diabetes	0	+2

If not diabetic, see below

	≤75	76–81	82–88	89–99	100–105	106–111	112–117	118–125	≥126
Nondiabetic, FBS (mg/dL)	−1.5	−1	−0.5	0	+0.5	+1	+1.5	+2	

Diabetic (above)

Total risk score =

Scores exceeding **40** are HIGH ABSOLUTE RISK category; 60th percentile relative risk score cutoffs by age-range are **29** for age 35–39; **32** for age 40–44; **36** for age 45–49; and **40** for age 50–54.

HDL = High-density lipoprotein; LDL = low-density lipoprotein; LVH = left ventricular hypertrophy; MI = myocardial infarction; SBP = systolic BP.

Table 15 COSEHC CV Risk Score for Women

Risk factor	Addition to risk score											Risk score
Age (years)	35–39	40–44	45–49	50–54	55–59	60–64	65–69	70–74				
Extra for	0	+5	+9	+14	+18	+23	+27	+32				
cigarette smoking	+13	+12	+11	+10	+10	+9	+9	+8				
SBP (mm Hg)	110–119	120–129	130–139	140–149	150–159	160–169	170–179	180–189	190–199	200–209	≥210	
	0	+1	+2	+3	+4	+5	+6	+7	+8	+9	+10	
Total cholesterol concentration (μmol/L)	<6.0	6.0–7.9	≥8.0									
	0	+1	+2									
Height (inches)	<57	57–<61	61–<65	65–<69	≥69							
	+6	+4	+3	+2	0							
Creatinine concentration (μmol/L)	<50	50–69	70–89	90–109	≥110							
	0	+1	+2	+3	+4							
Homocysteine (μmol/L)	≤6	6–7.2	7.3–8.4	8.5–9.6	9.7–11.9	12–13.2	13.3–14.4	14.5–15.9	≥16			
	-4	-3	-2	-1	0	+1	+2	+3	+4			
Uric acid	≤333 add 0		>333 add +4									
Microalbuminuria	Absent add 0		Present add +3									
Prior MI	No	0	Yes	+8								
Family history of MI Pre-55 ♂ or pre-65 ♀	No	0	Yes	+6								
Prior stroke	No	0	Yes	+8								

					If not diabetic see below				
LVH	**No**	**0**	**Yes**	**+3**					
Diabetes	**No**	**0**	**Yes**	**+9**					
Nondiabetic, FBS (mmol/L)	≤4.0	4.1–4.5	4.6–5.2	5.3–5.5	5.6–5.9	6.0–6.3	6.4–6.6	6.7–6.9	≥7.0
	−2	**−1**	**0**	**+1**	**+2**	**+3**	**+4**	**+5**	

Diabetic (above)
Total risk score =

Scores **exceeding 40 and 47** are HIGH and VERY HIGH **ABSOLUTE** RISK category, respectively. ASA recommended for scores exceeding 37. 60th percentile **RELATIVE** RISK SCORES by age-range are **18** for age 35–39; **21** for age 40–44; **27** for age 45–49; **31** for age 50–54; **36** for age 55–59; **41** for age 60–64.

Absolute risk score	**% dying from CVD in 5 years**
0	0.04
5	0.07
10	0.11
15	0.19
20	0.31
25	0.51
30	0.84
35	1.4
40	2.3
45	3.7
50	6.1
55	9.8
60	15.6
65	24.5
70	37.0

CVD = Cardiovascular disease; LVH = left ventricular hypertrophy; MI = myocardial infarction; SBP = systolic BP.

Table 16 COSEHC CV Risk Score for Men

Risk factor	Addition to risk score	Risk score
Being male	Add 12 points	+12
Age (years)	35–39: 0; 40–44: +4; 45–49: +7; 50–54: +11; 55–59: +14; 60–64: +18; 65–69: +22; 70–74: +25	
Extra for cigarette smoking	35–39: +9; 40–44: +7; 45–49: +7; 50–54: +6; 55–59: +6; 60–64: +5; 65–69: +4; 70–74: +4	
SBP (mm Hg)	110–119: 0; 120–129: +1; 130–139: +2; 140–149: +3; 150–159: +4; 160–169: +5; 170–179: +6; 180–189: +8; 190–199: +9; 200–209: +10; ≥210: +11	
Total cholesterol (mmol/L)	<5.0: 0; 5.0–5.9: +2; 6.0–6.9: +4; 7.0–7.9: +5; 8.0–8.9: +7; ≥9.0: +9	*If full profile unknown*
LDL cholesterol (mmol/L)	< 2.6: 0; 2.6–3.3: +1; 3.4–4.0: +3; ≥ 4.1: +4	
HDL cholesterol (mmol/L)	< 0.9: +4; 0.9–1.1: +2; 1.2–1.4: +1; >1.4: 0	
Triglyceride (mmol/L)	<1.7: 0; ≥1.7: +1	
Height (inches)	<63: +6; 63–<67: +4; 67–<71: +3; 71–<75: +2; ≥75: 0	
Creatinine (μmol/L)	<70: 0; 70–89: +1; 90–109: +2; 110–129: +3; ≥130: +4	
Homocysteine (μmol/L)	≤8.4: −4; 8.5–9.6: −3; 9.7–10.8: −2; 10.9–11.9: −1; 12–14.4: 0; 14.5–15.6: +1; 15.7–16.9: +2; ≥17: +3	
Uric acid	≤416 add 0; >416 add +2	
Microalbuminuria	**Absent** add 0; Present add +3	
Prior MI	**No** 0; **Yes** +8	
Family history of MI		

					OR, if not diabetic, see below				
Pre-55 ♂ or pre-65 ♀	**No**	0	**Yes**	**+6**					
Prior stroke	**No**	0	**Yes**	**+8**					
LVH	**No**	0	**Yes**	**+3**					
Diabetes	**No**	0	**Yes**	**+2**					
Nondiabetic, FBS (mmol/L)	≤4.0	4.0–4.4	4.5–4.9	5.0–5.5	5.6–5.9	6.0–6.4	6.5–6.9	≥7.0	
	−1.5	**−1**	**−0.5**	**0**	**+0.5**	**+1**	**+1.5**	**+2**	
								Diabetic (above)	**+2**
								Total risk score =	

Scores exceeding 40 and 47 are HIGH and VERY HIGH ABSOLUTE RISK category, respectively. ASA recommended for scores exceeding 37. 60th percentile RELATIVE risk score cutoffs by age-range are **29** for age 35–39; **32** for age 40–44; **36** for age 45–49; and **40** for age 50–54.

Absolute risk score	% dying from CVD in 5 years
0	0.04
5	0.07
10	0.11
15	0.19
20	0.31
25	0.51
30	0.84
35	1.4
40	2.3
45	3.7
50	6.1
55	9.8
60	15.6
65	24.5
70	37.0

CVD = Cardiovascular disease; LVH = left ventricular hypertrophy; MI = myocardial infarction; SBP = systolic BP.

Secondary Hypertension [238]

Cause	Signs and Symptoms	Confirmation
Oral contraceptives	Recent onset of hypertension	Cessation of oral contraceptive should be followed by normalization of BP within 6 months
	Average 5% increase in BP after 7 years	
Licorice intoxication	Eating large amounts of licorice	Cessation of licorice intake should cause normalization of BP within 1 month
	Pseudo-hyperaldosteronism	
Primary aldosteronism	Muscle cramps, weakness, polyuria, hypokalemia, metabolic alkalosis	Decreased PRA, increased urinary K^+, increased serum aldosterone, decreased serum K^+, positive saline suppression test, aldosterone IPRA ratio >25
Pheochromocytoma	Sustained hypertension, intermittent hypertension, headaches, sweating, palpitation, pallor, tachycardia, orthostatic hypotension	24-hour urinary or serum catecholamines, VMA, CT scan, MIBG scan, MRI scan, clonidine suppression test, PET scan, metanephrines
Hyperparathyroidism	Bone pain, constipation, fatigue	Hypercalcemia, hypophosphatemia, increased parathyroid hormone
Thyroid disease	Hyperthyroidism, hypothyroidism	Free thyroxine index, free trüodothyronine index, thyroid-stimulating hormone
Acromegaly	Physical findings	Growth hormone level
Decongestants	Tachycandia, sudden increased BP	History of OTC medications
Stress, anxiety, depression	Tachycardia, sweating	Clinical history, anxiolytics and antidepressants, weight loss
Obesity	Increase weight	Sleep study, arterial blood gases, PFRs
Burns	Second and third degree	
Sleep apnea	Obesity, snoring, apnea, daytime somnolence	Increased urinary 17-hydroxycorticosteroids and 17-ketosteroids and urine and plasma cortisol, loss of diurnal variation of serum cortisol, dexamethasone suppression test
Cushing's syndrome	Moon face, central obesity, hirsutism, hypokalemia, diabetes	

Cause	Signs and Symptoms	Confirmation
Coarctation of the aorta	Headache, lower extremity claudication, leg BP 20 mm Hg lower than arm BP, reduced femoral pulse, abnormal chest x-ray	Arteriography of aorta, chest CT or MRI
Renal disease	Dysuria, nocturia, hematuria, RBC casts, recurrent UTI, edema	Creatinine, BUN, urinalysis, nuclear medicine GFR, ultrasound, renal biopsy
Renovascular hypertension	Recent-onset, accelerated hypertension, abdominal bruit, DBP $\geqslant$110 mm Hg resistant to treatment, atherosclerotic and fibromuscular dysplasia subtypes	Arteriography, renal vein renins, PRA, nuclear medicine GFR and renogram, captopril test (captopril renal scan), renal artery Doppler scan, MRA
Miscellaneous drugs or toxins*	Hypertension or attenuation of antihypertensive drug action	Discontinue medications; serum and urine studies
Neurologic disorders	Brain tumors, head injury, quadraplegia, GBS, baroreceptor dysfunction, autonomic insufficiency	Clonidine, Nitroglycerin, HS
Peri-operative CV surgery	Transient BP increase	Observation
SIADH	Increase volume and weight hypoanemia	Increased intravascular volume, hyponatremia, t UNa$^+$, and Uosmols

*NSAIDs, sympathomimetics, cocaine, alcohol, erythropoietin, cyclosporin, tacrolimus, anabolic steroids, cortisone, caffeine, ephedrine, MDMA, methylphenidate, nicotine, phencyclidine, phenylephrine, phenylpropanolamine, ergotamine, bromocriptine, metoclopramide, TCA, lead, mercury, cadmium, arsenic, digitalis, disulfiram, lithium, herbals, thallium

BP Measurement

Indirect measurement of BP [6, 7, 120, 238]
Equipment
Sphygmomanometer (aneroid or mercury manometer).

Methodology
1. The patient should be seated for 5 minutes in a quiet, comfortable environment, with the arm free of restrictive clothing or other materials and supported at heart level. The patient should avoid exertion, temperature extremes, eating, caffeine, or smoking for 1 hour before BP measurement.
2. The observer (clinician) should be at eye level of the meniscus of the mercury column or centered in front of the gauge; avoid strained posture.
3. The appropriate cuff size should be selected. The cuff bladder should be 20% wider than the diameter of the extremity. The bladder length should be approximately twice the recommended width.
4. The deflated cuff should be placed at least 2.5 cm above the antecubital space. The cuff should fit smoothly and snugly around the arm, with the bladder centered directly over the brachial artery.
5. Palpate for the brachial pulse. To estimate SBP, rapidly inflate the cuff until the brachial pulse can no longer be felt.
6. Place the bell of the stethoscope over the previously palpated brachial artery. Rapidly inflate the cuff to 30 mm Hg above the point at which the brachial pulse disappears; deflate the cuff at the rate of 2–3 mm Hg/s.
7. Record SBP as the first Korotkoff sound and DBP as the fifth Korotkoff sound.
8. Allow 1–2 minutes between BP determinations.
9. BP should then be determined in the upright posture after the patient has been standing for 2 minutes with pulse rate. The arm should be positioned at heart level, with the forearm at the horizontal level of the fourth intercostal space.
10. On the initial visit, BP readings should be performed in both arms and in the thigh. Subsequent BP determinations should be performed in the arm with the higher reading if there is more than a 10-mm Hg discrepancy in BP reading.

Korotkoff sounds [7]
Phase I: Marked by the first appearance of faint, clear tapping sounds which gradually increase in intensity. Phase I should be used as the SBP.
Phase II: Period during which a murmur or swishing sound is heard.
Phase III: Period during which sounds are crisper and increase in intensity.
Phase IV: Period marked by the distinct, abrupt muffling of sound (soft, blowing quality is heard).
Phase V: The point at which sounds disappear. Phase V should be used as the DBP (except on rare occasions, e.g., aortic insufficiency).

Common mistakes in BP measurement [5, 7, 238]
1. Failure to keep the person in the supine position for 5 minutes before measuring the BP.
2. Failure to keep the arm at the level of the heart.

3. If Korotkoff sounds cannot be heard, failure to completely deflate the cuff before determining BP and failure to wait 1–2 minutes before doing further determinations.
4. Observer error, because of hearing impairment, bias (preferring some digits over others), or unconscious bias toward under-reading or over-reading BP depending on dividing line of normal.
5. Failure to keep the eyes at the level of the mercury manometer.
6. Deflating cuff too rapidly. The cuff should be deflated at a rate of 2–3 mm Hg/s.
7. Failure to use appropriate cuff size. Use of a regular adult cuff for obese patients leads to a high BP reading. Use a large adult cuff or thigh cuff for obese persons; use a child's cuff for children. The cuff should cover two-thirds of the arm above the antecubital space.
8. Failure to position the cuff correctly. The cuff should be placed 2–3 cm above the antecubital space.
9. Failure to provide a conducive environment: comfortable room temperature and quiet surroundings free of noises and distracting stimuli.
10. Missing the heartbeat during auscultation in patients with excessive bradycardia.
11. Patient has consumed alcohol, caffeine, smoked recently, or is under stress.

Masked hypertension definition, impact, outcomes (*J Clin Hyperten* 2007; 9: 956–963)

The phenomenon of masked hypertension (MH) is defined as a clinical condition in which a patient's office BP level is <140/90 mm Hg but ambulatory or home BP readings are in the hypertensive range. The prevalence in the population is about the same as that of isolated office hypertension; about one in seven or eight persons with a normal office BP level may fall into this category. The high prevalence of MH would suggest the necessity for measuring out-of-office BP in persons with apparently normal or well-controlled office BP. Reactivity to daily life stressors and behavioral factors such as smoking, alcohol use, contraceptive use in women, and sedentary habits can selectively influence MH. MH should be searched for in individuals who are at increased risk for CV complications including patients with kidney disease or diabetes. Individuals with MH have been shown to have a greater-than-normal prevalence of organ damage, particularly with an increased prevalence of metabolic risk factors, left ventricular (LV) mass index, carotid intima/media thickness (IMT), and impaired large artery distensibility compared with patients with a truly normal BP level in and out of the clinic or office. In addition, outcome studies have suggested that MH increases CV risk, which appears to be close to that of in-office and out-of-office hypertension.

Incidence of CV events in white-coat, masked, and sustained hypertension vs. true normotension: a meta-analysis (*J Hypertens* 2007; 25: 2193–2198)

In this meta-analysis, a search for individual studies was made in which the adjusted relative risk of incident CV events was assessed in patients with WCHT, masked, and sustained hypertension vs. normotension in the same study population. For each type of hypertension, the weighted overall hazard ratio (HR) and 95% confidence intervals (CI) were calculated.

Results: Seven studies were identified, involving a total of 11 502 participants. Four studies were performed in the population, two in primary care and one in specialist care. Two studies were exclusively on treated hypertensive patients; individuals on antihypertensive treatment were included in all the other studies except one. Cutoff BP was 140/90 mmHg for office BP in all studies and 135/85 mmHg (83 in one study) for out-of-office BP. The average age of the study populations was 63 years; 53% were men. The endpoint consisted of CV death in one study and of various aggregates of fatal and nonfatal CV events in the others. During an average follow-up of 8.0 years, there were 912 first CV events. The overall adjusted HR vs. normotension was 1.12 (95% CI 0.84–1.50) for WCHT (p = 0.59), 2.00 (1.58–2.52) for MH (p < 0.001), and 2.28 (1.87–2.78) for sustained hypertension (p < 0.001).

Conclusion: The meta-analysis indicates that the incidence of CV events is not significantly different between WCHT and true normotension, whereas the outcome is worse in patients with masked or sustained hypertension.

Role of ambulatory blood pressure monitoring in the management of hypertension (*Am J Health Syst Pharm* 2008; 65: 209–218)

Ambulatory blood pressure monitoring (ABPM) is a fully automated technique in which multiple BP measurements are taken at regular intervals (usually every 15–30 minutes) over a 24–48-hour period, providing a continuous BP record during the patient's normal daily activities. Some experts advocate the use of 24-hour ABPM for all first diagnoses of hypertension and for treatment decision-making. The use of ABPM can improve BP monitoring so that treatment can be optimized more rapidly and more patients can achieve BP targets with appropriate therapy. ABPM may lead to better patient outcomes while requiring less-intensive drug regimens to maintain BP control and reduce treatment costs. By more accurately and reliably measuring BP, especially circadian changes, ABPM has been shown to predict CV morbidity and mortality and end-organ damage. ABPM is especially beneficial for patients whose hypertension is difficult to diagnose, including the elderly, patients with diabetes, and individuals with resistant hypertension. ABPM is also beneficial for predicting disease severity and prognosis among patients with chronic renal disease, a condition associated with significant CV risk. Furthermore, ABPM has helped differentiate the 24-hour antihypertensive efficacy of antihypertensive agents among and within differing drug classes and is also useful in drug development for determining optimal dosing. ABPM is an effective method for the accurate diagnosis and management of hypertension and may positively affect clinical outcomes of patients with other risk factors for CV events.

Hypertension–Atherosclerotic Syndrome [238]

Hypertension is not just a disorder of increased intra-arterial pressure. Rather, it is part of a syndrome of commonly associated genetic and/or acquired metabolic functional and structural abnormalities, including dyslipidemia, insulin resistance, hyperinsulinemia, impaired glucose tolerance, hyperglycemia, DM, central or portal obesity, renal function abnormalities, microalbuminuria, abnormal vascular and cardiac smooth muscle proliferation, metabolism, hypertrophy, and hyperplasia, abnormal cellular cation transport or membranopathy, endocrine changes, coagulation abnormalities, hyperuricemia, inflammation, oxidative stress, autoimmune dysfunction, and ED. These abnormalities can lead to acceleration of arterial damage, atherosclerosis, and a greater incidence of atherosclerotic CV complications. This metabolic and structural syndrome of vascular disease exists in both treated and untreated hypertensive patients and in children of hypertensive parents [147]. In fact, hypertensive patients who have been treated to normal BP still have a higher CV event rate than their normotensive counterparts (Figure 23). This could be due to the other risk factors that coexist as part of the hypertensive syndrome or perhaps due to the adverse metabolic and structural side effects associated with the diuretics and BBs used in many of the earlier hypertension trials. Recognition of this concept should lead to a more rational and logical approach to the treatment of hypertension [5, 147, 238].

Prevalence of insulin resistance

- 63% in type 2 diabetes
- 57% in patients with low high-density lipoprotein (HDL) cholesterol
- 54% in hypertriglyceridemia
- 41% in impaired glucose tolerance
- 37% in hyperuricemia
- 29% in hypertension
- 25% in hypercholesterolemia.

(Adapted from Bonora E, Kiechel S, Willeit J, et al. Prevalence of insulin resistance in metabolic disorders: The Bruneck Study. Diabetes 1998; 47: 1643–1649.)

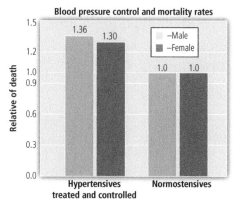

Blood pressure control and mortality rates

Hypertensive patients who have been treated and controlled still have a higher mortality rate than normotensive subjects of 30%

Adapted from Havik RJ et al. *Hypertension* 1989; 13 (suppl 1): 1-22–1-32.

Figure 23 Blood Pressure Control and Mortality Rates in Treated vs Normotensive Patients.

Vascular changes and CV risk factors in borderline hypertensive patients (BP 130/94 mm Hg) vs. normotensive patients

- Vascular resistance   +22%
- Vessel structural changes   +11%
- Total cholesterol   +8%
- HDL cholesterol   −7%
- Triglycerides   +42%
- Insulin   +43%
- Glucose   +4%
- Insulin resistance   +29%

(From Julius S, Jamerson K, Mejia A, et al. The association of borderline hypertension with target organ changes and higher coronary risk: Tecumseh Blood Pressure study. *JAMA* 1990; 264: 354–358.)

Normotensive Hypertension and Hypertension Syndromes [147, 238]

- Hypertension is associated with a constellation of metabolic, biochemical, functional, structural, and clinical abnormalities in over 70% of cases.
- These abnormalities precede development of hypertension by years or decades and worsen with progression of hypertension levels.
- Normotensive adults and children with a positive family history of hypertension have a CV risk profile that is similar to hypertensive patients.
- Early detection, CV risk factor control, lifestyle modification, and nonpharmacologic and pharmacologic therapy are mandatory to reduce CV events.

The following metabolic and structural abnormalities have been demonstrated in the "*Normotensive Hypertensive*" and in the *Hypertension Syndrome* [147, 238].

1. Endothelial dysfunction
2. Abnormal ventricular and arterial compliance (AC)—both proximal C-1 and distal C-2 AC
3. Abnormal glucose/carbohydrate metabolism
4. Insulin resistance (>50%)
5. Endocrine and neurohormonal dysfunction (SNS, RAAS, PRA, aldosterone, and endothelin)
6. Renal function abnormalities (Na+, uric acid, CrCl, MAU, NAG, B2M)
7. Thrombotic/coagulation abnormalities (PAI-1, platelets, fibrinogen, Von Willibrand factor, and thromboxane A2)
8. LVH, LV mass index, and diastolic dysfunction (>50%)
9. Dyslipidemia (80%)
10. Central/portal obesity
11. Hyperuricemia
12. Accelerated atherogenesis
13. Vascular inflammation, oxidative stress, and autoimmune dysfunction
14. Vascular smooth muscle hypertrophy/dystrophic changes and abnormal vascular remodeling with vascular smooth muscle hyperplasia (VSMH)
15. Increased pulse wave velocity (PWV) and increased augmentation index (AI)
16. Increased adhesion molecules (VCAM, ICAM, E-selectin) and leukotrienes
17. Increased growth factors (FBGF, VEGF)
18. Increased ET-1 (endothelin)
19. Increased oxidative stress (radical oxygen species) with reduced oxidative defense
20. Abnormal SBP and DBP response to exercise.

Prehypertension

Epidemiological evidence suggests a continuous relation of usual BP readings of 115/75 mm Hg and the risk of CVD [255]. The Framingham cohort had a stepwise increase in CV events in individuals with high baseline BP within the normotensive range [256]. It would appear that in patients without hypertension (BP <140/90 mm Hg), the BP levels parallel CVD risk in the same way as hypertension [257]. The normotensive patients with various risk factors and an increased global CV risk score may have a higher predicted CV risk than mildly hypertensive patients without the risk factors. In such cases, the absolute benefits of antihypertensive drug therapy could be much greater than for the uncomplicated hypertensive patient. Overall, the disease burden may actually be greater in the normotensive population as they are greater in number than the hypertensive population [257].

Nonpharmacological reduction in BP should be the initial and preferred means of treatment in the prehypertensive patient as will be discussed in detail in Part 3. Small but significant falls in BP have been found in several meta-analysis using nonpharmacological treatments [258–261]. If drug therapy is used in this population, diuretics and the nonselective or cardioselective BBs should be avoided due to their adverse metabolic effects. Preferred drugs are ACEI, ARB, and CCB. The RI, vasodilating BBs, and alpha/beta-blockers are also good choices. Two recent studies have documented that treatment of prehypertensive patients with RAAS agents delayed the onset of stage I hypertension and prolonged the hypertension-free period [262–263]. Evaluation of global CV risk is preferred to determine the need for treatment rather than simply looking at BP level in the absence of other CV risk factors such as DM or dyslipidemia.

Part 3
Treatment of Hypertension

Handbook of Hypertension. By M.C. Houston. Published 2009 by Blackwell Publishing,
ISBN: 978-1-4051-8250-8

Nonpharmacologic Treatment of Hypertension[1]

Nonpharmacologic therapy should be an initial and adjunctive therapy to drug therapy and should be continued during drug therapy to enhance efficacy, reduce dose and number of drugs, limit adverse effects, and promote CV health. An initial trial of 3–6 months should be instituted in patients who have mild elevations in BP without significant risk factors or high-risk global CV risk calculation, end-organ damage, DM, renal insufficiency, CHF, CHD, previous MI or CVA, or other compelling indications. In a compliant patient, these measures can be an effective means of BP reduction (see Hypertension Guidelines: JNC 7, ESH/ESC, BHS, JBS, CHS).

1. Weight reduction (to ideal body weight [IBW]): About 60% of hypertensive patients are at least 20% over IBW. A weight loss of about 4–5 kg will result in a reduction in BP of 7/5 mm Hg in obese and nonobese patients. Weight loss also potentiates the effects of other lifestyle modifications and also drug therapy. Weight reduction should decrease adipose tissue, not lean muscle mass. Reduction in visceral obesity (waist circumference) is particularly important in reducing CV risk. Weight loss improves cardiac output (CO), decreases left ventricular filling pressure (LVFP) and intravascular volume, reduces insulin levels, improves insulin sensitivity, lowers catecholamine levels, and decreases systemic vascular resistance (SVR), sodium retention, sympathetic nervous system activity, plasma renin activity (PRA), and serum aldosterone levels. In addition, weight loss reduces HS-CRP (high-sensitivity C-reactive protein), cytokines (tumor necrosis factor-alpha [TNF-a], interleukins [ILs]) as well as other inflammatory markers and decreases oxidative stress. However, only about 13% of patients will maintain their weight reduction at 36 months.

2. Discontinuation of smoking will reduce vasoconstriction, sympathetic nervous system activity, norepinephrine (NE) levels, RAAS activity, carbon monoxide levels, platelet aggregation, coagulation risk, oxidative stress, and inflammatory markers.

3. Discontinuation or limitation of caffeine will reduce vasoconstriction, PRA, NE levels, and PWV and improve central aortic compliance.

4. Limitation of alcohol: More than one drink per day such as 8 oz of wine, 2 oz of hard liquor, or 24 oz of beer elevates BP, PRA, aldosterone, and cortisol. There appears to be a "U-Shaped" curve for alcohol consumption and BP levels as well as CV risk. Alcohol consumption should be kept below 3 g/day or 20 g/week.

5. Aerobic and resistance exercise and physical training: A combination of aerobic and resistance training for at least 60 min/day should be performed. The aerobic exercises should be for 30 min/day to 60–80% of maximal aerobic capacity (MAC) for age: MAC = MHR (maximal heart rate) = (220 − age). Resistance training should be for 30 min/day alternating muscle groups each day such as upper or lower body exercises. Resistance training may initially elevate BP if not done under supervision with lighter weights. However, progressive resistance training under supervision will improve lean muscle mass, improve insulin sensitivity, and lower BP. Once the patient has optimal CV conditioning, the BP will fall about 11.3/7.5 mm Hg, and CHD reduction is achieved. About 4200 kJ/week achieves maximal reduction in CHD risk. Exercise increases eNOS, NO, improves ED, increases coronary artery blood flow, and reduces SVR and insulin resistance.

---

[1] References at the end of this book are numbers [151, 213–215, 238, 253, 254].
References at the end of this section are numbers [1–51].

TREATMENT OF
HYPERTENSION

6. Other behavioral modifications: Stress management, biofeedback, relaxation, Yoga, Pilates, psychotherapy, hypnosis, transcendental meditation, spirituality, and religion may also lower BP.

7. Discontinuation of concomitant medications that increase BP:
   (a) Oral contraceptives
   (b) NSAIDs and COX-2 inhibitors: interfere with diuretics, BBs, ACEIs, and ARBs
   (c) Antihistamines/decongestants: phenylpropanolamine, ephedrine, phenylephrine, and pseudoephedrine
   (d) Corticosteroids, mineralocorticoids, and anabolic steroids
   (e) Sympathomimetics and amphetamine-like drugs
   (f) Carbenoxolone or licorice
   (g) Tricyclic antidepressants
   (h) Monoamine oxidase (MAO) inhibitors
   (i) Ergot alkaloids
   (j) Diet pills and "energy" pills
   (k) Toxins: lead, cadmium, thallium, mercury, arsenic
   (l) Erythropoietin compounds
   (m) Cyclosporin and tacrolimus
   (n) Caffeine
   (o) Alcohol (over 3 g/day of ETOH)
   (p) Nicotine
   (q) Bromocriptine
   (r) Metoclopramide
   (s) Digitalis
   (t) Disulfuram
   (u) Lithium
   (v) Some herbals.

8. Assurance, patient education, frequent follow-up, and improved patient compliance.

9. Optimal nutrition with selected vitamins, minerals, antioxidants, and nutraceutical supplements [151, 238, 253, 254]. See next section for detailed discussion.

Nutrition, Vitamins, Minerals, Antioxidants, Dietary, and Nutraceutical Supplements in the Prevention and Treatment of Hypertension[2]

Introduction

New and future treatment guidelines for lower target BP levels in the general hypertensive population as well as in specific hypertensive populations will demand a combination of nonpharmacologic and pharmacologic therapy [7, 27]. Hypertensive patients with DM, renal insufficiency, proteinuria, CHF, CHD, and those with previous MI, CVA, or transient ischemic attacks (TIA) often require three to four antihypertensive medications to reach a BP of 140/90 mm Hg or less [7, 27]. Lower recommended target BP goals of 130/80 mm Hg or perhaps 110/70 mm Hg cannot be attained without aggressive use of balanced drug and nondrug treatments. Optimal nutrition and diet, sodium restriction, nutraceutical supplements, achieving IBW, exercise (aerobic and resistance training), restriction of caffeine and alcohol, and cessation of all tobacco products are crucial ingredients of this combination approach if BP and subsequent TOD are to be reduced [253, 254].

Hypertension, nutrition and vascular biology

Hypertension is a consequence of the interaction of our environment and genetics. Macronutrients and micronutrients are crucial in the regulation of BP, subsequent TOD, and atherosclerosis (AS). Nutrient–gene interactions, oxidative stress, inflammation, and subsequent gene expression have either positive or negative influences on vascular biology (VB) in humans. ED and vascular smooth muscle (VSM) dysfunction are the initiating and perpetuating factors in essential hypertension. The correct combination of macronutrients and micronutrients will significantly influence prevention and treatment of hypertension and subsequent vascular complications. Treatment should be directed at the blood vessel as well as the BP. This approach includes identification of and optimal management of CV risk factors, concurrent medical diseases, oxidative stress, and inflammation in order to reduce AS and TOD. Calculation of global CV risk is mandatory to determine timing, need for treatment, type and aggressiveness of therapies. TOD reduction is dependent on both hypertensive and nonhypertensive mechanisms.

Nutritional needs have been imposed on the population during our evolution from a preagricultural, hunter-gatherer milieu to a highly technological agricultural industry that is dependent on mechanical processing for our food supply [18, 48, 253, 254]. The paleolithic diet consisted of low sodium, high potassium and magnesium, high fiber, low fat, high lean animal protein, low refined carbohydrate, and low cholesterol. This dietary intake was composed of fruits, vegetables, berries, nuts, fish, fowl, wild game, and other nutrient-dense foods. However, the modern diet of processed, chemically altered, fast, fried, and frozen food has resulted in an epidemic of nutritionally related diseases such as hypertension, hyperlipidemia, DM, metabolic syndrome, and obesity.

---

[2]References at the end of this book are numbers [151, 213–215, 238, 253, 254].
References at the end of this section are numbers [1–51].

Nutrition trials and hypertension

Reduction in BP and reductions in CV morbidity and mortality have been demonstrated in numerous short- and long-term clinical hypertension nutritional trials [4, 5, 12, 44, 45, 47]. Up to 50% of hypertensive patients in the appropriate stage and risk category may be initially treated with lifestyle modifications based on global hypertensive guidelines [27, 213–215]. However, specific patients with high global CV risk or those with existing CVD, cerebrovascular disease, renal insufficiency, or other TOD, DM, metabolic syndrome or multiple CV risk factors usually require immediate drug therapy in conjunction with lifestyle modifications [27].

Combined nutrients present in food, especially fruits and vegetables, as well as single and combined nutraceutical, nutrient or dietary supplementation have been demonstrated to reduce BP (Table 17) [43, 238, 253, 254].

DASH diets

The combined low sodium Dietary Approaches to Stop Hypertension (DASH-II) diet [4, 45] reduced BP 11.5/6.8 mm Hg within 2 weeks, maintained this BP for the duration of the 2-month study, and improved the quality of life. This level of BP reduction is equivalent to that achieved with pharmacologic monotherapy. All of the DASH diets will be discussed later in this book.

Sodium [253, 254]

A reduction in sodium intake to 2400 mg/day lowers BP an average of 4–6 mm Hg systolic and 2–3 mm Hg diastolic BP in salt-sensitive hypertensive patients [3]. Reduced sodium intake also reduces renal dysfunction, proteinuria, CVD, CHD, MI, CHF, CVA, vascular hypertrophy, LVH, diastolic dysfunction, platelet dysfunction, and sympathetic nervous system activity. Further reductions of BP can be achieved with progressive restriction from 150 mmol to 100 mmol to 50 mmol of dietary sodium per day in the DASH-II diet [45]. The ratio of sodium to potassium, magnesium, and calcium is important, as well as the total sodium intake. A sodium to potassium ratio of 1:1 is optimal. Decreasing intake of refined carbohydrates enhances the effect of sodium restriction and BP. Reduction in TOD is also independent of BP reduction.

Table 17 Lifestyle Changes and SBP Meta-analysis of Clinical Diet Trials

Intervention	Reduction in SBP (mm Hg)
↑ Mg^{++}	0–1
↑ Ca^{++}	2
↑ K^+	4
↓ ETOH	4
Fish oil	6
↓ Na^+	6
↓ Weight	8
Exercise	10
DASH diet	12

DASH = Dietary Approaches to Stop Hypertension; SBP = systolic blood pressure.

Potassium [253, 254]

The magnitude of BP reduction with dietary supplementation of 60–120 mEq/day of potassium is 4.4 mm Hg systolic and 2.5 mm Hg diastolic BP in hypertensive patients [3, 49]. In addition, potassium may reduce CV events and CVA independent of BP reductions and will decrease the risk of cardiac arrhythmias, renal insufficiency, insulin resistance, and glucose intolerance. The recommended dietary intake is a K^+/Na^+ ratio of 5:1. Potassium is best obtained from fruits and vegetables and other whole foods rather than oral supplements if possible. Potassium intake must be limited in patients with renal insufficiency. The mechanisms for BP reduction include natriuresis, baroreflex sensitivity modulation, reduction in SVR, decreased sensitivity to NE and A-II, increase in Na/K ATPase and DNA synthesis in vascular smooth muscle cell (VSMC), with decrease in VSM hypertrophy and increase in bradykinin and urinary kallikrein.

Magnesium [253, 254]

Magnesium supplementation in the range of 500–1000 mg/day reduces SBP 2.7 mm Hg and DBP 3.4 mm Hg [51]. The most effective magnesium is one that is chelated to an amino acid to improve absorption and reduce the incidence of diarrhea. Magnesium is a direct vasodilator which lowers SVR, reduces arrhythmias, improves insulin resistance, decreases LVH, and improves arterial compliance. The mechanism is blockade of calcium influx into VSM cells and increases levels of the vasodilating prostaglandin E1 (PGE1). Magnesium binds in a necessary and cooperative manner with potassium to reduce SVR. Magnesium intake must be limited in patients with renal insufficiency.

Calcium [253, 254]

A recent meta-analysis of the effect of calcium supplementation in hypertensive patients demonstrated a reduction in SBP of 4.3 mm Hg and DBP of 1.5 mm Hg [9]. Calcium is particularly effective in patients with a high sodium intake and when given in a natural form with potassium and magnesium [36, 41, 50]. Blacks, elderly, diabetic, salt-sensitive, pregnant and postmenopausal women, and low-renin hypertensive patients have the best response. Vitamin D intake must be balanced with the calcium intake.

Protein [253, 254]

High intake of nonanimal protein (1 g/kg/day) (Intersalt Study and Intermap Study) is associated with a lower BP [3, 19]. Hydrolyzed whey protein [29] and sardine muscle extract [28] significantly lower BP in humans through an ACEI mechanism. Sardine muscle protein at 3 g/day reduced BP 9.7/5.3 mm Hg. Whey protein must be hydrolyzed to be effective in lowering BP. Doses of 30 g/day reduce BP by 11/7 mm Hg within 7 days. Bonito protein is also a natural ACEI which decreases BP 10.2/7 mm Hg at 1.5 g/day. In addition, protein reduces SNS activity, induces natriuresis, inhibits tyrosine kinase, reduces VSM hypertrophy, lowers superoxide anion, and decreases aldosterone. The ingestion of 40 g of soybean protein lowers BP about 4.3/2.1 mm Hg. Fermented soy is recommended. Soy protein improves arterial compliance and activates peroxisome proliferator-activated receptors (PPARs).

Fats [253, 254]

Consumption of omega-3 fatty acids (polyunsaturated fatty acids – PUFA) such as EPA (eicosapentaenoic acid) and DHA (docosahexanoic acid) significantly reduces mean BP in humans by 5.8–8.1 mm Hg [8, 32, 37, 42]. DHA is more effective than EPA in lowering BP. Combined with omega-9 fatty acids (olive oil) (monounsaturated [MUFA] oleic acid), low saturated fat, elimination of trans-fatty acids, and increased GLA (gamma linolenic acid), these dietary changes may have dramatic effects on BP, VB, and AS. The omega-3 to omega-6 fatty acid ratio should be 1:1 to 4:1 with consumption of cold-water fish (cod, tuna, mackerel, salmon) or EPA/DHA supplements (3–4 g/day). The olive oil dose (MUFA) is 40 g of extra-virgin olive oil per day (4 tablespoons) [20]. MUFA in these doses reduce BP 8/6 mm Hg and improve glucose intolerance. The GLA dose should be about 50% of the total daily intake of DHA and EPA. GLA increases PGE1 and PGE2 which vasodilate. GLA also reduces aldosterone, reduces adrenal AT1R affinity and density, and decreases SNS and RAAS activity. Gamma/Delta Vitamin E at about 100 IU should be consumed with these doses of DHA, EPA, and GLA to reduce oxidative stress in the cell membranes. Omega-3 fatty acids increase eNOS and NO, improve insulin sensitivity, act as PPAR alpha-agonists, improve ED, reduce NE, decrease calcium influx, suppress ACE activity, and transforming growth factor (TGF) beta expression trans fats will elevate BP.

Garlic [253, 254]

The prospective double-blinded placebo-controlled studies utilizing the correct form (wild garlic is best) and dose of garlic demonstrate only minimal decreases in SBP of 5–8 mm Hg or mean BP of 2–3 mm Hg. However, garlic may have numerous other beneficial vascular effects as it is a natural ACEI and CCB, and also increases NO and BK and decreases the sensitivity to NE, vasodilates by reducing SVR, and improves arterial stiffness [11].

Seaweed [253, 254]

Wakame seaweed in doses of 3.3 g/day significantly lowers BP in hypertensive humans within 4 weeks due to ACEI activity [38]. The average reduction in BP was 14/5 mm Hg. Long-term use in Japan appears to be safe.

Fiber [253, 254]

Clinical trials with various types of fiber to reduce BP have been inconsistent [3, 25]. The average BP reduction in prospective studies using 60 g/day of oatmeal fiber, 3 g of betaglucan per day, glucomannan, or 7 g of psyllium per day is 7.5 mm Hg/5.5 mm Hg. Fiber improves insulin sensitivity and ED, increases renal sodium loss, and decreases SNS activity.

Vitamin C [253, 254]

Vitamin C at doses of 250–500 mg BID lowers BP, especially in hypertensive patients with initially low plasma ascorbate levels [16, 21, 39]. Vitamin C improves ED, increases aortic compliance, nitric oxide, and PGI2 levels, is a potent antioxidant, decreases SVR, and has a mild diuretic effect. The BP falls an average of 7/4 mm Hg. The greater the initial BP and the lower the plasma ascorbate level, the greater the response. Combinations with other antioxidants and vitamins may have synergistic antihypertensive effects.

Vitamin B-6 [253, 254]

Supplemental vitamin B-6 at 5 mg/kg/day reduced BP 14/10 mm Hg over 4 weeks in one small human study [6]. Vitamin B-6 reduces central sympathetic nervous system activity, acts as a central alpha-agonist (i.e., clonidine), a CCB, and a diuretic. Pyridoxine also improves insulin sensitivity, and carbohydrate metabolism reduces SNS activity and end-organ responses to glucocorticoids and mineralocorticoids, which, in turn, improves BP. Daily doses should probably not exceed 200 mg to avoid neuropathy.

Vitamin E [253, 254]

The efficacy of vitamin E to lower BP in humans has been mixed. A recent study (*J Hypertension* 2007; 227: 227–234) did not show improvement on mixed tocopherols.

Vitamin D [253, 254]

Vitamin D deficiency leads to insulin resistance hypertension and VSMC hypertrophy. Replacement of vitamin D lowers BP, decreases HR, PRA, A-II. Doses of 5000 IU/day of Vitamin D3 are recommended until the plasma level is about 80 ng/mL.

Resveratrol

Resveratrol reduces central aortic pressure by 7.4 mm Hg with the consumption of 250 mL of regular or dealcoholized red wine (*Am J Hypertension* 2005; 18: 1161).

Dark chocolate and cocoa [253, 254]

One hundred grams of dark chocolate reduced SBP by 6.4 mm Hg. Meta-analysis indicates average reductions for 4.7/2.8 mm Hg (*Am J Clin Nutr* 2005; 81: 611 and *Arch Intern Med* 2007; 167: 626).

Lycopene [253, 254]

Paran et al. [40] evaluated 30 subjects with grade I hypertension given tomato lycopene extract for 8 weeks. The BP fell 9/7 mm Hg within 8 weeks. Lycopene is found in high concentrations in tomatoes, tomato products, guava, watermelon, papaya, and apricots.

Co-Enzyme Q-10 (ubiquinone) [253, 254]

Enzymatic assays show a deficiency of Co-Enzyme Q-10 (Co-Q-10) in 39% of essential hypertensive patients vs. only a 6% deficiency in controls [34]. Human studies demonstrate significant and consistent reductions in BP averaging 15/10 mm Hg in all of the reported prospective clinical trials [13–15, 31, 33]. Doses of 100–225 mg/day (1–2 mg/kg/day) to achieve a therapeutic plasma level of about $-3\,\mu g/mL$ are effective within 4–8 weeks in reducing BP. The BP remains steady at this level but returns to baseline at 2 weeks following discontinuation of Co-Q-10. Co-Q-10 reduces SVR, catecholamine, and aldosterone levels, improves insulin sensitivity and endothelial function, and increases nitric oxide levels [13, 14, 33]. No adverse effects have been noted at these doses with chronic use. Patients have been able to stop or reduce the number of antihypertensive drugs by one to three drugs with chronic ingestion of Co-Q-10. A reputable, certified absorbable form, with excellent bioavailability and documented measurement of plasma levels are important clinical considerations.

Alpha-lipoic acid [253, 254]
Alpha-lipoic acid 200 mg BID with acetyl-L-carnitine 500 mg BID reduced BP 7/3 mm Hg in patients with metabolic syndrome and hypertension, and increased brachial artery diameter (*J Clin Hypertension* 2007; 9: 249).

L-Arginine [253, 254]
L-Arginine is the natural predominant precursor for vascular nitric oxide. Administration of 10 g orally per day using a combination of food such as nuts and/or as a nutritional supplement significantly reduces BP in human subjects by 6.2/6.8 mm Hg, improves ED, PAD, and blood flow [30, 46].

Taurine [253, 254]
Taurine, a sulfonic beta-amino acid, is significantly reduced in the urine of essential hypertensive patients [2]. Administration of 6 g of taurine per day lowers BP 9/4 mm Hg [22]. Taurine induces a sodium-water diuresis, vasodilation, increases atrial natriuretic factor (ANF), reduces sympathetic nervous system activity and aldosterone levels, improves insulin sensitivity, and reduces homocysteine levels.

Celery [253, 254]
Celery has antihypertensive properties due to 3-*N*-butyl phthalide, apigenin, and other substances that act like ACEI or CCB. Four large celery sticks per day or the equivalent in celery juice, oil, or celery seed extract reduces BP in animals and humans [10, 17, 26, 34, 35].

Pycnogenol [253, 254]
Pycnogenol of 200 mg/day reduces BP 7/2 mm Hg, increases NO, and reduces thromboxane B2. It has a mild ACEI activity (*Nutr Res* 2001; 21: 1251).

Melatonin [253, 254]
Melatonin of 2.5 mg at night reduced BP 6/4 mm Hg (*Hypertension* 2004; 43: 192).

Zinc [253, 254]
Low levels of zinc are associated with hypertension, CHD, DM, and insulin resistance. Zinc inhibits gene expression and transcription via NFK-B (NF Kappa-B) and AP-I (activated protein-I) which effects membrane ion exchange. There exists a close relationship between zinc, calcium, sodium, magnesium, and potassium especially with modulation of the neurohormonal systems (SNS and RAAS). About 25–50 mg/day is recommended.

Combinations
Combinations of various nutraceutical or dietary supplements, vitamins, minerals, and antioxidants may further enhance BP reduction, reduce oxidative stress and inflammation, and improve vascular function and structure [24]. Optimal doses and combinations are yet to be determined, but future research will provide important data.

Finally, the addition of lifestyle modification with low-dose combination antihypertensive drugs provides additive or synergistic BP reduction to achieve these lower BP goals, improves risk factors, metabolic parameters, vascular structure and function, and allows for lower doses and number of drugs with reduced side effects to maximize reductions in TOD.

Natural antihypertensive compounds categorized by antihypertensive class

As has been discussed previously, many of the natural compounds such as food, nutraceutical and dietary supplements, vitamins, antioxidants, or minerals function in a similar fashion to a specific class of antihypertensive drugs (Table 18). Although the potency of these natural compounds may be less than or equal to the antihypertensive drug and the onset of action slower when used in combination with either the drugs or other nutraceutical agents, the antihypertensive effect is magnified. In addition, many of these natural compounds have varied, additive, or synergistic mechanisms of action in lowering BP.

Table 18 Natural Antihypertension Compounds Categorized by Antihypertensive Class

Intervention
Diuretics
Hawthorne berry
Vitamin B-6 (pyridoxine)
Taurine
Celery
GLA
Vitamin C (ascorbic acid)
K^+
Mg^{++}
Ca^{++}
Protein
Fiber
Co-Enzyme Q-10
L-Carnitine
Beta-blockers
Hawthorne Berry
Central alpha-agonists
Taurine
K^+
Zinc
Na^+ Restriction
Protein
Fiber
Vitamin C
Vitamin B-6
Co-Enzyme Q-10
Celery
GLA/DGLA
Garlic
Direct vasodilators
Omega-3 FA
MUFA (omega-9 FA)
K^+
Mg^{++}
Ca^{++}
Soy
Fiber
Garlic

(Continued)

Table 18 (*Continued*)

Intervention

Flavonoids
Vitamin C
Vitamin E
Co-Enzyme Q-10
L-Arginine
Taurine
Celery
ALA
Calcium channel blockers
ALA
Vitamin C (ascorbic acid)
Vitamin B-6 (pyridoxine)
Magnesium (Mg^{++})
NAC
Vitamin E
Hawthorne berry
Celery
Omega-3 fatty acids (EPA and DHA)
Calcium
Garlic
Angiotensin converting enzyme inhibitors
Garlic
Seaweed—various (Wakame, etc.)
Tuna protein/muscle
Sardine protein/muscle
Hawthorne berry
Bonito fish (dried)
Pycnogenol
Casein
Hydrolyzed whey protein
Sour milk
Gelatin
Sake
Essential fatty acids (Omega-3 FA)
Chicken egg yolks
Zein
Dried salted fish
Fish sauce
Zinc
Hydrolyzed wheat germ isolate
Angiotensin receptor blockers
Potassium (K$^+$)
Fiber
Garlic
Vitamin C
Vitamin B-6 (Pyridoxine)
Co-Enzyme Q-10
Celery
GLA and DGLA

ALA = alpha-lipoic acid; DGLA = dihomo gamma linolenic acid; DHA = docosahexanoic acid; EPA = eicosapentaenoic acid; GLA = gamma linolenic acid; MUFA = monounsaturated fatty acid; NAC = N-acetyl cysteine.

Nutritional Intervention, Prevention, and Treatment of Hypertension Trials and Consensus Reports

There are many prospective nutritional studies that have demonstrated improvement in BP as well as CV events. These are outlined as follows [238, 253, 254].

1. Health Professionals Follow-Up Study: CVA reduction (K+ intake)
2. Health Professionals Follow-Up Study: CHD/MI reduction
3. Multiple Risk Factor Intervention Trial (MRFIT): CHD reduction
4. Lyon Diet Heart Study: CHD/MI reduction
5. Trials of Hypertension Prevention (TOHP-I and -II): BP prevention
6. Trial of Nonpharmacologic Intervention in Elderly (Tone): BP reduction
7. Treatment of Mild Hypertension Study (TOMHS): BP reduction
8. Dietary Approaches to Stop Hypertension (DASH-I): BP reduction
9. Dietary Approaches to Stop Hypertension (DASH-II-Na+): BP reduction
10. Neonatal Sodium Restriction Study: BP prevention × 15 years
11. Mediterranean Diet: BP reduction
12. Inter map: BP reduction (nonanimal protein)
13. JNC 7: BP reduction
14. AHA Nutritional Committee (BP reduction)
15. Cardiovascular Risk Reduction Dietary Intervention Trial (CRRDIT)
16. INTERSALT: BP reduction
17. Nurses Health Study (NHS)
18. US Male Health Study (USMHS)
19. National Diet Heart Study (NDHS)
20. Vanguard Study
21. Premier Trial

Further Reading on Nutrition and Dietary Supplements

1. Ackermann RT, Mulrow CD, Ramirez G, et al. Garlic shows promise for improving some cardiovascular risk factors. *Arch Intern Med* 2001; 161: 813–824.
2. Ando K, Fujita T. Etiological and physiopathological significance of taurine in hypertension. *Nippon Rinsho* 1992; 50: 374–381.
3. Appel LJ. The role of diet in the prevention and treatment of hypertension. *Curr Atheroscler Rep* 2000; 2: 521–528.
4. Appel LJ, Moore TJ, Obarzanek E, et al. A clinical trial of the effects of dietary patterns on blood pressure. *N Engl J Med* 1997; 336: 1117–1124.
5. Ascherio A, Rimm EB, Hernan MA, et al. Intake of potassium, magnesium, calcium and fiber and risk of stroke among US men. *Circulation* 1998; 98: 1198–1204.
6. Aybak M, Sermet A, Ayyildiz MO, Karakilcik AZ. Effect of oral pyridoxine hydrochloride supplementation on arterial blood pressure in patients with essential hypertension. *Arzneimittelforschung* 1995; 45: 1271–1273.
7. Bakris GL. A practical approach to achieving recommended blood pressure goals in diabetic patients. *Arch Intern Med* 2001; 161: 2661–2667.
8. Bao DQ, Mori TA, Burke V, et al. Effects of dietary fish and weight reduction on ambulatory blood pressure in overweight hypertensives. *Hypertension* 1998; 32: 710–717.
9. Bucher HC, Cook RJ, Guyatt GH, et al. Effects of dietary calcium supplementation on blood pressure. A meta-analysis of randomized controlled trials. *JAMA* 1996; 275: 1016–1022.
10. Castleman M. *The Healing Herbs: The Ultimate Guide to the Curative Power of Nature's Medicines.* Emmaus, PA: Rodale Press, 1991: 105–107.
11. Clouatre D. *European Wild Garlic: The Better Garlic.* San Francisco: Pax Publishing, 1995.
12. De Lorgeril M, Salen P, Martin JL, et al. Mediterranean diet, traditional risk factors and the rate of cardiovascular complications after myocardial infarction: Final report of the Lyon Diet Heart Study. *Circulation* 1999; 99: 779–785.
13. Digiesi V, Cantini F, Bisi G, et al. Mechanism of action of coenzyme Q10 in essential hypertension. *Curr Ther Res* 1992; 51: 668–672.
14. Digiesi V, Cantini F, Brodbeck B. Effect of coenzyme Q10 on essential hypertension. *Curr Ther Res* 1990; 47: 841–845.
15. Digiesi V, Cantini F, Oradei A, et al. Coenzyme Q-10 in essential hypertension. *Mol Aspects Med* 1994; 15: 8257–8263.
16. Duffy SJ, Gokce N, Holbrook M, et al. Treatment of hypertension with ascorbic acid. *Lancet* 1999; 354: 2048–2049.
17. Duke JA. *The Green Pharmacy Herbal Handbook.* Emmaus, PA: Rodale Press, 2000: 68–69.
18. Eaton SB, Eaton SB III, Konner MJ. Paleolithic nutrition revisited: A twelve-year retrospective on its nature and implications. *Eur J Clin Nutr* 1997; 51: 207–216.
19. Elliott P, Dennis B, Dyer AR, et al. Relation of dietary protein (total, vegetable, animal) to blood pressure: INTERMAP epidemiologic study. Presented at the 18th Scientific Meeting of the International Society of Hypertension, Chicago, IL, August 20–24, 2000.

20. Ferrara LA, Raimondi S, d'Episcopa I, et al. Olive oil and reduced need for antihypertensive medications. *Arch Intern Med* 2000; 160: 837–842.

21. Fotherby MD, Williams JC, Forster LA, et al. Effect of vitamin C on ambulatory blood pressure and plasma lipids in older persons. *J Hypertens* 2000; 18: 411–415.

22. Fujita T, Ando K, Noda H, et al. Effects of increased adrenomedullary activity and taurine in young patients with borderline hypertension. *Circulation* 1987; 75: 525–532.

23. Gaby AR. The role of co-enzyme Q-10 in clinical medicine: Part II. Cardiovascular disease, hypertension, diabetes mellitus and infertility. *Altern Med Rev* 1996; 1(3): 168–175.

24. Galley HF, Thornton J, Howdle PD, et al. Combination oral antioxidant supplementation reduces blood pressure. *Clin Sci* 1997; 92: 361–365.

25. He J, Welton PK. Effect of dietary fiber and protein intake on blood pressure. A review of epidemiologic evidence. *Clin Exp Hypertens* 1999; 21: 785–796.

26. Heinerman J. *Heinerman's New Encyclopedia of Fruits and Vegetables.* Paramus, NJ: Prentice Hall, 1995: 93–95.

27. Joint National Committee on Prevention, Detection, Evaluation, and Treatment of High Blood Pressure: The sixth report of the Joint National Committee on the prevention, detection, evaluation, and treatment of high blood pressure. *Arch Intern Med* 1997; 157: 2413–2446.

28. Kawasaki T, Seki E, Osajima K, et al. Antihypertensive effect of valyl-tyrosine, a short chain peptide derived from sardine muscle hydrolyzate, on mild hypertensive subjects. *J Hum Hypertens* 2000; 14: 519–523.

29. Kawase M, Hashimoto H, Hosoda M, et al. Effect of administration of fermented milk containing whey protein concentrate to rats and healthy men on serum lipids and blood pressure. *J Dairy Sci* 2000; 83: 255–263.

30. Kelly JJ, Williamson P, Martin A, Whitworth JA. Effects of oral l-arginine on plasma nitrate and blood pressure in cortisol-treated humans. *J Hypertens* 2001; 19: 263–268.

31. Kendler BS. Nutritional strategies in cardiovascular disease control: An update on vitamins and conditionally essential nutrients. *Prog Cardiovasc Nurs* 1999; 14: 124–129.

32. Knapp HR, Fitzgerald GA. The antihypertensive effects of fish oil: A controlled study of polyunsaturated fatty acid supplements in essential hypertension. *N Engl J Med* 1989; 320: 1037–1043.

33. Langsjoen P, Willis R, Folkers K. Treatment of essential hypertension with coenzyme Q10. *Mol Aspects Med* 1994; 15: 8265–8272.

34. Le OT, Elliott WJ. Dose response relationship of blood pressure and serum cholesterol to 3-*N*-butyl phthalide, a component of celery oil. *Clin Res* 1991; 39: 750A. Abstract.

35. Le OT, Elliott WJ. Mechanisms of the hypotensive effect of 3-*N*-butyl phthalide (BUPH): A component of celery oil. *J Am Hypertens* 1992; 40: 326A. Abstract.

36. McCarron DA. Calcium metabolism in hypertension. *Keio J Med* 1995; 44: 105–114.

37. Morris M, Sacks F, Rosner B. Does fish oil lower blood pressure? A meta-analysis of controlled trials. *Circulation* 1993; 88: 523–533.

38. Nakano T, Hidaka H, Uchida J, et al. Hypotensive effects of wakame. *J Jpn Soc Clin Nutr* 1998; 20: 92.

39. Ness AR, Chee D, Elliot P. Vitamin C and blood pressure — an overview. *J Hum Hypertens* 1997; 11: 343–350.

40. Paran E, Engelhard Y. Effect of tomato's lycopene on blood pressure, serum lipoproteins, plasma homocysteine and oxidative stress markers in grade I hypertensive patients. *Am J Hypertens* 2001; 14: 141A. Abstract P-333.

41. Preuss HG. Diet, genetics and hypertension. *J Am Coll Nutr* 1997; 16: 296–305.

42. Frisco D, Paniccia R, Bandinelli B, et al. Effect of medium-term supplementation with a moderate dose of n-3 polyunsaturated fatty acids on blood pressure in mild hypertensive patients. *Thromb Res* 1998; 91: 105–112.

43. Reaven P, Parthasarathy S, Grasse BJ, et al. Effects of oleate-rich and linoleate-rich diets on the susceptibility of low density lipoprotein to oxidative modification in mildly hypercholesterolemic subjects. *J Clin Invest* 1993; 91: 668–676.

44. Resnick LM, Oparil S, Chait A, et al. Factors affecting blood pressure responses to diet: The Vanguard Study. *Am J Hypertens* 2000; 13: 956–965.

45. Sacks FM, Svetkey LP, Vollmer WM, et al. Effects on blood pressure of reduced dietary sodium and the dietary approaches to stop hypertension (DASH) diet. *N Engl J Med* 2001; 344: 3–10.

46. Siani A, Pagano E, Lacone R, et al. Blood pressure and metabolic changes during dietary l-arginine supplementation in humans. *Am J Hypertens* 2000; 13: 547–551.

47. The Treatment of Mild Hypertension Research Group. The Treatment of Mild Hypertension Study: A randomized, placebo-controlled trial of a nutritional hygienic regimen along with various drug monotherapies. *Arch Intern Med* 1991; 151: 1413–1423.

48. Weder AB. Your mother was right: Eat your fruits and vegetables. *Curr Hypertens Rep* 1999; 1: 11–12.

49. Whelton PK, He J. Potassium in preventing and treating high blood pressure. *Semin Nephrol* 1999; 19: 494–499.

50. Whiting SJ, Wood R, Kim K. Calcium supplementation. *J Am Acad Nurse Pract* 1997; 9: 187–192.

51. Witteman JCM, Grobbee DE, Derk FHM, et al. Reduction of blood pressure with oral magnesium supplementation in women with mild to moderate hypertension. *J Clin Nutr* 1994; 60: 129–135.

The DASH Diets: DASH-I and DASH-II Sodium [4, 45]

Dietary approaches to stop hypertension

The DASH-I diet published in 1997 [4] was a landmark nutritional trial that demonstrated significant reduction in BP in hypertensive patients. The DASH-II sodium diet published in 2001 [45] confirmed the value of DASH-I, but proved that moderate to severe sodium restriction further enhanced BP reduction. These nutritional studies are so important in the nonpharmacologic management of hypertension that they will be presented in detail.

The DASH-I diet was a 2-month, multicenter, randomized, controlled prospective clinical trial of 379 subjects with borderline or stage I hypertension (SBP <160 mm Hg and DBP 80–95 mm Hg), no concomitant diseases and on no antihypertensive drugs. The average age was 45 years, two-thirds were minorities (60% blacks, 6% other races, and 34% whites). The design of the study and prescribed nutrition for the three treatment groups, which included control subjects, the fruit and vegetable (F + V) group and the combined diet (C) group, are shown in Figures 24 and 25. After a 3-week control diet in all subjects, randomization was to one of the three aforementioned treatment groups for 8 weeks. The sodium content remained the same in all three groups at 3 g/day. All diets were prepared and were well tolerated with a 93% adherence rate. There was no change in alcohol intake, weight, or sodium excretion during the study. Subjects met weekly with the investigators.

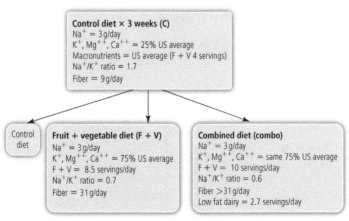

- Borderline or stage I hypertension (SBP<160, DBP 80–95)
- Age average 45 years; 2/3 minorities; $n = 379$
- No antihypertensive drugs, otherwise healthy
- Protocol

Control diet × 3 weeks (C)
$Na^+ = 3$ g/day
$K^+, Mg^{++}, Ca^{++} = 25\%$ US average
Macronutrients = US average (F + V 4 servings)
Na^+/K^+ ratio = 1.7
Fiber = 9 g/day

Control diet

Fruit + vegetable diet (F + V)
$Na^+ = 3$ g/day
$K^+, Mg^{++}, Ca^{++} = 75\%$ US average
F + V = 8.5 servings/day
Na^+/K^+ ratio = 0.7
Fiber = 31 g/day

Combined diet (combo)
$Na^+ = 3$ g/day
$K^+, Mg^{++}, Ca^{++} = $ same 75% US average
F + V = 10 servings/day
Na^+/K^+ ratio = 0.6
Fiber >31 g/day
Low fat dairy = 2.7 servings/day

8 weeks (all diets)

DBP = diastolic blood pressure; SBP = systolic blood pressure.

Figure 24 DASH-I Trial Design.

The results of this clinical trial demonstrated significant reductions in BP with a controlled diet including the described modifications of increasing whole grains, nuts, poultry, fish, fruits, vegetables, K^+, Mg^{++}, and Ca^{++}, while reducing intake of saturated and trans-fatty acids, red meat, sweets, sugars, and other refined carbohydrates. The hypertensive subjects on the combined diet had the greatest BP reduction of 11.4/5.5 mm Hg. Minority subjects, especially blacks, had greater reductions in BP compared to white subjects, and hypertensive subjects had greater BP reductions than normotensive subjects. Urinary Mg^{++} and K^+ increased in the "F + V" and "C" groups, whereas urinary Ca^{++} decreased in the "F + V" group. The urinary Na^+ remained constant in all three groups.

The reduction in BP occurred immediately, reaching near maximum levels at 2 weeks, but was sustained throughout the 8-week study. In addition, the quality of life improved in subjects on the "F + V" and "C" diets. The combined treatment group had reductions in BP that were equal to that obtained with pharmacologic treatment of mild hypertension. DASH-I emphasizes the importance of combined nutrients as they occur in natural food.

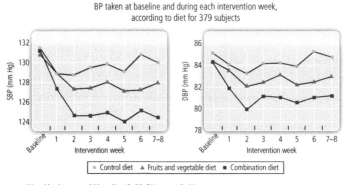

BP taken at baseline and during each intervention week, according to diet for 379 subjects

⬤ Control diet   ▲ Fruits and vegetable diet   ■ Combination diet

BP = blood pressure; DBP = diastolic BP; SBP = systolic BP.

Figure 25 Mean Systolic and Diastolic BP.

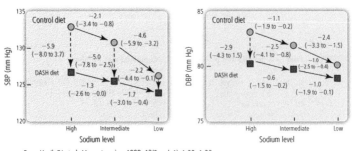

From Havik RJ et al. *Hypertension* 1989; 13(Suppl. 1): 1-22–1-32.
DBP = diastolic blood pressure; SBP = systolic blood pressure.

Figure 26 DASH-II Sodium Diet: Results.

The DASH-II diet took the DASH-I diet one step further, proving that moderate to severe Na$^+$ restriction reduced BP even more in all three study groups (Figure 26). This was a multicenter, randomized, controlled prospective study of 412 subjects on either a control diet or one of three DASH-Na$^+$ diets for 30 days (150, 100, or 50 mmol Na$^+$ intake). The SBP and DBP reductions were significant with each incremental decrease in Na$^+$ intake. The important conclusions and results of this study are shown. Hypertensive subjects, blacks, and women had the greatest BP reductions.

A comparison of the relative BP reduction in DASH-I and DASH-II in hypertensive subjects is shown in Table 19. The net BP reduction vs. the control patient reduction was greatest in the DASH-II combination, low Na$^+$ (50 mmol) diet ($-11.5/6.8$ mm Hg). The message from these two studies is clear. Hypertensive patients can achieve significant BP reductions that are equivalent to drug therapy when used in mild hypertensive patients by combining a more severe Na$^+$ restriction of 50 mmol/day with the combination DASH-I diet. These benefits are immediate, sustainable, inexpensive, increase nutrient levels, and improve the individual's quality of life.

DASH-I and DASH-II conclusions

- Reduction of sodium intake to 50 mmol/day from current recommendations of 100 mmol/day significantly reduces BP.
- DASH combination diet with low sodium intake of 50 mmol/day lowers BP more in combination than either singly.
- Level of dietary sodium had twice BP reducing effect with the control diet than with DASH diet (p < 0.001).
- BP reductions occurred in all patients regardless of age, gender, ethnicity, or BP level (normal).
- Hypertensive patients, blacks, and women had the greatest BP reductions.
- Low Na1 intake attenuated the hypotensive effects of K$^+$ and Ca$^+$.

Conclusion: Individuals with above-optimal BP, including stage I hypertension, can make multiple lifestyle changes that lower BP.

Key point: Patients with suboptimal BP who receive behavioral interventions plus DASH diet have only a 12% chance of developing hypertension at 6 months and 35% chance of having optimal BP at 6 months (3-to-1 odds of beneficial outcome).

Table 19 Summary of BP Reductions in DASH-I and DASH-II Na$^+$ Diets Hypertensive Patients and Overall

	SBP (mm Hg)	DBP (mm Hg)
DASH-I overall combination diet vs. control diet	-5	-3
DASH-I hypertensive patients combination diet vs. control diet	-10.7	-5.2
DASH-II overall combination low Na$^+$ DASH diet vs. control high Na$^+$ diet	$-8.9*$	-4.5
DASH-II hypertensive patients combination low Na$^+$ DASH diet vs. control high Na$^+$ diet	$-11.5*$	$-6.8*$

DASH = Dietary Approaches to Stop Hypertension; DBP = diastolic blood pressure; SBP = systolic blood pressure.
*p < 0.001.

The Premier Clinical Trial [211]

The premier clinical trial [211] evaluated lifestyle modifications on 810 subjects using an established recommendations, established plus DASH and advice only (Figures 27 and 28). The prevalence of optimal BP <120/80 mm Hg was 19% in the advice only group, 39% in the established group, and 35% in the established plus DASH group.

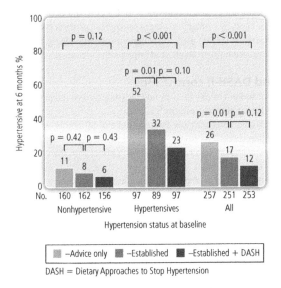

DASH = Dietary Approaches to Stop Hypertension

Figure 27 Percentage of Participants with Hypertension at 6 Months by Randomized Group Among Nonhypertensive, Hypertensive, and All Participants at Baseline.

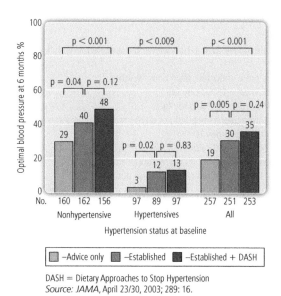

DASH = Dietary Approaches to Stop Hypertension
Source: JAMA, April 23/30, 2003; 289: 16.

Figure 28 Percentage of Participants with Optimal Blood Pressure at 6 Months by Randomized Group Among Nonhypertensive Participants at Baseline, Hypertensive at Baseline, and All Participants at Baseline.

Obesity

1. It is not safe to lose over 3.3 lb/week and the preferred weight loss is 1–2 lb/week.
2. Body fat is more important than body weight.
   Males should be <15% body fat
   Females should be <22% body fat.
3. The number of calories needed per day to maintain the same weight is your weight in pounds times 10.
   That is, 160 lb = 1600 calories
   1600 calories is your BMR (basal metabolic rate).
4. It takes a 3500-calorie deficit to lose one pound.
5. If body mass index (BMI) is over 27, there is a danger of developing significant health problems.
6. Four major factors contribute to obesity:
   (i) Genetics
   (ii) Metabolic factors
   (iii) Diet
   (iv) Physical inactivity.
7. Waist circumference over the value indicated below is associated with a high risk of disease and may be the single best predictor of obesity-related CVD and overall morbidity and mortality:
   Men over 40 inches
   Women over 35 inches.
8. Neck circumference also correlates with high disease risk.
   Men over 15.6 inches
   Women over 14.4 inches.
9. Obesity will increase the risk of morbidity and mortality of the following diseases:
   Hypertension
   Dyslipidemia
   Type 2 diabetes and insulin resistance
   CHD and MI
   Stroke
   Gallbladder disease
   Osteoarthritis
   Sleep apnea
   Respiratory problems
   Cancer of breast, prostate, colon, and endometrium
   Chronic kidney disease
   Microalbuminuria and proteinuria.
10. IBW calculation (depends on the body frame size):
    Women: 100 lb first 5 feet, then 5 lb for each additional inch of height
    Men: 106 lb first 5 feet, then 6 lb for each additional inch of height
    10% for large frame and delete 10% for small frame.

Exercise Activities and Kilocalories Used

Energy values in kilocalories per hour of selected activities:

Weight (pounds)	95	125	155	185	215	245
Slow walking	86	114	140	168	196	222
Fast walking	172	228	280	336	392	555
Hiking	285	342	420	504	588	666
Jogging	430	570	700	840	980	1110
Running	480	770	945	1134	1323	1499
Heavy work	194	256	315	378	441	500
Sweeping	108	142	175	210	245	278
Scrubbing	237	313	385	462	539	611
Tennis	301	399	490	588	686	777
Golf (walk)	237	313	385	462	539	611
Golf (in a cart)	151	200	245	294	343	389
Swimming (light laps)	344	456	560	672	784	888
Swimming (hard laps)	430	570	700	840	980	1110

Exercise: the prescription

Aerobic exercise should be combined with resistance training:

- Duration: 60 minutes per session/daily
  Warmup/Condition/Cooldown
  300 calories expenditure.
- Intensity: Percent of MHR for age—MHR = MAC
  Mild: 50–60% × (220 − age)
  Moderate: 70% × (220 − age)
  Heavy: 80% × (220 − age).
- Methods: walk, run, bicycle, swim, water-jog, treadmill, Nordic Ski Track, Health Rider
- Graduated supervised exercise regimen over 6–8 weeks of CV training
- CHD risk reduction plateaus at a level of 4200 kJ/week.

Approaches to Selection of Antihypertensive Therapy

1. Stepped-care approach: limited usefulness [4, 5, 9]
2. Demographic approach (race, sex, age)
3. Renin profile analysis: Laragh method is useful for "V" and "R" patients [11, 12, 218] (Table 20)
4. Subsets of hypertension: individualized therapy—recommended approach [4, 5, 9]
   (a) Pathophysiology: Membranopathy, ion transport defects, structural factors, smooth muscle hypertrophy (vascular, cardiac, cerebral, renal), functional factors, vasoconstrictive forces, and ED
   (b) Hemodynamics: SVR, CO, arterial compliance, organ perfusion, BP. Select the appropriate therapy to reverse the circulatory dysregulation
   (c) End-organ damage: Reduce risk factors for all end-organ damage
   (d) Concomitant medical diseases and problems: Select antihypertensive medications with favorable or neutral effects
   (e) Demographics: Race, age, gender
   (f) Quality of life effects of medications
   (g) Compliance with medication regimen
   (h) Total health care costs: Direct and indirect costs.

Table 20 Renin Profiling: The Laragh Method [218]

Hypertensive patients fall into two basic types	
V hypertension (volume)	**R hypertension (renin)**
PRA < 0.65 ng/mL/hr	PRA>0.65 ng/mL/hr
Direct renin level <5 μU/mL	Direct renin level >5 μU/mL
	Have progressively more renin-angiotensin-mediated vasoconstrictor hypertension
Have predominately sodium → volume-mediated hypertension	

Antihypertensive drugs also fall into two basic types	
V drugs	**R drugs**
Reduce sodium → volume factor: spironolactone, diuretics, ABs, or CCBs	Block plasma renin-angiotensin system: CEIs, ARBs, or BBs

Laragh Method

- Individual hypertensive patients differ in underlying pathophysiology and in response to drugs
- Individual hypertensive patients have V or R forms of hypertension
- Drugs act against either V or R forms of hypertension; therefore different patients respond to different drugs
- Targeted monotherapy is the ultimate realizable goal for treating most individual patients

ABs = alpha-blockers; ARBs = Angiotensin receptor blockers; BBs = beta-blockers; CCBs = calcium channel blockers; CEIs = converting enzyme inhibitors; PRA = plasma rennin activity.

Hemodynamics in Hypertension

$BP = CO \times SVR$

$CO = $ Stroke volume (SV) $\times$ HR

$SVR = $ Peripheral vascular resistance (PVR) + Renal vascular resistance (RVR)

Increased vasoconstriction with decreased arterial compliance are the hallmarks due to

1. Abnormalities in capacitance, oscillatory, and resistance arteries
2. Structural abnormalities in VSM
3. Imbalance between vasodilators and vasoconstrictors.

Hemodynamic progression of hypertension

1. Early hypertension: Increased CO with relative increase in SVR (inappropriately increased)
2. Established hypertension: Decreased CO and increased SVR
3. Late hypertension: Decreased CO (25%) and markedly increased SVR (25–30%). All patients with essential hypertension have elevated SVR as the primary hemodynamic abnormality. Even in the uncommon case in which the CO may be transiently increased, the SVR is inappropriately elevated. Antihypertensive therapy should reverse the hemodynamic abnormalities.

Hemodynamics: logical and preferred method to reduce BP

1. Reduce SVR
2. Preserve CO
3. Improve arterial compliance
4. Maintain organ perfusion.
   Achieving all the above by avoiding compensatory neurohumoral reflexes, such as reflex tachycardia, salt and water overload, and reflex vasoconstriction (NE, Ang-II, and antidiuretic hormone)
   Maintaining full 24-hour BP control
   Maintaining BP control under all circumstances: rest, exercise, stress, mental function, and during the diurnal variation.

Vascular/arterial compliance

1. Three vessel wall components contribute to vascular compliance:
   (a) Elastin: very elastic
   (b) Smooth muscle: immediate elasticity
   (c) Collagen: very stiff.
2. Vascular compliance is composed of three arterial functions:
   (a) Capacitive: large conduit arteries, store blood in systole
   (b) Oscillatory: small branch arteries, contribute to pressure oscillations and to reflected waves
   (c) Resistance: arterioles control blood flow and resistance function.
3. ED is first manifested in the elastin components of thin-walled arterioles (oscillatory and resistance). This raises resistance in these thin-walled arterioles prior to any effect on conduit arteries.

4. C2-oscillatory and resistance arteriolar compliance is reduced markedly in elderly hypertensives and diabetics. Early hypertensives, normotensive hypertensives, and normotensive children of hypertensive parents have reduced C2 compliance. A low C2-AC predicts an increased risk of future CV events.

5. C1-capacitance compliance is reduced more in isolated systolic hypertension (ISH) than in essential hypertension.

Hemodynamic Effects of Antihypertensive Drugs [4, 5, 9, 13–30]

The hemodynamic effects of antihypertensive drugs are shown in Table 21.

1. Reduce SVR, preserve CO, and improve arterial compliance and perfusion.[3]
   (a) CCBs
   (b) ACEIs
   (c) ARB
   (d) RIs
   (e) Vasodilating BBs
   (f) SARAs.
2. Reduce SVR, preserve CO, and perfusion; effects on arterial compliance unknown.[3]
   (a) Central alpha-agonists
   (b) ABs.
3. Reduce SVR, preserve CO, and perfusion, but worsen arterial compliance.
   (a) Direct vasodilators
   (b) BBs with ISA
   (c) Combined alpha/beta-blockers.
4. Reduce SVR, CO, and perfusion, and worsen arterial compliance.
   (a) Diuretics
   (b) Neuronal-inhibiting drugs.
5. Increase SVR and reduce CO, perfusion, and arterial compliance.
   (a) BBs without ISA

TREATMENT OF HYPERTENSION

---

[3]The best hemodynamic profile is achieved by CCBs, ACEI, ARB, RI, vasodilating BB, and SARAs. The central alpha-agonists, combined alpha/beta-blockers, and ABs are the next best. Diuretics and older first and second generation nonvasodilating BB have the worst hemodynamic profile.

Table 21 Hemodynamic Effects of Antihypertensive Drugs

	Diuretics	Beta-blockers	Calcium channel blockers	Angiotensin-converting enzyme inhibitors	ARBs	Central alpha-agonists	Alpha-blockers	Direct vasodilators	Alpha- and beta-blockers	BBs with ISA	Neuron inhibitors
SVR	↓/→	↑	→	↓	↓	↓	↓/→	↓	↓/→	→	→
CO	→	→	↑/→	↓	↓	↑	→/↑	↑	↓/→	↓/→	→
SV	→	→	↑/→	↓	↓	↑	→/↑	↑	↓/→	↓/→	→
HR	↑	→	→/↓	↑	↑	↓/→	→/↑	↑	↑/→	→/↑	→
RBF	↑	→	→	↓	↓	↑	↑	↑	↑/→	↑	→
RVR	↑	↑	→	↓	→	↑	↓	↓	↓/→	↓/↑	→
GFR	→	→	↓/→	↓	↓	↑/→	↑	↑	↑/→	↑	→
Cerebral blood flow	→	→	↑	↑	↑	↑/→	→/↑	↑	↑	↑	↓/↑
CABF	→	↑/→	↑	↑	↑	↑/→	→/↑	↑	↑	↑	↑
Intravascular volume	→	→	→	→	→	↓/→	→/↓	↑	↓/→	→	←
Arterial compliance	→	→	↑	↑	↑	?	?	↑	↑/↓	→	↓/↑
Perfusion	↓/→	→	→	↓	↓	↑	↑	↑	→	↑/→	→/↓
LVH	↓/→	↓/→	→	→	→	→	→	↓	→	↑	↓/↑
VSM hypertrophy	↑	↑	→	↑	↑	↑	↑	↑	→	→/↓	↓/↑
Exercise	→/↓	→	→/↑	↑	↑	↑	↑	↑	→/↓	→	→

↓ Reduced; ↑ increased; → no change; ? unknown.

CABF = coronary artery blood flow; CO = cardiac output; GFR = glomerular filtration rate; HR = hazard ratio; LVH = left ventricular hypertrophy; RBF = renal blood flow; RVR = renal vascular resistance; SV = stroke volume; SVR = systemic vascular resistance; VSM = vascular smooth muscle.

Part 4
Problems Associated
with Hypertension

Handbook of Hypertension. By M.C. Houston. Published 2009 by Blackwell Publishing,
ISBN: 978-1-4051-8250-8

Hypertension-Related End-Organ Damage [3, 31, 32]

1. Cerebrovascular
   (a) Cerebral infarctions: thrombotic or lacunar infarct
   (b) Intracranial hemorrhage: hemorrhagic CVA
   (c) Hypertensive encephalopathy
   (d) Dementia and cognitive dysfunction (vascular dementia and Alzheimer's disease)
2. Cardiac
   (a) CHD
       (i) Angina pectoris
       (ii) MI
   (b) CHF
       (i) Systolic CHF
       (ii) Diastolic CHF (diastolic failure and dysfunction)
   (c) LVH
   (d) Sudden death
3. Renal
   (a) Microalbuminuria and proteinuria
   (b) Chronic renal insufficiency
   (c) Chronic renal failure (ESRD)
4. Large artery disease
   (a) Carotid artery stenosis and obstruction
   (b) Lower extremity arterial disease or peripheral vascular disease and claudication
   (c) Aortic aneurysm and dissection
5. Progression of hypertension: accelerated and malignant hypertension
6. Retinopathy.

ASSOCIATED PROBLEMS

Life Expectancy and Blood Pressure (Man, 35 Years Old) [9, 32]

1. BP (mm Hg)   Life expectancy (years)
   120/80   76
   130/90   67.5
   140/95   62.5
   150/100   55
2. There is a positive correlation between BP level and total mortality.
3. The lower the SBP or DBP in either sex, the lower the mortality and the greater the BP, the higher the mortality.
4. For every 10-mm Hg rise in mean arterial pressure (MAP), there is a 40% rise in cardiovascular risk.
5. The higher the pulse pressure, the greater the morbidity and mortality.
6. SBP is a better predictor of cardiovascular and cerebrovascular morbidity and mortality than DBP in most patients, especially after 50 years.
7. Framingham and MRFIT studies indicate reductions in CV morbidity and mortality with BP reductions to perhaps as low as 110/70 mm Hg. Recent meta-analysis supports BP levels of 115/75 mm Hg [197] to optimize TOD reduction.

Systolic, Diastolic, and Pulse Pressure Concepts [152]

- SBP > DBP to predict CVD—qualified depending on age
- PP predicts CVD with absolute superiority in some populations
- DBP in elderly if excessively low (<60 mm Hg) is associated with increased risk of CVD.

The systolic, diastolic, and PP concepts are shown in Figures 29–33 and Tables 22–24

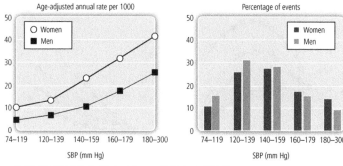

Framingham Heart Study: 38-year follow-up. Subjects aged 35–64 years.

Figure 29 Risk of cardiovascular events by level of systolic blood pressure [154]

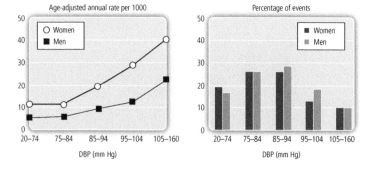

Figure 30 Risk of cardiovascular events by level of diastolic blood pressure [154]

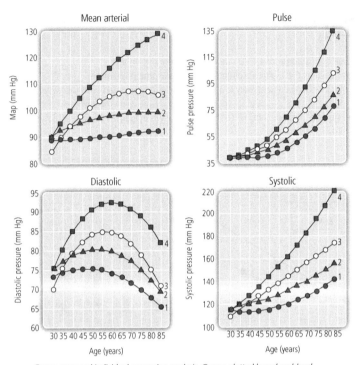

Group averaged individual regression analysis. Curves plotted based on blood pressure–predicated values at 5-year age intervals (age 30–85 years) from least-squares regression equations, developed from individual intercept, slope and quadratic term (curvature), coefficients averaged from individual least-squares mean regressions of each arterial pressure component by age, MAP, mean arterial pressure. Baseline mean SBP groupings: Group 1, SBP<120 mm Hg; Group 2, SBP 120–139mm Hg; Group 3 140–159 mm Hg; Group 4, SBP 160+ mmHg.

Figure 31 Arterial pressure components by age [153]

By level of systolic blood pressure (SBP) and diastolic blood pressure (DBP)

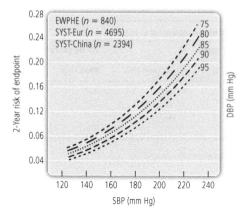

The 2-year probability of a cardiovascular endpoint was adjusted for active treatment, sex, age, previous cardiovascular complications, and smoking by Cox multiple regression with stratification for Trial (European Working Party on High Blood Pressure in the Elderly Trial, Systolic Hypertension in Europe Trial, and Systolic Hypertension in China Trial)

Figure 32 Risk associated with increasing SBP at fixed levels of DBP

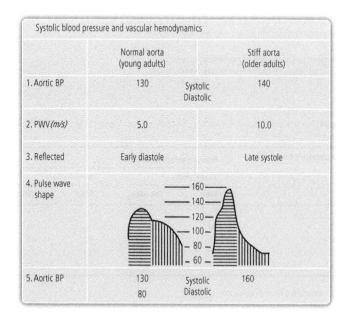

Figure 33 Isolated systolic hypertension (ISH)

Table 22 Increase in Risk of Cardiovascular Events per SD Increase in Blood Pressure Parameter [154] (30-Year Follow-Up)

Types of hypertension	Standardized increment in risk			
	35–64 years		65–94 years	
	Men (%)	Women (%)	Men (%)	Women (%)
Systolic	41*	51*	43*	23*
Mean arterial	41*	44*	42*	18*
Pulse pressure	29*	42*	36*	22*
Diastolic	35*	30*	33*	9**

Source: Framingham Study: According to Age and Sex.
*p <0.001; **p = NS.

Table 23 Risk of Cardiovascular Events by Type of Hypertension [154] (30-Year Follow-Up)

Types of hypertension	Age-adjusted risk ratio[a]			
	35–64 years		65–94 years	
	Men (%)	Women (%)	Men (%)	Women (%)
Isolated diastolic	1.8*	1.2***	1.2*	1.6***
Isolated systolic	2.4***	1.9****	1.9****	1.4****
Combined (%)	2.74***	2.2***	2.2***	1.6***

Source: Framingham Study: According to Age and Sex.

[a]Reference group consists of normotensive persons.
*p < 0.05; **p < 0.01; ***p < 0.001; ****p = NS.

Table 24 Risk of Cardiovascular Events by Pulse Pressure: Framingham Study [154] (30-Year Follow-Up)

Pulse pressure (mm Hg)	Age-adjusted rate/1000			
	35–64 years		65–94 years	
	Men	Women	Men	Women
2–39	9	4	2	17
40–49	13	6	16	19
50–59	16	7	32	22
60–69	22	10	39	25
70–182	33	16	58	32

Reg. = regression; RF = Risk Factor.
*p < 0.001

Part 5
The Clinical Trials of Hypertension

Handbook of Hypertension. By M.C. Houston. Published 2009 by Blackwell Publishing, ISBN: 978-1-4051-8250-8

Clinical Hypertension Trials and Antihypertensive Drug Therapy [32–43]

The pharmacologic treatment of stages I and II (mild to moderate) hypertension (DBP <110 mm Hg) has reduced only some end-organ damage in the diuretic/BB trials (Tables 25 and 26).

1. BP reduction has reduced consequences of pressure-related arteriolar disease:
   a. Intracranial hemorrhage and cerebral infarction
   b. CHF, systolic CHF[1]
   c. Progression of hypertension: accelerated and malignant
   d. Retinopathy
   e. Aortic aneurysm and dissection
   f. Hypertensive encephalopathy.
2. BP reduction has not achieved expected reduction in the diuretic/BB trials in:
   a. LVH
   b. Diastolic CHF
   c. Chronic renal insufficiency (CRI) and failure
3. BP reduction has not reduced consequences of atherosclerotic-related diseases to the predicted extent in diuretic/BB trials except in ALLHAT that was diuretic (chlorthalidone)-based rather than diuretic/BB-based therapy (compared to CCB or ACEI trials) [150].
   a. CHD
   b. Angina pectoris
   c. MI
   d. Sudden death
   e. Larger artery disease: carotid, lower extremities

BB monotherapy does not reduce CHD or MI in the elderly. However, the STONE, SYST-EUR, SYST-CHINA, HOT, STOP-2, CHEN-DU, INSIGHT, NORDIL, NIC-EH, CONVINCE, VHAS, PREVENT, ALLHAT, VALUE, ASCOT, and GLANT prospective clinical trials have shown significant reductions in CV and cerebrovascular morbidity and mortality with the CCBs, especially with amlodipine in ALLHAT, VALUE, and ASCOT.

CAPPP, STOP-2, ALLHAT, PROGRESS, HOPE, ANBP-2, and ASCOT have demonstrated significant reductions in CHD and MI as well as other CV and CVA morbidity and mortality with ACEI.

LIFE showed reductions in CVA and CVD morbidity and mortality with an ARB compared to a BB, and VALUE and MOSES reduced CVD with an ARB. RENAAL, IRMA, IDNT, and AASK showed renal protection with ARBs in hypertensive diabetes.

However, unmasking of asymptomatic CHF, study design, demographics, BP differences, or other factors may have accounted for this difference (see details on ALLHAT study). It should be noted that the primary endpoint of MI was equal among the three treatment groups.

CLINICAL TRIALS

---

[1] ALLHAT showed questionable superiority of chlorthalidone to amlodipine and lisinopril in preventing new onset nonfatal CHF in a high-risk elderly population.

Table 25 Completed Trials and Trials in Progress in Hypertension Treatment [160]

Trial details						Patient characteristics				Estimated events	
Acronym	Title	Patients (n)	Planned follow-up (years)	Randomized treatments (factorial assignments)	Completion date	Entry criteria	Age (years)	Entry blood pressure levels (mm Hg)			
								DBP	SBP	CHD	Stroke
AASK	African-American Study of Kidney Disease and Hypertension	1200	5	ACE, BB, DCA (more, less)	2001	HBP+RD	18–70	=95	Any	144	72
ABCD	Appropriate Blood Pressure Control In Diabetes Trial	950	5	ACE, DCA	1998	DM	=40< =70	Any	No ISH	119	59
ACTION	A Coronary Disease Trial Investigating Outcome with Nifedipine GITS	6000	5	DCA, plac	2003	CAD	>34	None	None	918	333
ADVANCE	Action in Diabetes and Vascular Disease	11 140	4.5	Perindopril + indapamide vs. plac	2006	DM	>30	None	None	—	—
ALLHAT	Antihypertensive Therapy and Lipid-Lowering Heart Attack Prevention Trial	40 000	6	ACE, AB, DCA, diur (chol, open)	2002	HBP+ CVD risk	>55	>89, <110	>139, <180	2580	2790
ANBP-2	Australian National Blood Pressure Study 2	6000	5	ACE, diur	2002	HBP	65–84	>89	>159	300	150
ASCOT	Anglo-Scandinavian Cardiac Outcomes Trial	18 000	5	DCA±ACE, BB±diur (chol, plac)	2003	HBP+ CVD risk	>39– 79	>89	>139	1150	400

BENEDICT	Bergamo Nephrology Diabetes Complication Trial	2400	3	ACE, NCA, plac	2001	DM	>39	>80	>139	200	100
CAPPP	Captopril Prevention Project	10800	5	ACE, BB/diur	1998	HBP	23–66	>99	Any	324	162
CHEN-DU	Nifedipine Trial										
CLEVER	Chinese Lacidipine Event Reduction Trial	10000	3	DCA, plac	2002	HBP+ CVD risk	50–79	95–115	160–210	200	400
CSG	Collaborative Study Group of Irbesartan										
CONVINCE	Controlled onset Verapamil Investigation for Cardiovascular Endpoints	15000	5	NCA, BB/diur	2001	HBP+ CVD risk	>54	>89, <110	>139, <190	1250	750
DIAB-HYCAR	Diabetes Hypertension Cardiovascular Morbidity-Mortality and Ramipril	4000	3	ACE, plac	1999	DM+prot	>50	Any	Any	300	150
ELSA	European Lacidipine Study of Atherosclerosis	2251	4	DCA, BB	2000	HBP	45–75	>94, <116	<149, <211	89	44
EUROPA*	European Trial on Reduction of Cardiac Events with Perindopril	10500	3	ACE, plac	2004	CAD	>18	Any	Any	964	350
FACET	Fosinopril and Amlodipine Cardiac Events Trial	380	3.5	CCB, ACE	1998	NIDDM+ HBP	—	>90	>140	—	—
GLANT	Study Group on Long-term Antihypertensive Therapy	1936		ACE, CCB		HBP	60+	90–114	>160	2	5
HDS	Hypertension in Diabetes Study	1148	8.2	ACE, BB, open (ins, sul, diet)	1998	HBP+ DM	25–75	>84	>149	244	122

(Continued)

Table 25 (Continued)

| Trial details | | Patients (n) | Planned follow-up (years) | Randomized treatments (factorial assignments) | Completion date | Entry criteria | Patient characteristics | | | Estimated events | |
| Acronym | Title | | | | | | Age (years) | Entry blood pressure levels (mm Hg) | | CHD | Stroke |
								DBP	SBP		
HOPE	Heart Outcomes Prevention Evaluation Study	9541	4.7	ACE, plac (vit E, plac)	2000	CVD risk	>54	Any	Any	1200	550
HOT	Hypertension Optimal Treatment Trial	19196	3.5	More, Less (asp, plac)	1997	HBP	50–80	>99, <116	Any	552	276
HYVET	Hypertension in the Very Elderly Trial	2100	5	ACE, diur, plac	2001	HBP	>89	>89, <110	>159, <220	683	341
IDNT	Irbesartan Diabetes Nephropathy Trial	1650	3	AIIA, dCA, plac	2000	DM + prot	30–70	>84	>134	124	62
INSIGHT	International Nifedipine GITS Study Intervention as a Goal for Hypertension Therapy	6592	3	dCA, diur	1999	HBP+ CVD risk	55–80	>94	>149	246	123
INVEST	International Verapamil/ Trandolapril Study	27000	2	NCA, BB	2001	HBP+ CAD	>49	None	None	581	268
LIFE	Losartan Intervention for Endpoint Reduction in Hypertension	9194	4	AIIA, BB	2001	HBP+ LVH	55–80	95–115	160–200	693	347
MIDAS	Multicenter Isradapine Diuretic Atherosclerosis Study	883		dCA, diur	1996	HBP	50–64	>96, <101	>149, <165	—	—

MOSES	Morbidity and Mortality After Stroke: Eprosartan vs. Nitrendipine in Secondary Prevention	1400	2.5	CCB, ARB	2004	Stroke during the past 24 months	Any	Any	Any	—	—
NICS-EH	National Intervention Cooperative Study in Elderly Hypertensives	1000	5	dCA, diur	1997	HBP	>59	<115	>159, <220	30	1
NORDIL OPERA	Nordic Diltiazem Study Omapatrilat in Persons with Enhanced Risk of Atherosclerotic Events	11 000 12 600	5	NCA, BB/diur Omapatrilat vs. plac	2002	HBP	50–69	>99	Any	360	180
PART-2	Prevention of Atherosclerosis with Ramipril	617	4	ACE, plac	1998	Athero	18–75	Any	Any	40	14
PATE	Practitioners Trial on the efficacy of Antihypertensive Treatment in the Elderly hypertension	1748	3	ACE, CCB	2000	HBP	>60	>84	>150	45	37
PEACE	Prevention of Events with Angiotensin Converting Enzyme Inhibition	8000	5	ACE, plac		CAD	>50	Any	Any	1224	444
PHYLLIS	Plaque Hypertension Lipid-Lowering Italian Study	450	3	ACE, plac (chol, plac)	2000	CIT	45–70	95–115	>150, <211	7	4
PRESERVE	Prospective Randomized Enalapril Study Evaluation Regression of Ventricular Enlargement	303	None	CCB, ACE	2001	>50 + LV mass	>50	>90	>150	—	—

(Continued)

Table 25 (Continued)

Trial details						Patient characteristics				Estimated events	
Acronym	Title	Patients (n)	Planned follow-up (years)	Randomized treatments (factorial assignments)	Completion date	Entry criteria	Age (years)	Entry blood pressure levels (mm Hg)			
								DBP	SBP	CHD	Stroke
PREVENT	Prospective Randomized Evaluation of Vascular Effects at Norvasc	825	5	dCA, plac	1997	ang CHD	30–80	Any	Any	20	6
PROGRESS	Perindopril Protection Against Recurrent Stroke Study	6000	5	ACE, plac	2000	Stroke or TIA	Any	Any	Any	600	300
PROTECT	Perindopril Regression of Vascular Thickening European Community Trial										
QUIET	Quinapril Ischemia Event Trial	1750	3	ACE, plac	1996	ang CHD	18–75	Any	Any	500	350
RENAAL	Randomized Evaluation of NIDDM with the All Antagonist Losartan	1500	4	ANA, plac	2002	DM	31–70	<110	<200	100	50
SCAT	Simvastatin/Enalapril Coronary Atherosclerosis Trial	460	5	ACE, plac (chol, plac)	1998	CAD		Any	Any	42	15
SCOPE	Study of Cognition and Prognosis in Elderly Patients with Hypertension	4000	2.5	AIIA, plac	2003	HBP	70–89	90–99	160–179	60	30

SHELL	Systolic Hypertension in the Elderly Lacidipine Long-Term Study	4800	3.5	dCA, diur	1999	HBP	>59	<95	>160	101	50
STONE	Shanghai Trial of Nifedipine in the Elderly	1632	2.5	CCB, plac	1995	HBP	60–79	Any	Any	—	—
STOP-2	Swedish Trial in Old Patients with Hypertension	6628	4	ACE, BB/diur, dCA	1998	HBP	70–84	>104	>179	318	167
SYST-EUR	SYST-EUR Multicentre Trial	4695	1.6	dCA, plac	1997	ISH	>59	<95	160–119	500	250
SYST-CHINA	Systolic Hypertension in China	2400	2.8	CCB, plac		ISH	>60				
VALUE*	Diovan Antihypertensive Long-term Use Evaluation	14400	6	AIIA, dCA	2004	HBP + CVD risk	>49	<115	<210	1450	869
VHAS	Verapamil in Hypertension Atherosclerosis Study	1414	2	NCA, diur	1996	HBP	40–65	>94	>159	40	20

AIIA = angiotensin II antagonist ang CHD = angiographic coronary heart disease; asp = aspirin; athero = atherosclerosis; CAD = coronary artery disease; chol = cholesterol lowering; CIT = carotid intimal thickness; dCA = dihydropyridine calcium antagonist; diur = diuretic; ins = insulin; less = less intensive blood pressure lowering; LVH = left ventricular hypertrophy; more = more intensive blood pressure lowering; NCA = non-dihydropyridine calcium antagonist; open = open control; plac = placebo; prot = proteinuria; RD = renal disease; sul = sulfonamide; vit E = vitamin E.

*Collaboration pending.

Table 26 Twenty-Three Controlled, Randomized, Clinical Trials with Diuretics and BBs in Mild-to-Moderate Hypertension and CHD (1979–1992)

No.	Trial (Date)	Initial number of patients	Blind	DBP (mm Hg)	Treatment	Mean duration (years)	CHD incidence
1.	HDFP (1979)[33]	10940	No	90–114	Referred care vs. stepped care	5	Decreased
2.	VA Cooperative II (1970)[34]	380	Double	90–114	Placebo vs. diuretics + reserpine + hydralazine	3.8	No difference
3.	Oslo (1980)[37]	785	No	90–109	None vs. diuretics + methyldopa + propranolol	10	Increased
4.	Australian (1980)[38]	3427	Double	95–110	Placebo vs. diuretics + methyldopa + propranotol + pindolol	4.1	No difference
5.	MRC (1984)[39]	17354	Single	90–109	Placebo vs. bendrofluazide or propranolol	5	No difference
6.	MRFIT (1982)[40]	8012	Open	90–114	Thiazide diuretics	7	No difference
7.	EWPHE (1985)[41]	840	Double	90–120	Placebo vs. thiazide diuretics + triamterene + methyldopa	4.8	No difference
8.	MPPCD (1985)[42]	1203	No	95–110	No drug vs. pindolol 1 propranolol, diuretics, hydralazine	5	Increased
9.	USPHS (1977)[45]	389	Double	90–115	Placebo vs. diuretics reserpine	7–10	No difference
10.	VA-NHLBI (1978)[46]	1012	Double	85–105	Placebo vs. chlorthalidone + reserpine	1–5	No difference
11.	IPPSH (1972)[47]	6357	Double	100–125	No treatment vs. oxprenolol	3–5	No difference
12.	HEP (1936)[48]	884	No	105–120	No treatment vs. atenolol + thiazide diuretics	8	No difference
13.	HAPPHY (1987)[49]	6500	No	100–130	Diuretics vs. atenolol or metoprolol	4	No difference
14.	MAPHY (1983)[50]	3234	No	100–130	Metoprolol vs. thiazide diuretics	5	Less in metoprolol vs. thiazides

	Study		N	BP	Comparison	Years	Outcome
15.	SHEP (1991)[51]	Double	4736	SBP >160; DBP <90	Placebo vs. thiazide diuretics + BBs	5	Decrease in nonfatal MI only
16.	STOP (1991)[52]	Double	1627	105–120	Moduretic, atenolol metoprolol, or pindolol	5	No difference
17.	VA COOP I (1967)[157]	Double	143	SBP >186 DBP >121	Placebo vs. diuretics, reseyme hydralazine	1.5	Reduced (severe HBP study)
18.	CARTER (1970)[161]	Double	97	SBP >160 DBP >110	Diuretics vs. placebo	4.0	CHD not reported, reduced CVA only
19.	BARRACLOUGH (1973)[162]	Double	116	109	Diuretics vs. placebo	2.0	Reduced (NS)
20.	HYPERTENSION-STROKE COOP (1974)[163]	Double	452	SBP >167 DBP >100	Diuretics vs. placebo	2.3	Reduced CVA, no CHD data
21.	Kuramoto (1989)[164]	Double	91	SBP >168; DBP >86	Diuretics vs. placebo	4.0	Reduced
22.	SHEP-P (1989)[165]	Double	551	SBP >172; DBP >75	Diuretics (low dose)	2.8	Reduced CVA, no CHD data
23.	MRC-II (1992)[166]	Double	4396	SBP >185; DBP >91	Diuretics (low dose) + BB OSP	5.8	Reduced in diuretic group but not BB group

EWPHE = European Working Party on Hypertension in the Elderly; HAPPHY = Heart Attack Primary Prevention in Hypertension; HDFP = Hypertension Detection and Follow-up Program; HEP = Hypertension in the Elderly; IPPPSH = International Prospective Primary Prevention Study in Hypertension; MAPHY = Metoprolol Atherosclerosis Prevention in Hypertension Trial; MPPCD = Multifactorial Primary Prevention of Cardiovascular Diseases; MRC = Medical Research Council Trial; MRFIT = Multifactorial Risk Factor Intervention Trial; SHEP = Systolic Hypertension in the Elderly Program; SHEP P = Pilot; STOP = Swedish Trial in Old Patients with Hypertension; USPHS = US Public Health Service Trial; VA–NHLBI = Veterans Administration–National Heart, Lung, and Blood Institute.

CLINICAL TRIALS

Treatment of Hypertension: Questions Posed[1]

1. What level of BP requires initiation of treatment and does this level vary depending on demographics, risk factors, and concomitant diseases?
2. What is the goal BP to optimally reduce target organ damage and does it vary depending on demographics, risk factors, and concomitant diseases?
3. Is there a difference among the various classes of antihypertensive drugs and CV, cerebrovascular, and renal outcomes?

---

[1]These questions will be addressed in this section on clinical trials in hypertension and drug treatment.

Clinical Hypertension Trials: Important Clinical Points

1. The risks of CV morbidity and mortality increase with rising BP level. (Figure 34).
2. Hypertension becomes more progressive and severe without intervention.
   a. Placebo study patients had more progression of hypertension (>15%).
   b. Drug treatment patients had little or no progression of hypertension (<1%).
3. Higher BP levels induce more vascular damage, arteriosclerosis, and atherosclerosis that is synergistic to additional risk factors such as hyperlipidemia, DM, or smoking.
4. Elderly hypertensives or those with more CV risk factors or with CV or renal disease will show more benefit sooner on any drug treatment at equal BP reduction compared to younger patients and those without concomitant CV or renal disease.
5. Renal outcomes in most of the large prospective clinical hypertension trials have been largely ignored or not reported adequately.
6. The major recent meta-analysis trials (randomized controlled trials on hypertension) have been selective in analysis of data and excluded many trials. Conclusions therefore may not only be biased but also invalid [156–160].
7. All the diuretic/BB trials done before 1985 used high-dose diuretic, hydrochlorothiazide (HCTZ) over 50 mg/day; later studies used low doses of 12.5–25 mg of HCTZ.
8. Before the SHEP study in 1989, the criteria for entry into clinical trials and definition of BP control were based on DBP and not on SBP. It is now clear that SBP is more important in predicting CV risk in most patients (especially those over 55 years).

Within each decade of age, the proportional difference in the risk of vascular death associated with a given absolute difference in usual BP is about the same down to at least 115 mm Hg usual SBP and 75 mm Hg usual DBP, below which there is

CLINICAL TRIALS

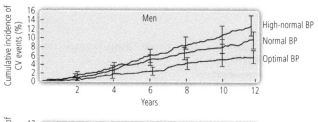

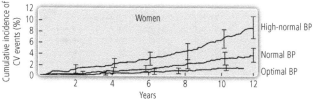

Optimal BP: <120/80 mm Hg: normal BP: 120–129/80–84 mm Hg: high-normal BP: 130–139/85–89 mm Hg.
Source: Vasan RS et al. *N Engl J Med* 2001; 345: 1291–1297.

Figure 34 Impact of High-Normal BP on CV risk.

little evidence. At ages 40–69 years, each difference of 20 mm Hg usual SBP (or, approximately equivalently, 10 mm Hg usual DBP) is associated with more than a twofold difference in the stroke death rate and with twofold differences in the death rates from CHD and other vascular causes. All these proportional differences in vascular mortality are about half as extreme at ages 80–89 years as at ages 40–49 years, but the annual absolute differences in risk are greater in old age. The age-specific associations are similar for men and women suffering from cerebral hemorrhage and cerebral ischemia. For predicting vascular mortality from a single BP measurement, the average of SBP and DBP is slightly more informative than either only SBP or only DBP, and PP is much less informative (Figure 35).

Throughout middle and old age, usual BP is strongly and directly related to vascular (and overall) mortality, without any evidence of a threshold down to at least 115/75 mm Hg.

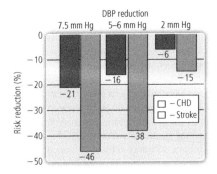

Source: Cook NR et al. *Arch Intern Med* 1995; 155: 701–709.

Figure 35 Implications of Small Reductions in DBP for Primary Prevention.

Table 27 Meta-Analysis of 18 Randomized placebo Controlled Diuretic-Beta-Blocker Clinical Trials in Hypertension [157, 202–204, 206]

Total of over 47,000 hypertensive patients

Outcome drug regimen	Dose	No. of trials	Events, active treatment/control	RR (95% CI)	RR (95% CI) 0.4 / 0.7 / 1.0
Stroke					Treatment better / Treatment worse
Diuretics	High	9	88/232	0.49 (0.39–0.62)	
Diuretics	Low	4	191/347	0.66 (0.55–0.78)	
β-blocker		4	147/335	0.71 (0.59–0.86)	
HDFP	High	1	102/158	0.64 (0.50–0.82)	
Coronary heart disease					
Diuretics	High	11	211/331	0.99 (0.83–1.18)	
Diuretics	Low	4	215/363	0.72 (0.61–0.85)	
β-blocker		4	243/459	0.93 (0.80–1.09)	
HDFP	High	1	171/189	0.90 (0.73–1.10)	

Diuretic high = high dose > 50 mg HCTZ
Diuretic low = low dose < 50 mg HCTZ (12.5–25 mg HCTZ)

Note the following from Table 27.

1. BBs and diuretics both significantly reduced stroke, but diuretics were more effective at either high or low dose compared to BBs (34–54 vs. 29%). BBs are inferior to all other antihypertensive drug classes in reducing CVA.

2. Diuretics at high doses did not reduce CHD. But diuretics at low doses reduced CHD by 28%; BBs did not reduce CHD.

3. This meta-analysis is selective and does not include all 23 reported studies on the previous pages. It includes only 18 of 23 studies. It excludes study numbers 6, 8, 11, 13, and 14. Three studies did not report the CHD events [18, 20, 22].

4. Older patients benefited more and sooner than younger patients with equal BP reductions.

Diuretic/BB Clinical Trials in Mild-to-Moderate Hypertension and CHD: Summary

CHD mortality increased
Oslo   1980
MPPCD   1985

Sudden death increased (abnormal electrocardiogram [ECG])
MRFIT   1982
HDFP   1979

CHD mortality decreased
HDFP   1979
SHEP   1991 (SBP >160)
MRC-2   1992 (diuretic group only, not BB group)
MAPHY   1988 (BB better than diuretic, no placebo)

No Difference in CHD Mortality Between Control vs. Treatment or Aggressive vs. Less Aggressive Treatment
VA Cooperative   1970
Barraclough   1973
USPHS   1977
VA-NHLBI   1978
Australian   1980
MRC   1984
MRFIT   1982
EWPHE   1985
IPPPSH   1972
HEP   1986
HAPPHY   1987
STOP   1991

Summary of clinical trials with diuretics
1. Diuretics (nonloop diuretics) are equally effective in reducing BP compared to most other antihypertensive drug classes. Indapamide may have slightly more antihypertensive effects compared to HCTZ at equivalent doses.
2. Low-dose and not high-dose diuretics are preferred (i.e., HCTZ or chlorthalidone at 6.25–25 mg/day, or indapamide at 0.625–2.5 mg/day). Chlorthalidone is about 1.5 times more potent than HCTZ. Chlorthalidone, 15 mg, is equivalent to HCTZ, 25 mg. However, indapamide may be preferred due to less hypokalemia, less hyperglycemia, less hyperuricemia, better reduction in LVH, and reno-protective effects. Indapamide may improve GFR and is effective in patients with lower GFR.
3. CVA is reduced about 38–51%, which is similar to other antihypertensive drug classes but superior to BBs.
4. CHD and MI are reduced by about 28% with low-dose diuretics in some studies, but high-dose diuretics (with the exception of indapamide) do not reduce CHD or MI. There is a suboptimal reduction in CHD in most clinical trials with the exception of ALLHAT. There may also be increased risk for sudden

death due to cardiac arrhythmias in predisposed patients with CHD, electrolyte disorders (hypokalemia or hypomagnesemia), or those on digitalis. The diuretic/ BB combination in ASCOT was inferior in all CV event reduction compared to CCB/ACEI combination.

5. Renal insufficiency, reduction in GFR, end-stage renal disease (ESRD), and proteinuria are not improved as much with diuretic monotherapy compared to ACEI and ARB therapy and may be nephrotoxic with chronic use. These nephrotoxic effects do not apply to indapamide.

6. CHF is reduced about 52%. However, LVH is not reduced as much as with ACEI, ARB, and CCB drugs.

7. New onset type 2 DM and hyperglycemia are more common with diuretics (except indapamide) than with other antihypertensive drug classes, except for the BBs that are equally diabetogenic or perhaps worse than diuretics.

8. Diuretics promote atherogenesis compared to other agents as evidenced by increases in carotid intima/media thickness (IMT) and coronary artery calcification by electron beam computed tomography (EBT). These atherogenic effects do not apply to indapamide, which is anti-atherogenic.

9. Metabolic and biochemical abnormalites are common and include hypokalemia, hypomagnesemia, hyperglycemia, hyperuricemia and gout, hyperhomocysteinemia, hyperlipidemia, increased PAI-1, metabolic alkalosis, hypercalcemia, hyponatremia, and insulin resistance. HCTZ also increases CRP and thus has vascular inflammatory effects.

10. Increased risk of renal cell cancer and colonic cancer.

11. No improvement in structure or function of arterioles with chronic therapy; endothelial dysfunction and abnormalities of arterial compliance remain despite normalization of BP.

12. High adverse effect profile and low compliance rate with chronic use.

Summary of clinical trials with BBs

1. BP reduction is inferior to other agents in all populations, but especially in the black and elderly population. Central arterial pressure is not reduced as much as the brachial arterial pressure, and the reduction is inferior compared to other antihypertensive drugs.

2. CVA is reduced but less compared to diuretics, CCB, ACEI, and ARBs. The reduction in CVA is about 29%.

3. CHD and MI are not significantly reduced with BB monotherapy in the treatment of hypertension (7% NS). However in patients with known CHD, the future event rate and progression of CHD is reduced.

4. CHF is reduced and prevented. BBs are indicated for CHF patients.

5. Patients post-MI should receive non-ISA BBs or combined alpha/beta-blockers.

6. Renal protection and reduction in proteinuria may be inferior to ACEI, ARB, and CCB, but perhaps better than thiazide and thiazide-like diuretics.

7. The adverse effects are high and the compliance rates are low.

8. Metabolic abnormalities such as dyslipidemia (reduction in HDL and elevation of triglycerides) hyperglycemia, and insulin resistance are common.

9. Drug-induced new onset type 2 DM and glucose intolerance occur most frequently with diuretics (HCTZ and chlorthalidone) and BBs due to insulin resistance. Both induce type 2 DM individually, but the combination is additive or synergistic.

Meta-Analysis of Randomized Controlled Clinical Hypertension Trials with Antihypertensive Drug Therapy

Several recent meta-analysis studies have been published, which review the clinical CV and cerebrovascular outcomes in the treatment of hypertension using various classes of new antihypertensive drugs [156, 158, 159, 197, 202–206] and compare these results to the diuretic/BB trials.

Meta-analysis may provide clinical results that are suggestive of CV outcomes and specific influences by antihypertensive drug class, but by no means are these results definitive. Numerous flaws exist in such analysis:

1. Study selection bias and incomplete review of published clinical trials.
2. Statistical analysis of varied study designs, sample size different demographics, inclusion and exclusion criteria, defined primary and secondary outcomes, and initial and posttreatment BP levels. Concomitant CV risk factors, specific drugs used as well as doses and administration frequency, confounders of all types such as concomitant nonantihypertensive therapy, varied definitions of outcomes, and subject adherence to assigned treatment.
3. Lack of critical analysis of the validity of the reported results of such trials with blanket assumption of accuracy and then subsequent inclusion in the meta-analysis renders conclusions circumstantial.

1. The summary of these meta-analyses suggests the following reductions in clinical CV outcomes compared to placebo:
   a. CHF reduced 52%
   b. CVA reduced 38–42%
   c. MI/CHD reduced 16–20%
   This assumes a SBP reduction of 10–12 mm Hg and a DBP reduction of 5–6 mm Hg.
2. Regarding specific drug classes, there appears to be no significant difference in CHF, CVA, CHD, or MI outcomes. Despite trends in favor of one drug class over another, none of these reached statistical significance. For example, the DHP-CCB reduced ischemic CVA more than other classes of antihypertensive drugs. Total mortality was equal among drug classes as well.
   These meta-analyses will be reviewed in detail below (Tables 28–33 and Figures 36–48).

Meta-analysis by Pahor et al. [159]
- This review included nine trials of 27 743 subjects.
- The trial selection was biased and incomplete. It included trials that were of small sample size and inappropriate for such a meta-analysis.
- The results and conclusions are invalid and open to major criticism.
- The incidence of CVA and the total mortality were equal among drug classes.
- The suggestion that MI, CHF, and CV events were higher with CCBs is not valid due to biased study selection, inclusion of short-acting CCB trials, small sample studies with inability to define outcomes that are statistically significant, and inclusion of inappropriate studies. Subsequent larger prospective clinical trials as well as better and more accurate meta-analysis totally refute this meta-analysis.
- See reference for details. This is, at best, a mediocre meta-analysis with inappropriate biased inferential conclusions.

Table 28 Trials Included in the First Round of Analyses [158]

Acronym	Main treatments compared	Type of data provided	Number of patients	Disease history	Mean age (years)	Proportion of male patients (%)
Trials comparing active treatment and placebo						
HOPE[36]	Ramipril vs. placebo	Tabular	9297	CHD, CVD, or DM + CVDRF	66	73
PART2[37]	Ramipril vs. placebo	IPD	617	CHD or CVD	61	82
QUIET[39]	Quinapril vs. placebo	Tabular	1750	CHD	58	82
SCAT[40]	Enalapril vs. placebo	Tabular	460	CHD	61	89
PREVENT[38]	Amlodipine vs. placebo	IPD	825	CHD	57	80
SYST-EUR[41]	Nitrendipine vs. placebo	IPD	4695	HBP	70	33
Trials comparing more intensive and less intensive BP-lowering strategies						
ABCD[28]	Target DBP 75 vs. <90 mm Hg	Tabular	470	HBP + DM	58	67
HOT[42]	Target DBP <80 vs. <85 or <90 mm Hg*	Tabular	18790	HBP	62	53
UKPDS-HDS[34,35]	Target DBP <85 vs. <105 mm Hg	IPD	1148	HBP + DM	56	55
Trials comparing regimens based on different drug classes						
CAPPP[29]	Captopril vs. BB (not specified) or diuretic (not specified)	Tabular	10985	HBP	53	53
STOP[233]	Enalapril or lisinopril vs. felodipine or isradipine vs. atenolol or metoprolol or pindolol or HCTZ + amiloride	Tabular	6614	HBP	76	33
UKPDS-HDS[34,35]	Captopril vs. atenolol	IPD	758	HBP + DM	56	54
INSIGHT[30]	Nifedipine GITS vs. HCTZ + amiloride	Tabular	6321	HBP + CVD RF	65	46
NICS-EH[31]	Nicardipine vs. trichlormethiazide	IPD	429	HBP	70	33
NORDIL[32]	Diltiazem vs. BB (not specified) or diuretic (not specified)	Tabular	10881	HBP + DM	60	49
VHAS[43,44]	Verapamil vs. chlorthalidone	Tabular	1414	HBP	54	49
ABCD-hypertensive[28]	Enalapril vs. nisoldipine	Tabular	470	HBP + DM	58	67

CVD RF = Other cardiovascular disease risk factor; GITS = gastrointestinal transport system, IPD = individual participant data.
*Felodipine was the first-line drug used in all randomized groups in HOT.

CLINICAL TRIALS

113

Table 29 BP Differences, Proportion Remaining on Randomized Treatments, and Proportion Achieving BP Goals [159]

Acronym	SBP/DBP at entry (mm Hg)	BP differences (treatment-control)* between randomized groups during follow-up (mm Hg)		Proportion remaining on randomized treatment or achieving BP goal (%)		Duration of follow-up (years)
		SBP	DBP	Study treatment	Control*	
Trials comparing active treatment and placebo						
HOPE	139/79	−3	−1	71	73	5
PART-2	133/79	−6	−4	72	75	4
QUIET	123/74	NA	NA	72	75	2
SCAT	130/78	−4	−3	NA	NA	5
PREVENT	129/79	−5	−4	69	78	3
SYST-EUR	174/86	−10	−5	72	66	2
Trials comparing more intensive and less intensive BP-lowering strategies						
ABCD-hypertensive†	155/98	−6	−8	49	89	5
HOT‡	169/105	−3	−3	55	80	4
UKPDS-HDS§	160/94	−10	−5	56	91	8
*Trials comparing regimens based on different drug classes**						
CAPPPH	161/99	+3	+1	67	86	6
STOP-2	194/98	<3	<1	64	62	5
UKPDS-HDS	160/94	+1	+2	78	65	8
INSIGHT	173/99	<1	<1	60	67	4
NICS-EH	172/94	0	+2	92	94	4
NORDIL	173/106	+3	<1	77	93	5

VHAS	169/102	<1	<1	78	77	2
ABCD-hypertensive[†]	155/98	<1	<1	45	40	5

NA = not available.

*In all studies except ABCD, group randomized to BB and/or diuretic therapy designated control.

[†]Group randomized to calcium antagonist designated control, Group randomized to ACEI designated treatment. Mean BP levels achieved: 132/78 mm Hg in more intensive vs. 138/86 mm Hg in less intensive groups.

[‡]Most intensive BP lowering regimen (target DBP <80 mm Hg) designated treatment, less intensive regimens designated control. Mean BP levels achieved: 140/81 mm Hg in more intensive vs. 143/84 mm Hg in less intensive groups.

[§]Mean BP levels achieved: 144/62 mm Hg in more intensive vs. 154/87 mm Hg in less intensive group. _BP difference (2/2 mm Hg) present between randomized groups at study entry.

Table 30 Characteristics of Trials in Hypertension Comparing Different Active Treatments [136]

Characteristics	Trials								
	UKPDS[16,27]*	STOP[26]	CAPPP[4]	NORD1L[9]	INSIGHT[8]	ALLHAT[10]	MIDAS[3]	NICS[5]	VHAS[53†]
Masking type	Open	Open	Open	Open	Double	Double	Double	Double	Open
Number of patients	1148	6614	10985	10881	6321	24335	883	414	1414
Treatment									
Reference	Atenolol <180/105	HCTZ/A or β-blockers	Diuretic or β-blockers	Thiazide or β-blockers	HCTZ/A	Chlorthalidone	HCTZ	Trichlormethiazide	Chlorthalidone
Experimental	<Captopril <150/85	ACEIs DHPs	Captopril	Diltiazem (SR)	Nifedipine (GITS)	Doxazosin	Isradipine	Nicardipine (SR)	Verapamil (SR)
Age (mean [SD], years)	56(8)	76(..)	53(8)	60(7)	65(7)	67(8)	59(9)	70(7)	53(7)
Mean systolic/diastolic blood pressure (mm Hg)									
At entry	160/94	194/98	161/99	173/106	167/96	145/831	150/97	172/94	169/102
Difference during follow-up[§]	−1/−1	−0.3/+0.5	−3/−1	−3.1/+0.2	~0/~0	−2/+1	−3.5/~0	−0.7/−1.2	−1.0/+0.4
Proportion of patients (%)									
Women	45	67	47	51	54	47	22	67	51
Cardiovascular complications	::	~20	4	−8	~20	45	~4	~28	5
DM	100	11	5	7	21	36	::	::	411
Follow-up (years)									
Median	8.4	::	::	::	::	3.3	3.0	4.3	2.0
Mean	::	5.0	6.1	4.5	3.5	::	::	::	::

ACEIs = angiotensin-converting enzyme inhibitors; DHPs = dihydropyridine calcium-channel blockers (felodipine or isradipine); GITS = gastro-intestinal therapeutic system; HCTZ = hydrochlorothiazide; HCTZ/A = hydrochlorothiazide plus amiloride; SR = sustained release. Acronyms of trials are explained in the appendix.
*UKPDS compared captopril with atenolol and tested two levels of control of SBP/DBP.
†In VHAS, study drug was given in a double-blind fashion during the initial 6 months and thereafter in an open way.
§Negative values indicate tighter BP control on old drug classes.

Table 31 Pooled Estimates of Advantage of New vs. Old Antihypertensive Drugs with Respect to Cause-Specific Mortality [156]

	Zeten's p-value*	Pooled estimates of advantage of new vs. old drugs expressed in percent[†]		
		Estimate (SD)	95% CIs	p
Cause of death[‡]				
Stroke				
CCBs	0.95	−5.3 (17.9)	−31.4 to 30.7	0.79
ACEIs	0.89	−5.6 (18.6)	−32.5 to 31.8	0.79
CCBs and ACEIs	0.99	−5.4 (14.0)	−26.8 to 22.5	0.70
MI				
CCBs	0.13	22.6 (16.6)	−92 to 65.8	0.19
ACEIs	032	−6.3 (15.1)	−28.9 to 23.4	0 68
CCBs add ACEIs	0.12	7.9 (12.1)	−13.6 to 35.0	0.53
Sudden death				
CCBs	0.46	−8.8 (18.4)	−34.5 to 26.8	0.64
ACEIs	0.07	3.8 (19.3)	−26.5 to 46.7	0.89
CCBs and ACEIs	0.12	−5.3 (15.1)	−28.0 to 25.1	0.74
MI plus sudden death				
CCBs	0.92	7.9 (12.2)	−13.8 to 35.2	0.53
ACEIs	0.07	−2.5 (11.6)	−21.4 to 20.9	0.85
CCBs and ACEIs	0.20	2.5 (9.3)	−13.8 to 22.1	0.81

*The hypothesis of heterogeneity across the reviewed trials was rejected for all fatal outcomes.
[†]Negative values indicate better outcome on the new drugs.
[‡]The reviewed trials are those listed in Table 1 with the exception of ALLHAT, because CV mortality was unavailable from the published report. Cause-specific CV mortality was also not reported for MIDAS-3, M1CS-5, and VHAS-63.

Table 32 Variance Explained by Initial BP and BP Difference [156]

	Variance explained and corresponding probability					
	Overall model		Initial BP		BP difference	
	R^2	p	R^2	p	R^2	p
Outcome						
CV mortality						
Systolic	0.47	0.002	0.11	0.05	0.36	0.0004
Diastolic	0.42	0.005	0.10	0.08	0.32	0.001
CV events						
Systolic	0.66	<0.0001	0.006	0.56	0.65	<0.0001
Diastolic	0.51	0.002	~0	0.99	0.51	0.001
Stroke						
Systolic	0.71	<0.0001	0.004	0.48	0.71	<0.0001
Diastolic	0.66	0.0001	0.007	0.55	0.65	<0.0001
Stroke						
Systolic	0.55	0.001	0.02	0.37	0.53	0.0005
Diastolic	0.54	0.001	0.09	0.06	0.45	0.002

Every metaregression model included BP at entry and BP difference between study groups as independent variables and was weighted by the inverse of the variance odds ratios.

Table 33 Observed Odds Ratios and Odds Ratios Predicted by Differences in SBP in Metaregression [156]

	Observed odds ratio* (95% CI)	Predicted mean odds ratio (95% CI)[†]	Difference (% [95% CI])[‡]	p[§]
ALLHAT[10]				
CV events	1.24 (1.15–1.33)	1.14 (0.98–1.32)	−8.4 (−27.0 to 7.4)	0.32
Stroke	1.18 (0.99–1.39)	1.06 (0.92–1.22)	−11.3 (−38.1 to 10.3)	0.33
MI	1.01 (0.88–1.16)	1.13 (0.98–1.31)	10.7 (−8.2 to 26.2)	0.25
CAPPP[4]				
CV mortality	0.80 (0.58–1.09)	0.99 (0.81–1.22)	19.8 (−16.1 to 44.6)	0.24
CV events	1.10 (0.95–1.27)	1.23 (1.03–1.46)	10.3 (−11.5 to 27.9)	0.33
Stroke	1.29 (1.03–1.61)	1.14 (0.96–1.34)	−13.4(−49.0 to 13.8)	0.37
MI	1.01 (0.80–1.26)	1.21 (1.02–1.44)	17.0 (−9.8 to 37.2)	0.19
HOPE[7]				
CV mortality	0.73 (0.62–0.86)	0.86 (0.74–0.99)	14.4 (−5.7 to 30.6)	0.15
CV events	0.76 (0.67–0.85)	0.82 (0.75–0.91)	8.4 (−6.2 to 21.0)	0.24
Stroke	0.68 (0.52–0.86)	0.77 (0.69–0.85)	11.1 (−12.3 to 29.6)	0.32
MI	0.79 (0.69–0.90)	0.85 (0.77–0.93)	7.2 (−8.6 to 20.6)	0.35
NORDIL[5]				
CV mortality	1.16 (0.89–1.50)	1.00 (0.81–1.22)	−16.1 (−60.8 to 16.2)	0.37
CV events	1.04 (0.91–1.20)	1.24 (1.04–1.47)	15.5 (−4.8 to 31.9)	0.13
Stroke	0.81 (0.65–1.01)	1.14 (0.97–1.35)	28.8 (6.8 to 45.5)	0.01
MI	1.19 (0.95–1.48)	1.22 (1.02–1.46)	3.0 (−28.1 to 26.5)	0.83
PART-2/SCAT[12,15]				
CV mortality	0.47 (0.21–0.98)	0.83 (0.73–0.95)	43.3 (−19.8 to 73.2)	0.14
CV events	0.64 (0.44–0.94)	0.78 (0.70–0.86)	17.3 (−22.8 to 44 3)	0.35
MI	0.63 (0.38–1.05)	0.80 (0.73–0.88)	21.2 (−31.1 to 52.7)	0.36

*Odds ratio reported in the published articles.
[†]Mean odds ratio (95% CI) predicted try metaregression lines (Figures 4 and 5).
[‡]Difference between predicted minus observed ddds ratio (95% CI) expressed in percent of predicted odds ratio.
[§]Significance of difference between observed and predicted odds ratios.

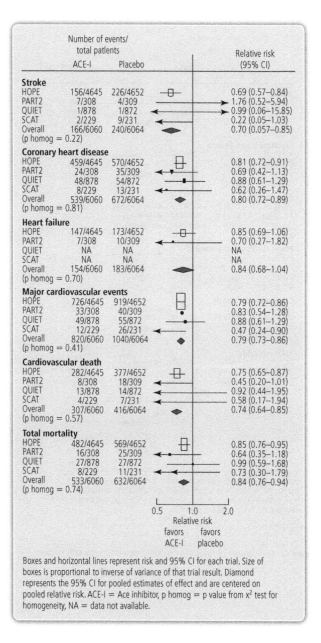

| | Number of events/ total patients | | Relative risk |
	ACE-I	Placebo	(95% CI)
Stroke			
HOPE	156/4645	226/4652	0.69 (0.57–0.84)
PART2	7/308	4/309	1.76 (0.52–5.94)
QUIET	1/878	1/872	0.99 (0.06–15.85)
SCAT	2/229	9/231	0.22 (0.05–1.03)
Overall	166/6060	240/6064	0.70 (0.057–0.85)
(p homog = 0.22)			
Coronary heart disease			
HOPE	459/4645	570/4652	0.81 (0.72–0.91)
PART2	24/308	35/309	0.69 (0.42–1.13)
QUIET	48/878	54/872	0.88 (0.61–1.29)
SCAT	8/229	13/231	0.62 (0.26–1.47)
Overall	539/6060	672/6064	0.80 (0.72–0.89)
(p homog = 0.81)			
Heart failure			
HOPE	147/4645	173/4652	0.85 (0.69–1.06)
PART2	7/308	10/309	0.70 (0.27–1.82)
QUIET	NA	NA	NA
SCAT	NA	NA	NA
Overall	154/6060	183/6064	0.84 (0.68–1.04)
(p homog = 0.70)			
Major cardiovascular events			
HOPE	726/4645	919/4652	0.79 (0.72–0.86)
PART2	33/308	40/309	0.83 (0.54–1.28)
QUIET	49/878	55/872	0.88 (0.61–1.29)
SCAT	12/229	26/231	0.47 (0.24–0.90)
Overall	820/6060	1040/6064	0.79 (0.73–0.86)
(p homog = 0.41)			
Cardiovascular death			
HOPE	282/4645	377/4652	0.75 (0.65–0.87)
PART2	8/308	18/309	0.45 (0.20–1.01)
QUIET	13/878	14/872	0.92 (0.44–1.95)
SCAT	4/229	7/231	0.58 (0.17–1.94)
Overall	307/6060	416/6064	0.74 (0.64–0.85)
(p homog = 0.57)			
Total mortality			
HOPE	482/4645	569/4652	0.85 (0.76–0.95)
PART2	16/308	25/309	0.64 (0.35–1.18)
QUIET	27/878	27/872	0.99 (0.59–1.68)
SCAT	8/229	11/231	0.73 (0.30–1.79)
Overall	533/6060	632/6064	0.84 (0.76–0.94)
(p homog = 0.74)			

Relative risk favors ACE-I   favors placebo

Boxes and horizontal lines represent risk and 95% CI for each trial. Size of boxes is proportional to inverse of variance of that trial result. Diamond represents the 95% CI for pooled estimates of effect and are centered on pooled relative risk. ACE-I = Ace inhibitor, p homog = p value from x^2 test for homogeneity, NA = data not available.

Figure 36 Comparisons of ACE-Inhibitor-based Therapy with Placebo.

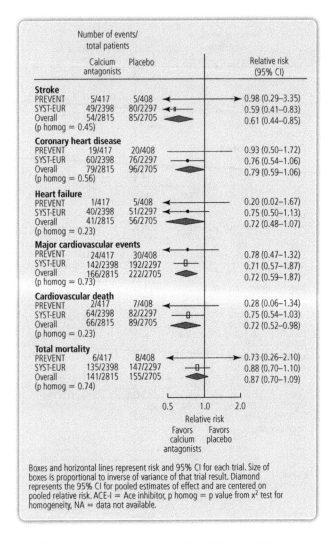

Boxes and horizontal lines represent risk and 95% CI for each trial. Size of boxes is proportional to inverse of variance of that trial result. Diamond represents the 95% CI for pooled estimates of effect and are centered on pooled relative risk. ACE-I = Ace inhibitor, p homog = p value from x^2 test for homogeneity, NA = data not available.

Figure 37 Comparisons of Calcium-Antagonist-based Therapy with Placebo.

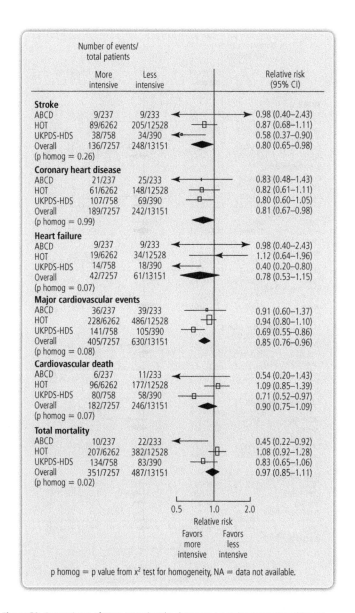

	Number of events/ total patients			Relative risk (95% CI)
	More intensive	Less intensive		
Stroke				
ABCD	9/237	9/233		0.98 (0.40–2.43)
HOT	89/6262	205/12528		0.87 (0.68–1.11)
UKPDS-HDS	38/758	34/390		0.58 (0.37–0.90)
Overall	136/7257	248/13151		0.80 (0.65–0.98)
(p homog = 0.26)				
Coronary heart disease				
ABCD	21/237	25/233		0.83 (0.48–1.43)
HOT	61/6262	148/12528		0.82 (0.61–1.11)
UKPDS-HDS	107/758	69/390		0.80 (0.60–1.05)
Overall	189/7257	242/13151		0.81 (0.67–0.98)
(p homog = 0.99)				
Heart failure				
ABCD	9/237	9/233		0.98 (0.40–2.43)
HOT	19/6262	34/12528		1.12 (0.64–1.96)
UKPDS-HDS	14/758	18/390		0.40 (0.20–0.80)
Overall	42/7257	61/13151		0.78 (0.53–1.15)
(p homog = 0.07)				
Major cardiovascular events				
ABCD	36/237	39/233		0.91 (0.60–1.37)
HOT	228/6262	486/12528		0.94 (0.80–1.10)
UKPDS-HDS	141/758	105/390		0.69 (0.55–0.86)
Overall	405/7257	630/13151		0.85 (0.76–0.96)
(p homog = 0.08)				
Cardiovascular death				
ABCD	6/237	11/233		0.54 (0.20–1.43)
HOT	96/6262	177/12528		1.09 (0.85–1.39)
UKPDS-HDS	80/758	58/390		0.71 (0.52–0.97)
Overall	182/7257	246/13151		0.90 (0.75–1.09)
(p homog = 0.07)				
Total mortality				
ABCD	10/237	22/233		0.45 (0.22–0.92)
HOT	207/6262	382/12528		1.08 (0.92–1.28)
UKPDS-HDS	134/758	83/390		0.83 (0.65–1.06)
Overall	351/7257	487/13151		0.97 (0.85–1.11)
(p homog = 0.02)				

0.5   1.0   2.0
Relative risk

Favors more intensive   Favors less intensive

p homog = p value from x² test for homogeneity, NA = data not available.

Figure 38 Comparisons of More Intensive Blood Pressure Lowering Strategies with Less Intensive Strategies.

CLINICAL TRIALS

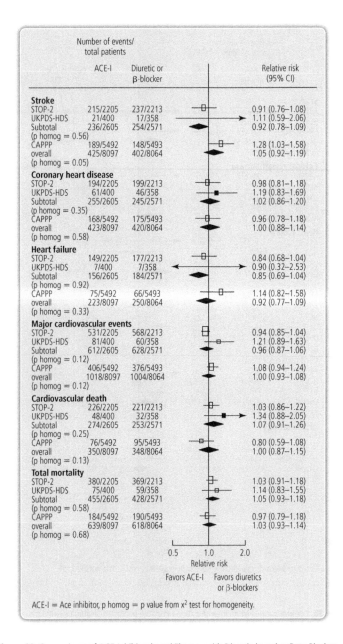

Figure 39 Comparisons of ACE-Inhibitor-based Therapy with Diuretic-based or Beta-Blocker Therapy.

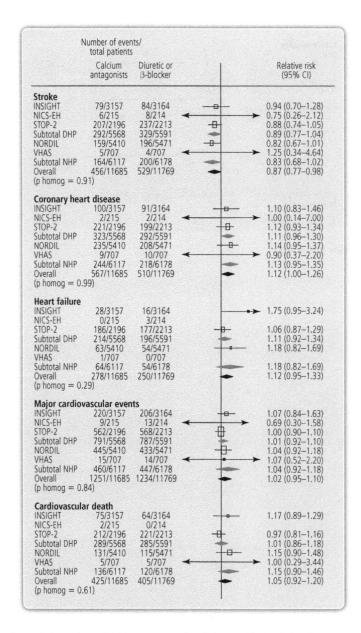

	Number of events/ total patients		Relative risk (95% CI)
	Calcium antagonists	Diuretic or β-blocker	
Stroke			
INSIGHT	79/3157	84/3164	0.94 (0.70–1.28)
NICS-EH	6/215	8/214	0.75 (0.26–2.12)
STOP-2	207/2196	237/2213	0.88 (0.74–1.05)
Subtotal DHP	292/5568	329/5591	0.89 (0.77–1.04)
NORDIL	159/5410	196/5471	0.82 (0.67–1.01)
VHAS	5/707	4/707	1.25 (0.34–4.64)
Subtotal NHP	164/6117	200/6178	0.83 (0.68–1.02)
Overall	456/11685	529/11769	0.87 (0.77–0.98)
(p homog = 0.91)			
Coronary heart disease			
INSIGHT	100/3157	91/3164	1.10 (0.83–1.46)
NICS-EH	2/215	2/214	1.00 (0.14–7.00)
STOP-2	221/2196	199/2213	1.12 (0.93–1.34)
Subtotal DHP	323/5568	292/5591	1.11 (0.96–1.30)
NORDIL	235/5410	208/5471	1.14 (0.95–1.37)
VHAS	9/707	10/707	0.90 (0.37–2.20)
Subtotal NHP	244/6117	218/6178	1.13 (0.95–1.35)
Overall	567/11685	510/11769	1.12 (1.00–1.26)
(p homog = 0.99)			
Heart failure			
INSIGHT	28/3157	16/3164	1.75 (0.95–3.24)
NICS-EH	0/215	3/214	
STOP-2	186/2196	177/2213	1.06 (0.87–1.29)
Subtotal DHP	214/5568	196/5591	1.11 (0.92–1.34)
NORDIL	63/5410	54/5471	1.18 (0.82–1.69)
VHAS	1/707	0/707	
Subtotal NHP	64/6117	54/6178	1.18 (0.82–1.69)
Overall	278/11685	250/11769	1.12 (0.95–1.33)
(p homog = 0.29)			
Major cardiovascular events			
INSIGHT	220/3157	206/3164	1.07 (0.84–1.63)
NICS-EH	9/215	13/214	0.69 (0.30–1.58)
STOP-2	562/2196	568/2213	1.00 (0.90–1.10)
Subtotal DHP	791/5568	787/5591	1.01 (0.92–1.10)
NORDIL	445/5410	433/5471	1.04 (0.92–1.18)
VHAS	15/707	14/707	1.07 (0.52–2.20)
Subtotal NHP	460/6117	447/6178	1.04 (0.92–1.18)
Overall	1251/11685	1234/11769	1.02 (0.95–1.10)
(p homog = 0.84)			
Cardiovascular death			
INSIGHT	75/3157	64/3164	1.17 (0.89–1.29)
NICS-EH	2/215	0/214	
STOP-2	212/2196	221/2213	0.97 (0.81–1.16)
Subtotal DHP	289/5568	285/5591	1.01 (0.86–1.18)
NORDIL	131/5410	115/5471	1.15 (0.90–1.48)
VHAS	5/707	5/707	1.00 (0.29–3.44)
Subtotal NHP	136/6117	120/6178	1.15 (0.90–1.46)
Overall	425/11685	405/11769	1.05 (0.92–1.20)
(p homog = 0.61)			

Figure 40 Comparisons of Calcium-Antagonist-based Therapy with Diuretic-based or Beta-Blocker-based Therapy (*Continued*).

CLINICAL TRIALS

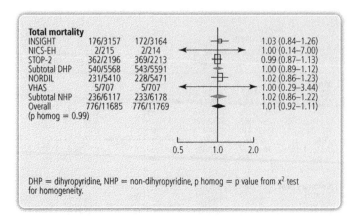

Total mortality				
INSIGHT	176/3157	172/3164		1.03 (0.84–1.26)
NICS-EH	2/215	2/214		1.00 (0.14–7.00)
STOP-2	362/2196	369/2213		0.99 (0.87–1.13)
Subtotal DHP	540/5568	543/5591		1.00 (0.89–1.12)
NORDIL	231/5410	228/5471		1.02 (0.86–1.23)
VHAS	5/707	5/707		1.00 (0.29–3.44)
Subtotal NHP	236/6117	233/6178		1.02 (0.86–1.22)
Overall	776/11685	776/11769		1.01 (0.92–1.11)
(p homog = 0.99)				

DHP = dihyropyridine, NHP = non-dihyropyridine, p homog = p value from x^2 test for homogeneity.

Figure 40 (*Continued*)

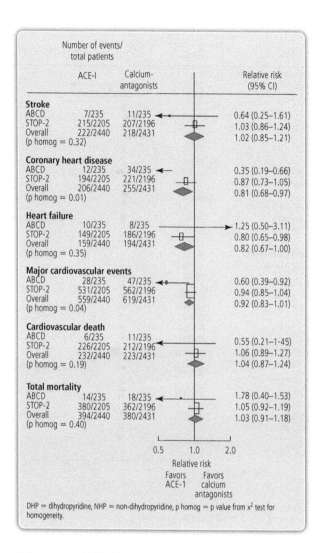

Number of events/
total patients

	ACE-I	Calcium-antagonists		Relative risk (95% CI)
Stroke				
ABCD	7/235	11/235		0.64 (0.25–1.61)
STOP-2	215/2205	207/2196		1.03 (0.86–1.24)
Overall	222/2440	218/2431		1.02 (0.85–1.21)
(p homog = 0.32)				
Coronary heart disease				
ABCD	12/235	34/235		0.35 (0.19–0.66)
STOP-2	194/2205	221/2196		0.87 (0.73–1.05)
Overall	206/2440	255/2431		0.81 (0.68–0.97)
(p homog = 0.01)				
Heart failure				
ABCD	10/235	8/235		1.25 (0.50–3.11)
STOP-2	149/2205	186/2196		0.80 (0.65–0.98)
Overall	159/2440	194/2431		0.82 (0.67–1.00)
(p homog = 0.35)				
Major cardiovascular events				
ABCD	28/235	47/235		0.60 (0.39–0.92)
STOP-2	531/2205	562/2196		0.94 (0.85–1.04)
Overall	559/2440	619/2431		0.92 (0.83–1.01)
(p homog = 0.04)				
Cardiovascular death				
ABCD	6/235	11/235		0.55 (0.21–1·45)
STOP-2	226/2205	212/2196		1.06 (0.89–1.27)
Overall	232/2440	223/2431		1.04 (0.87–1.24)
(p homog = 0.19)				
Total mortality				
ABCD	14/235	18/235		1.78 (0.40–1.53)
STOP-2	380/2205	362/2196		1.05 (0.92–1.19)
Overall	394/2440	380/2431		1.03 (0.91–1.18)
(p homog = 0.40)				

0.5   1.0   2.0
Relative risk
Favors   Favors
ACE-1   calcium
            antagonists

DHP = dihydropyridine, NHP = non-dihydropyridine, p homog = p value from χ^2 test for homogeneity.

Figure 41 Comparisons of ACE-Inhibitor-based Therapy with Calcium-Antagonist-based Therapy.

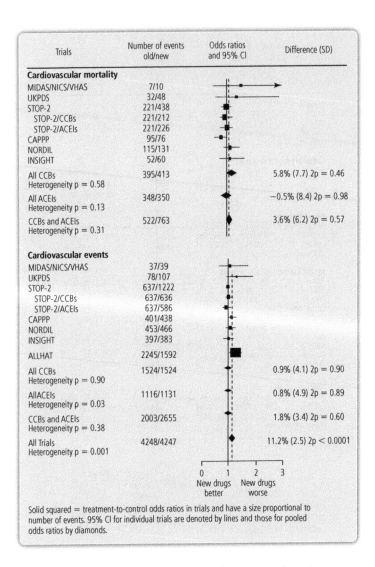

Trials	Number of events old/new	Odds ratios and 95% CI	Difference (SD)
Cardiovascular mortality			
MIDAS/NICS/VHAS	7/10		
UKPDS	32/48		
STOP-2	221/438		
STOP-2/CCBs	221/212		
STOP-2/ACEIs	221/226		
CAPPP	95/76		
NORDIL	115/131		
INSIGHT	52/60		
All CCBs Heterogeneity p = 0.58	395/413		5.8% (7.7) 2p = 0.46
All ACEIs Heterogeneity p = 0.13	348/350		−0.5% (8.4) 2p = 0.98
CCBs and ACEIs Heterogeneity p = 0.31	522/763		3.6% (6.2) 2p = 0.57
Cardiovascular events			
MIDAS/NICS/VHAS	37/39		
UKPDS	78/107		
STOP-2	637/1222		
STOP-2/CCBs	637/636		
STOP-2/ACEIs	637/586		
CAPPP	401/438		
NORDIL	453/466		
INSIGHT	397/383		
ALLHAT	2245/1592		
All CCBs Heterogeneity p = 0.90	1524/1524		0.9% (4.1) 2p = 0.90
AllACEIs Heterogeneity p = 0.03	1116/1131		0.8% (4.9) 2p = 0.89
CCBs and ACEIs Heterogeneity p = 0.38	2003/2655		1.8% (3.4) 2p = 0.60
All Trials Heterogeneity p = 0.001	4248/4247		11.2% (2.5) 2p < 0.0001

0   1   2   3
New drugs   New drugs
better   worse

Solid squared = treatment-to-control odds ratios in trials and have a size proportional to number of events. 95% CI for individual trials are denoted by lines and those for pooled odds ratios by diamonds.

Figure 42 Effects of Antihypertensive Treatment on Cardiovascular Mortality and All Cardiovascular Events in Trials Comparing Old with New Drugs.

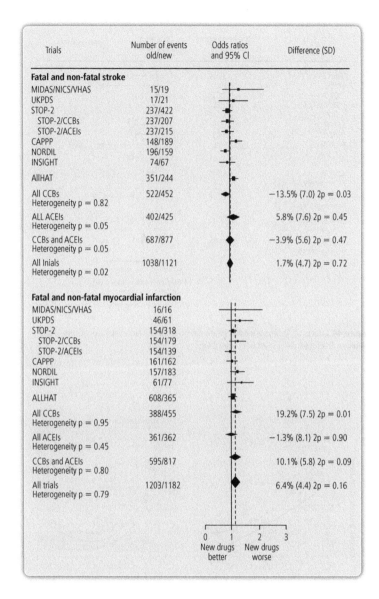

Trials	Number of events old/new	Odds ratios and 95% CI	Difference (SD)
Fatal and non-fatal stroke			
MIDAS/NICS/VHAS	15/19		
UKPDS	17/21		
STOP-2	237/422		
STOP-2/CCBs	237/207		
STOP-2/ACEIs	237/215		
CAPPP	148/189		
NORDIL	196/159		
INSIGHT	74/67		
AllHAT	351/244		
All CCBs Heterogeneity p = 0.82	522/452		−13.5% (7.0) 2p = 0.03
ALL ACEIs Heterogeneity p = 0.05	402/425		5.8% (7.6) 2p = 0.45
CCBs and ACEIs Heterogeneity p = 0.05	687/877		−3.9% (5.6) 2p = 0.47
All Inials Heterogeneity p = 0.02	1038/1121		1.7% (4.7) 2p = 0.72
Fatal and non-fatal myocardial infarction			
MIDAS/NICS/VHAS	16/16		
UKPDS	46/61		
STOP-2	154/318		
STOP-2/CCBs	154/179		
STOP-2/ACEIs	154/139		
CAPPP	161/162		
NORDIL	157/183		
INSIGHT	61/77		
ALLHAT	608/365		
All CCBs Heterogeneity p = 0.95	388/455		19.2% (7.5) 2p = 0.01
All ACEIs Heterogeneity p = 0.45	361/362		−1.3% (8.1) 2p = 0.90
CCBs and ACEIs Heterogeneity p = 0.80	595/817		10.1% (5.8) 2p = 0.09
All trials Heterogeneity p = 0.79	1203/1182		6.4% (4.4) 2p = 0.16

0 1 2 3
New drugs better   New drugs worse

Figure 43 Effects of Antihypertensive Treatment on Fatal and Non-Fatal Stroke and Myocardial Infarction in Trials Comparing Old with New Drugs.

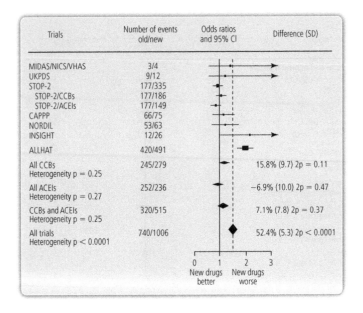

Figure 44 Effects of Antihypertensive Treatment on Fatal and Non-Fatal Congestive Heart Failure in Trials Comparing Old with New Drugs.

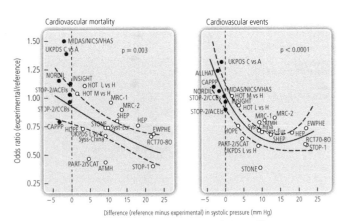

Odds ratios were calculated for experimental versus reference treatment. Blood pressure differences were calculated by subtracting achieved levels in experimental groups from those in reference groups. Negative differences indicate tighter blood pressure control on reference treatment. Regression lines were plotted with 95% CI and werer weighted for the inverse of individual odds ratios. Closed symbols denote trials that compared new with old drugs. Acronyms and references of trials are in the appendix.

Figure 45 Relation Between Odds Ratios for Cardiovascular Mortality and All Cardiovascular Events, and Corresponding Differences in Systolic Blood Pressure [156].

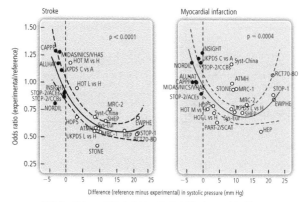

Fatal and non-fatal myocardial infarction includes sudden death. Odds ratios were calculated for experimental versus reference treatment. Blood pressure differences were calculated by subtracting achieved levels in experimental groups from those in reference groups. Negative differences indicate tighter blood pressure control on reference treatment. Regression lines were plotted with 95% CI and were weighted for the inverse of individual odds ratios. Closed symbols denote trials that compared new with old drugs.

Figure 46 Relation Between Odds Ratios for Fatal and Non-Fatal Myocardial Infarction, and Corresponding Differences in Systolic Blood Pressure [156].

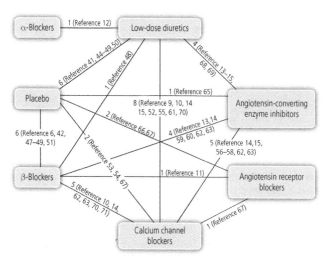

Each first-line drug treatment is a node in the network. The links between the nodes are trials or pairs of trial arms. The numbers along the link lines indicate the number of trials or pairs of trial arms for that link in the network. Reference numbers indicate the trials contributing to each link. A trial such as the Antihypertensive and Lipid-Lowering Treatment to Prevent Heart Attack Trial[12,15] (ALLHAT) with multiple arms appears along several links (diuretic-angiotensin-converting enzyme (ACE) inhibitors, diuretics-calcium channel blockers (CCBs), ACE inhibitors-CCBs, and diuretics-α-blockers). High-dose diuretics trials were excluded.

JAMA, MAY 21, 2003; 289, (19).

Figure 47 Network Meta-analysis of First-Line Antihypertensive Drug Treatment.

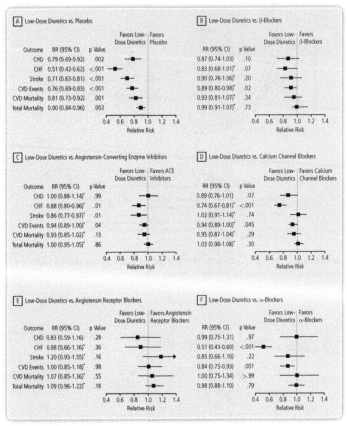

*β-blockers (p < .05), angiotensin-converting enzyme inhibitors (p < .05), calcium channel blockers (p < .05), and angiotensin-receptor blockers (p < .05) were significantly better than placebo for that outcome. α-Blockers were not significantly better than placebo for any outcome (>.05). ACE – angiotensin-converting enzyme; CHD – indicates coronary heart disease; CHF – congestive heart failure; CI – confidence interval; CVD – cardiovascular disease; and RR-relative risk.

Adapted from JAMA. May 21. 2003; 289 (19).

Figure 48 Network Meta-analysis of First-Line Treatment Strategies in Randomized Controlled Clinical Trials in Hypertension.

Meta-Analysis by BP Lowering Treatment Trialists Collaboration [158]

This overview included a total of 74 696 patients (15 trials).

1. Four placebo-controlled ACEI trials with 12 124 patients.
   CVA reduced 30%
   CHD reduced 20%
   CV events reduced 21%
2. Two placebo-controlled CCB trials with 5 520 patients.
   CVA reduced 39%
   CV events reduced 28%
3. More intensive BP reduction in three trials with 20 408 patients reduced events more than less intensive treatment.
   CVA reduced 20% more
   CHD reduced 19% more
   Major CV events reduced 15% more
4. Eight trials comparing different drug classes with 37 872 patients showed no significant differences among any CV outcomes.
5. Mean age of 62 years and 53% male subjects in the 15 included trials.

Staessen, Wang, and Thijs Meta-Analysis: Summary of Clinical Trials in Hypertension and Clinical Outcomes [156]

A reduction in SBP of 10–12 mm Hg and a reduction in DBP of 5–6 mm Hg result in the following reductions in CV endpoints based on meta-analysis studies of 27 trials on over 136 124 patients [156].

CHF	reduced	52%
CVA	reduced	38–42%
CHD and MI	reduced	16–21%

The conclusion was that results of the outcome trials for antihypertensive drugs can be explained by BP differences between randomized groups. All antihypertensive drugs had similar long-term efficacy and safety.

It was suggested that CCBs provided more reduction in CVA (13.5%, 95% CI 1.3–24.2, $p = 0.03$) and less reduction in the risk of MI (19.2%, CI 3.5–37.3, $p = 0.01$). The CVA reduction trend was confirmed in ALLHAT (NS) and in a recent meta-analysis, but the MI risk was not confirmed in ALLHAT (CCB) (amlodipine = chlorthalidone= lisinopril).

Specific BP reduction related to outcomes:

• SBP reduction of 10 mm Hg and DBP reduction 4 mm Hg:
  CVA decreased 30%
  MI decreased 23%
• DBP reduction (if DBP was predominant) of 5–6 mm Hg:
  CVA decreased 38%
  MI decreased 16%

Further Reading: Health Outcomes Analysis for Clinical Hypertension Trials

1. Joint National Committee on Prevention, Detection, Evaluation and Treatment of High Blood Pressure. The Sixth Report of the Joint National Committee on Prevention, Detection, Evaluation, and Treatment of High Blood Pressure. *Arch Intern Med* 1997; 157: 2413–2446.
2. Joint National Committee on Detection, Evaluation, and Treatment of High Blood Pressure. The Fifth Report of the Joint National Committee on Detection, Evaluation, and Treatment of High Blood Pressure (JNC V). *Arch Intern Med* 1993; 153: 154–183.
3. Psaty BM, Smith NS, Siscovick DS, et al. Health outcomes associated with antihypertensive therapies used as first-line agents: A systematic review and meta-analysis. *JAMA* 1997; 277: 739–745.
4. Veterans Administration Cooperative Study Group on Antihypertensive Agents. Effects of treatment on morbidity in hypertension: Results in patients with diastolic blood pressures averaging 115 through 129 mm Hg. *JAMA* 1967; 202: 116–122.
5. Veterans Administration Cooperative Study Group on Antihypertensive Agents II. Effects of treatment: Results in patients with diastolic blood pressure averaging 90 through 114 mm Hg. *JAMA* 1970; 213: 1143–1152.
6. Medical Research Council Working Party. MRC trial of treatment of mild hypertension: Principal results. *BMJ* 1985; 291: 97–104.
7. Hypertension Detection and Follow-up Program Co-operative Group. The effect of treatment on mild hypertension: Results of the Hypertension Detection and Follow-up Program. *N Engl J Med* 1982; 307: 976–980.
8. Hypertension Detection and Follow-up Program Co-operative Group. Five-year findings of the Hypertension Detection and Follow-up Program, III: Reduction in stroke incidence among persons with high blood pressure. *JAMA* 1982; 247: 633–638.
9. Brown MJ, Palmer CR, Castaigne A, et al. Morbidity and mortality in patients randomized to double-blind treatment with a long-acting calcium channel blocker or diuretic in the international nifedipine GITS study: Intervention as a Goal in Hypertension Treatment (INSIGHT). *Lancet* 2000; 356: 366–372.
10. Hansson L, Hedner T, Lund-Johansen P, et al. Randomised trial of effects of calcium antagonists compared with diuretics and beta-blockers on cardiovascular morbidity and mortality in hypertension: The Nordic Diltiazem (NORDIt) study. *Lancet* 2000; 356: 359–365.
11. Dahlof B, Devereux RB, Kjeldsen SE, et al. Cardiovascular morbidity and mortality in the Losartan Intervention For Endpoint reduction in hypertension study (LIFE): A randomised trial against atenolol. *Lancet* 2002; 359: 995–1003.
12. ALLHAT Officers and Coordinator for the ALLHAT Collaborative Research Group. Major cardiovascular events in hypertensive patients randomized to doxazosin vs. chlorthalidone: The Antihypertensive and Lipid-lowering Treatment to Prevent Heart Attack Trial (ALLHAT). *JAMA* 2000; 283: 1967–1975.
13. Hansson L, Lindholm LH, Niskanen L, et al. Effect of angiotensin-converting-enzyme inhibition compared with conventional therapy on cardiovascular morbidity and mortality in hypertension: The Captopril Prevention Project (CAPPP) randomized trial. *Lancet* 1999; 353: 611–616.

CLINICAL TRIALS

14. Hansson L, Lindholm LH, Ekbom T, et al. Randomized trial of old and new antihypertensive drugs in elderly patients: Cardiovascular mortality and morbidity the Swedish Trial in Old Patients with Hypertension-2 study. *Lancet* 1999; 354: 1751–1756.
15. ALLHAT Officers and Coordinators for the ALLHAT Collaborative Research Group. Major outcomes in high-risk hypertensive patients randomized to angiotensin converting enzyme inhibitor or calcium-channel blocker vs. diuretic: The Antihypertensive and Lipid Lowering Treatment to Prevent Heart Attack Trial (ALLHAT). *JAMA* 2002; 288: 2981–2997.
16. Pahor M, Psaty BM, Alderman MH, et al. Health outcomes associated with calcium antagonists compared with other first line antihypertensive therapies: A meta-analysis of randomised controlled trials. *Lancet* 2000; 356: 1949–1954.
17. Blood Pressure Lowering Treatment Trialists' Collaboration. Effects of ACE inhibitors, calcium antagonists, and other blood pressure lowering drugs: Results of prospectively designed overviews of randomised trials. *Lancet* 2000; 356: 1955–1964.
18. MacMahon S, Neal B. Differences between blood pressure lowering drugs. *Lancet* 2000; 356: 352–353.
19. Lumley T. Network meta-analysis for indirect treatment comparisons. *Stat Med* 2002; 21: 2313–2324.
20. MacMahon SW, Cutler JA, Furberg CD, Payne GH. The effects of drug treatment for hypertension on morbidity and mortality from cardiovascular disease: A review of randomized controlled trials. *Prog Cardiovasc Dis* 1986; 29(suppl. 1): 99–118.
21. Collins R, Peto R, MacMahon S, et al. Blood pressure, stroke, and coronary heart disease. Part 2, Short-term reductions in blood pressure: Overview of randomised drug trials in their epidemiologic context. *Lancet* 1990; 335: 827–838.
22. Mulrow CD, Cornell JA, Herrera CR, Kadri A, Farnett L, Aguilar C. Hypertension in the elderly: Implications and generaliability of randomized trials. *JAMA* 1994; 272: 1932–1938.
23. Hebert PR, Moser M, Mayer J, Glynn RJ, Hennekens CH. Recent evidence on drug therapy of mild to moderate hypertension and decreased risk of coronary heart disease. *Arch Intern Med* 1993; 153: 578–581.
24. Cutler JA, Psaty BM, MacMahon S, Furberg CD. Public health issues in hypertension control: What has been learned from clinical trials. In: Laragh JH, Brenner BM, eds. *Hypertension: Pathophysiology, Diagnosis and Management*, 2nd edn. New York, NY: Raven Press, 1995: 253–279.
25. Carter AB. Hypotensive therapy in stroke survivors. *Lancet* 1970; 1: 485–489.
26. Hegeland A. Treatment of mild hypertension: A five-year controlled drug trial: The Oslo Study. *Am J Med* 1980; 69: 725–732.
27. Liu L, Wang JG, Gong L, et al. Comparison of active treatment and placebo in older Chinese patients with isolated systolic hypertension. *J Hypertens* 1998; 16: 1823–1829.
28. Multiple Risk Factor Intervention Trial Research Group. Multiple Risk Factor Intervention Trial: Risk factor changes and mortality results. *JAMA* 1982; 248: 1465–1477.
29. Miettinen TA, Huttunen JK, Naukkarinen V, et al. Multifactorial primary prevention of cardiovascular diseases in middle-aged men: Risk factor changes, incidence and mortality. *JAMA* 1985; 254: 2097–2102.

CLINICAL TRIALS

30. Wolff FW, Lindeman RD. Effects of treatment in hypertension: Results of a controlled study. *J Chronic Dis* 1966; 19: 227–240.
31. Sprackling ME, Mitchell JRA, Short AH, Watt G. Blood pressure reduction in the elderly: A randomised controlled trial of methyldopa. *BMJ* 1981; 283: 1151–1153.
32. The IPPPSH Collaborative Group. Cardiovascular risk and risk factors in a randomized trial of treatment based on the beta-blocker oxprenolol: The International Prospective Primary Prevention Study in Hypertension (IPPPSH). *J Hypertens* 1985; 3: 379–392.
33. SCOPE Trial Investigators. Primary results of SCOPE. Presented at the International Society of Hypertension, Prague, Czech Republic, June 27, 2002.
34. Hansson L, Lithell H, Skoog I, et al. Study on cognition and prognosis in the elderly (SCOPE). *Blood Press* 1999; 8: 177–183.
35. Barraclough M, Joy MD, MacGregor GA, et al. Control of moderately raised blood pressure: Report of a co-operative randomized controlled trial. *BMJ* 1973; 3: 434–436.
36. Hypertension-Stroke Cooperative Study Group. Effect of antihypertensive treatment on stroke recurrence. *JAMA* 1974; 229: 409–418.
37. Smith WM. Treatment of mild hypertension: Results of a ten-year intervention trial. *Circ Res* 1977; 40(5 suppl. 1): I98–I105.
38. Perry Jr HM, Goldman AI, Lavin MA, et al. Evaluation of drug treatment in mild hypertension: VA-NHLBI feasibility study. *Ann N Y Acad Sci* 1978; 304: 267–288.
39. Anonymous. The Australian therapeutic trial in mild hypertension: Report by the Management Committee. *Lancet* 1980; 1: 1261–1267.
40. Kuramoto K, Matsushita S, Kuwajima I, Murakami M. Prospective study on the treatment of mild hypertension in the aged. *Jpn Heart J* 1981; 22: 75–85.
41. Amery A, Birkenhager W, Brixko P, et al. Mortality and morbidity from the European working party on high blood pressure in the elderly trial. *Lancet* 1985; 1: 1349–1354.
42. Coope J, Warrender TS. Randomised trial of treatment of hypertension in elderly patients in primary care. *BMJ* 1986; 293: 1145–1151.
43. Wilhelmsen I, Berglund G, Elmfeldt D, et al. Beta-blockers versus diuretics in hypertensive men: Main results from the HAPPHY trial. *J Hypertens* 1987; 5: 561–572.
44. Perry Jr MH, Smith WM, McDonald RH, et al. Morbidity and Mortality in the Systolic Hypertension in the Elderly Program (SHEP) pilot study. *Stroke* 1989; 20: 4–13.
45. SHEP Cooperative Research Group. Prevention of stroke by antihypertensive drug treatment in older persons with isolated systolic hypertension: Final results of the Systolic Hypertension in the Elderly Program (SHEP). *JAMA* 1991; 265: 3255–3264.
46. Kostis JB, Davis BR, Cutler J, et al. Prevention of heart failure by antihypertensive drug treatment in older persons with isolated systolic hypertension. *JAMA* 1997; 278: 212–216.
47. Dahlof B, Lindholm LH, Hansson L, Schersten B, Ekbom T, Wester PO. Morbidity and mortality in the Swedish Trial in Old Patients with Hypertension (STOP-Hypertension). *Lancet* 1991; 338: 1281–1285.
48. Medical Research Council Working Party. Medical Research Council trial of treatment of hypertension in older adults: Principal results. *BMJ* 1992; 304: 405–412.

CLINICAL TRIALS

49. The Dutch TIA Trial Study Group. Trial of secondary prevention with atenolol after transient ischemic attack or nondisabling ischemic stroke. *Stroke* 1993; 24: 543–548.

50. PATS Collaborating Group. Post-Stroke Antihypertensive Treatment Study: A preliminary report. *Chin Med J (Engl)* 1995; 108: 710–717.

51. Eriksson S, Olofsson BO, Wester PO. Atenolol in secondary prevention after stroke. *Cerebrovasc Dis* 1995; 5: 21–25.

52. Borhani NO, Mercuri M, Borhani PA, et al. Final outcome results of the Multicenter Isradipine Diuretic Atherosclerosis Study (MIDAS): A randomized controlled trial. *JAMA* 1996; 276: 785–791.

53. Staessen JA, Fagard R, Thijs L, et al. Randomized double-blind comparison of placebo and active treatment for older patients with isolated systolic hypertension. The Systolic Hypertension in Europe Trial Investigators. *Lancet* 1997; 350: 757–764.

54. Staessen JA, Thijs L, Birkenhager WH, Bulpitt CJ, Fagard R. Update on the Systolic Hypertension in Europe (SYST-EUR) Trial. *Hypertension* 1999; 33: 1476–1477.

55. Rosei EA, Dal Palu C, Leonetti G, et al. Clinical results of the Verapamil in Hypertension and Atherosclerosis Study (VHAS). VHAS Investigators. *J Hypertens* 1997; 15: 1337–1344.

56. Estacio RO, Jeffers BW, Hiatt MR, Biggerstaff SL, Gifford N, Schrier RW. The effect of nisoldipine as compared with enalapril on cardiovascular outcomes in patients with non-insulin-dependent diabetes and hypertension. *N Engl J Med* 1998; 338: 645–652.

57. Schrier RW, Estacio RO. Additional follow-up from the ABCD trial in patients with type 2 diabetes and hypertension. *N Engl J Med* 2000; 343: 1969.

58. Tatti P, Pahor M, Byington RP, et al. Outcome results of the Fosinopril versus Amlodipine Cardiovascular Events Trial (FACET) in patients with hypertension and non-insulin dependent diabetes mellitus. *Diabetes Care* 1998; 21: 597–603.

59. UK Prospective Diabetes Study Group. Tight blood pressure control and risk of macro-vascular and micro-vascular complications in type 2 diabetes: UKPDS 38. *BMJ* 1998; 317: 703–713.

60. UK Prospective Diabetes Study Group. Efficacy of atenolol and captopril in reducing risk of macro-vascular and micro-vascular complications in type 2 diabetes: UKPDS 39. *BMJ* 1998; 317: 713–720.

61. National Intervention Cooperative Study in Elderly Hypertensives Study Group. Randomized double-blind comparison of a calcium antagonist and a diuretic in elderly hypertensives. *Hypertension* 1999; 34: 1129–1133.

62. Agodoa LY, Appel L, Bakris GL, et al. Effect of ramipril vs. amlodipine on renal outcomes in hypertensive nephrosclerosis. *JAMA* 2001; 285: 2719–2728.

63. Wright Jr JT, Bakris G, Green T, et al. Effect of blood pressure lowering and antihypertensive drug class on progression of hypertensive kidney disease: Results from the AASK trial. *JAMA* 2002; 288: 2421–2431.

64. Wright J, for the AASK Study Group Investigators. The African-American Study of Kidney Disease and Hypertension. Presented at the American Society of Hypertension, New York, NY, May 18, 2002.

65. PROGRESS Collaborative Group. Randomised trial of perindopril-based blood pressure-lowering regimen among 6105 individuals with previous stroke or transient ischaemic attack. Lancet 2001; 358: 1033–1041.

66. Parving HH, Lehnert H, Brochner-Mortensen J, et al., for the Irbesartan in Patients with Type 2 Diabetes and Microalbuminuria Study. The effect of irbesartan on the development of diabetic nephropathy in patients with type 2 diabetes. *N Engl J Med* 2001; 345: 870–878.

67. Lewis EJ, Hunsicker LG, Clarke WR, et al. Reno-protective effect of angiotensin-receptor antagonist irbesartan in patients with nephropathy due to type 2 diabetes. *N Engl J Med* 2001; 345: 851–860.

68. The ANBP2 Investigators. Primary results of the Australian National Blood Pressure 2 Trial. Presented at the International Society of Hypertension, Prague, Czech Republic, June 23–27, 2002.

69. Wing LMH, Reid CM, Ryan P, et al. For the Second Australian National Blood Pressure Study Group. A comparison of outcomes with angiotensin-converting enzyme inhibitors and diuretics for hypertension in the elderly. *N Engl J Med* 2003; 348: 583–592.

70. Black HR, Grimm JRH, Hansson L, et al. Controlled Onset Verapamil Investigation of Cardiovascular Endpoints: CONVICE primary results. Presented at the American Society of Hypertension, New York, NY, May 18, 2002.

71. Zanchetti Z, Bond G, Hennig M, et al. Calcium antagonist lacidipine slows down progression of asymptomatic *caroitd* atherosclerosis: Principal results of the European Lacidipine Study on Atherosclerosis (ELSA): A randomized, double-blind, long-term trial. *Circulation* 2002; 106: 2422–2427.

72. Sewester CS, Dombek CE, Olin BR, Scott JA, Hebel SK, Novak KK, eds. *Drug Facts and Comparisons*. St. Louis, MO: Wolters Kluwer Co, 1996.

73. Berlin JA, Laird NM, Sacks HS, Chalmers TC. A comparison of statistical methods for combining event rates from clinical trials. *Stat Med* 1989; 8: 141–151.

74. Bucher HC, Guyatt GH, Griffith LE, Walter SD. The results of direct and indirect treatment comparisons in meta-analysis of randomized controlled trials. *J Clin Epidemiol* 1997; 50: 683–691.

75. Ekbom T, Dahlof B, Hansson L, Lindholm SH, Schersten B, Wester PO. Antihypertensive efficacy and side effects of three beta-blockers and a diuretic in elderly hypertensives: A report from the STOP-Hypertension study. *J Hypertens* 1992; 10: 1525–1530.

76. Alderman MH, Furberg CD, Kostis JB, et al. Hypertension guidelines: Criteria that might make them more clinically useful. *Am J Hypertens* 2002; 15: 917–923.

77. Yusuf S, Wittes J, Friedman L. Overview of results of randomized clinical trials in heart disease I: Treatments following myocardial infarction. *JAMA* 1988; 260: 2088–2093.

78. Soriano JB, Hoes AW, Meems L, Grobbee DE. Increased survival with beta-blockers: Importance of ancillary properties. *Prog Cardiovasc Dis* 1997; 39: 445–456.

79. Heidenreich PA, McDonald KM, Hastie T, et al. Meta-analysis of trials comparing b-blockers, calcium antagonists, and nitrates for stable angina. *JAMA* 1999; 281: 1927–1936.

80. Heidenreich PA, Lee TT, Massie BM. Effect of beta-blockers on mortality in patients with heart failure: A meta-analysis of randomized clinical trials. *J Am Coll Cardiol* 1997; 30: 27–34.

81. Lechat P, Packer M, Chalon S, Cucherat M, Arab T, Boissel JP. Clinical effects of beta-adrenergic blockade in chronic heart failure: A meta-analysis of double-blind, placebo-controlled, randomized trials. *Circulation* 1998: 98: 1184–1191.

CLINICAL TRIALS

82. Task Force on the Management of Stable Angina Pectoris. Management of stable angina pectoris: Recommendations of the Task Force of the European Society of Cardiology. *Eur Heart J* 1997; 18: 394–413.

83. Gibbons RJ, Chatterjee K, Daley J, et al. ACC/AHA/ACP-ASIM guidelines for the management of patients with chronic stable angina: Executive summary and recommendations. *Circulation* 1999; 99: 2829–2848.

84. Ryan TJ, Antman EM, Brooks NH, et al. 1999 Update: ACC/AHA guidelines for the management of patients with acute myocardial infarction: Executive summary and recommendations. *Circulation* 1999; 100: 1016–1030.

85. Braunwald E, Antman EM, Beasley JW, et al. ACC/AHA guidelines for the management of patients with unstable angina and non-ST-segment elevation myo-cardial infarction: Executive summary and recommendations. *Circulation* 2000; 102: 1193–1209.

86. Williams SV, Fihn SD, Gibbons RJ. Guidelines for the management of patients with chronic stable angina: Diagnosis and risk stratification. *Ann Intern Med* 2001; 135: 530–547.

87. The Heart Outcomes Prevention Evaluation Study Investigators. Effects of an angiotensin-converting-enzyme inhibitor, ramipril, on cardiovascular events in high-risk patients. *N Engl J Med* 2000; 342: 145–153.

88. Flather MD, Yusuf S, Kober L, et al. Long-term ACE-inhibitor therapy in patients with heart failure or left-ventricular dysfunction: A systematic overview of data from individual patients. ACE-Inhibitor Myocardial Infarction Collaborative Group. *Lancet* 2000; 355: 1575–1581.

89. Garg R, Yusuf S. Overview of randomized trials of angiotensin-converting enzyme inhibitors on mortality and morbidity in patients with heart failure. Collaborative Group on ACE Inhibitor Trials. *JAMA* 1995; 273: 1450–1456.

90. Pahor M, Psaty BM, Alderman MH, Applegate WB, Williamson JD, Furberg CD. Therapeutic benefits of ACE inhibitors and other antihypertensive drugs in patients with type 2 diabetes. *Diabetes Care* 2000; 23: 888–892.

91. Cupples LA, D'Agostino RB. Some risk factors related to the annual incidence of cardiovascular disease and death using pooled repeated biennial measurements: Framingham Heart Study, 30-year follow-up. In: Kannel WB, Wolf PA, Garrison RJ, eds. *The Framingham Study: An Epidemiological Investigation of Cardiovascular Disease*. Bethesda, MD: National Institutes of Health, 1987. NIH No. 87-2703.

92. Song F, Altman DG, Glenny AM, Deeks JJ. Validity of indirect comparisons for estimated efficacy of competing interventions: Empirical evidence from published meta-analyses. *BMJ* 2003; 326: 472.

93. Blackwelder WC. "Proving the null hypothesis" in clinical trials. *Control Clin Trials* 1982; 3: 345–353.

94. Blackwelder WC, Chang MA. Sample size graphs for "proving the null hypothesis." *Control Clin Trials* 1984; 5: 97–105.

95. Neaton JD, Grimm Jr RH, Prineas RJ, et al. Treatment of Mild Hypertension Study (TOMHS): Final results. Treatment of Mild Hypertension Research Group. *JAMA* 1993; 270: 713–724.

Combination Meta-Analysis of 354 Randomized Trials [220]

Design
Meta-analysis of 354 randomized, double-blind, placebo-controlled trials of thiazides, BBs, ACEI, ARBs, and CCBs in fixed dose.

Conclusions
Combination of low-dose drug treatment increases efficacy and reduces adverse effects. From the average BP in people who have strokes (150/90 mm Hg), three drugs at half standard dose are estimated to lower BP by 20 mm Hg systolic and 11 mm Hg diastolic thereby reducing the risk of stroke by 63% and ischemic heart disease events by 46% at age 60–69 years.

Key points
- The efficacies of five categories of drugs are similar at standard doses and only 20% lower at half standard doses; adverse effects are much less common at half standard dose than at standard dose.
- The drugs are effective for all pretreatment levels of BP.
- Reductions in BP with drugs in combinations are additive; adverse effects are less than additive.
- Using three BP lowering drugs in low-dose combination would reduce stroke by two-thirds and heart disease by half.

Prospective Clinical Trials in Hypertension Comparing CCBs to Other Antihypertensive Therapy: Total of 29 Trials [160]

1. Placebo-controlled published trials (six trials)
   I. IDNT: Irbesartan Diabetes Nephrology Trial
   II. PREVENT: Prospective Randomized Evaluation of Vascular Effects of Norvasc Trial
   III. STONE: Shanghai Trial of Nifedipine in the Elderly
   IV. SYST-EUR: Systolic Hypertension in Europe Trial
   V. CHEN-DU: Nifedipine Trial in China
   VI. SYST-CHINA: Systolic Hypertension in China Trial
2. Placebo-controlled trials recently published (three trials)
   I. CLEVER: China's Lacidipine Event Reduction Trial
   II. BENEDICT: Bergamo Nephrology Diabetes Complication Trial
   III. ACTION: A Coronary Disease Trial Investigating Outcome with Nifedipine GITS
3. Comparison of different antihypertensive drug classes: Published trials (15 trials)
   I. AASK: African-American Study of Kidney Disease and Hypertension
   II. ABCD: Appropriate Blood Pressure Control in Diabetes Trial
   III. ALLHAT: Antihypertensive and Lipid-Lowering Treatment to Prevent Heart Attack Trial
   IV. CONVINCE: Controlled Onset Verapamil Investigation of Cardiovascular Endpoints
   V. INSIGHT: International Nifedipine GITS Study: Intervention as a Goal in Hypertension Trial
   VI. NICS-EH: National Intervention Cooperative Study in Elderly Hypertensives
   VII. NORDIL: Nordic Diltiazem Study
   VIII. STOP-2: Swedish Therapy in Old Patients with Hypertension
   IX. VHAS: Verapamil in Hypertension and Atherosclerosis Study
   X. MIDAS: Multicenter Isradipine Diuretic Atherosclerosis Study
   XI. HOT: Hypertension Optimal Treatment Trial
   XII. PATE: Practioners Trial on the Efficacy of Antihypertensive Treatment in the Elderly
   XIII. GLANT: Study Group on Long-term Antihypertensive Therapy
   XIV. FACET: Fosinopril and Amlodipine Cardiac Events Trial
   XV. PRESERVE: Prospective Randomized Enalapril Regression Study
4. Comparison of different antihypertensive drug classes: Recently published trials (five trials)
   I. ELSA: European Lacidipine Study of Atherosclerosis
   II. INVEST: International Verapamil Trandolapril Study
   III. SHELL: Systolic Hypertension in the Elderly Lacidipine Long-Term Study
   IV. ASCOT: Anglo-Scandinavian Cardiac Outcomes Trial
   V. VALUE: Valsartan Antihypertensive Long-Term Use Evaluation.

Clinical Hypertension Trials with CCBs

1. **STONE:** Shanghai Trial of Nifedipine in the Elderly
2. **SYST-EUR:** Systolic Hypertension in Europe Trial
3. **CHEN-DU:** Nifedipine Trial in China
4. **SYST-CHINA:** Systolic Hypertension in China Trial
5. **HOT:** Hypertension Optimal Treatment Trial
6. **NICS-EH:** National Intervention Cooperative Study in Elderly Hypertensives
7. **INSIGHT:** International Nifedipine GITS Study: Intervention as a Goal in Hypertension Trial
8. **NORDIL:** Nordic Diltiazem Study
9. **CONVINCE:** Controlled Onset Verapamil Investigation of Cardiovascular Endpoints
10. **PREVENT:** Prospective Randomized Evaluation of Vascular Effects of Norvasc Trial
11. **VHAS:** Verapamil in Hypertension and Atherosclerosis Study
12. **PATE:** Practitioners Trial on the Efficacy of Antihypertensive Treatment in the Elderly (Japan)
13. **ALLHAT:** Antihypertensive Therapy and Lipid-Lowering Heart Attack Prevention Trial
14. **STOP-2:** Swedish Therapy in Old Patients with Hypertension
15. **IDNT:** Irbesartan Diabetes Nephrology Trial
16. **AASK:** African-American Study of Kidney Disease and Hypertension
17. **ABCD:** Appropriate Blood Pressure Control in Diabetes Trial
18. **ELSA:** European Lacidipine Study of Atherosclerosis
19. **INVEST:** International Verapamil Trandolapril Study
20. **SHELL:** Systolic Hypertension in the Elderly Lacidipine Long-Term Study
21. **MIDAS:** Multicenter Isradipine Diuretic Atherosclerosis Study
22. **GLANT:** Study Group on Long-Term Antihypertensive Therapy
23. **FACET:** Fosinopril and Amlodipine Cardiac Events Trial
24. **PRESERVE:** Prospective Randomized Enalapril Regression Study
25. **ACTION:** A Coronary Disease Trial Investigating Outcome with Nifedipine GITS
26. **ASCOT:** Anglo-Scandinavian Cardiac Outcomes Trial
27. **VALUE:** Valsartan Antihypertensive Long-Term Use Evaluation
28. **CLEVER:** China's Lacidipine Event Reduction Trial
29. **BENEDICT:** Bergamo Nephrology Diabetes Complication Trial

1. STONE [126]
   - Single blind
   - 1632 men and women (Chinese)
   - age 60–79
   - 3-year study with 30-month mean follow-up
   - Nifedipine tablets 10 mg (not GITS)
   - Placebo controlled
   - Add-on treatment: captopril or HCTZ.

Number and significance of high-incidence endpoints

| | Original treatment assignment | | |
| | Number of events | | |
	Placebo	Nifedipine	p value
All events	77	32	0.0001
CV events	59	24	0.0001
Strokes	36	16	0.0030
Severe arrhythmia	13	2	0.0007
Non-CV events	18	8	0.0366
All deaths	26	15	0.0614
CV deaths	14	11	0.4870

2. SYST-EUR [127]
   - Study Dates: 1990–1996, 198 centers
   - 4695 patients, age >60 years (average 70)
   - Two-thirds female
   - BP: SBP 160–219 mm Hg
     DBP <95 mm Hg
   - Drugs
     Nitrendipine 10–40 mg qd (two-thirds on monotherapy)
     Enalapril 5–20 mg qd
     HCTZ 12.5–25 mg qd

SYST-EUR Results

	Placebo	Treatment
SBP (mm Hg)	13	23
DBP (mm Hg)	2	7

	Placebo (1000 pt. yrs)	Treatment (1000 pt. yrs)	% Reduction (p)
Total CVA	13.7	7.9	42 (0.003)
Nonfatal CVA	10.1	5.7	44 (0.007)
Cardiac total events	20.5	15.1	26 (0.03)
Nonfatal cardiac events	12.6	8.5	33 (0.03)
CV total	33.9	23.3	31 (0.001)
CV mortality	13.5	9.8	27 (0.07)
CHF events	8.7	6.2	29 (0.12)
MI	8.0	5.5	30 (0.12)
MI deaths	2.6	1.2	56 (0.08)

Conclusions of SYST-EUR Study

1. Treatment of elderly patients with isolated systolic hypertension with nitrendipine reduces the rate of CV and cerebrovascular complications.
2. Treatment of 1000 patients for 5 years prevents 29 CVA or 53 major CV endpoints.
3. There was no increase in bleeding or cancer with nitrendipine compared with placebo.
4. Diabetic hypertensives had dramatic reductions in total mortality CV events, CVA, and coronary events on CCB that was superior to diuretics and BB in SHEP (Figure 49).

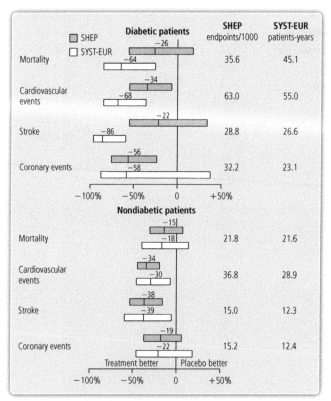

Outcomes in the Systolic Hypertension in the Elderly Program (SHEP) Trial. For these comparisons, the endpoints were standardized according to the definitions used in the SHEP trial. The Two right-hand columns show the number of events per 1000 patient-years in the placebo groups in the two trials. The bars indicate the 95% confidence intervals. The numbers above the bars indicate the benefit of the active treatment as compared with placebo. (From Tuomilehto J, Rastenyte D, Birkenhäger W, et al. Effects of calcium-channel blockade in older patients with diabetes and systolic hypertension *N Engl J Med* 1999; 340: 677–684 with permission).

Figure 49 Outcomes for SYS-EUR and SHEP.

Clinical Hypertension Trials with CCBs (*Continued*)

3. CHEN-DU Nifedipine Trial
   - 683 hypertensive patients
   - CV events at 6 years reduced from 14 to 5.2% (p = 0.05) in treated group
4. Systolic Hypertension in China Trial (SYST-CHINA) [128]
   - 2400 patients over 60 with ISH
   - Nitrendipine vs. placebo. Some received captopril or HCTZ
   - Goal SBP <150 or 20 mm Hg decrease
   - Median follow-up: 2 years 10 months

SYST-CHINA Results

- All-cause mortality reduced 79%
- CV mortality reduced 32%
- Total fatal and nonfatal CV events reduced 37%
- Congestive heart failure reduced 58%
- CVA reduced 58%
- No difference in MI
- No difference in fatal cancer
5. Hypertension Optimal Treatment (HOT) Trial 1
    - 18 700 patients, 26 countries, age 50–80
    - DBP 100–115 mm Hg
    - Randomized to three treatment groups

DBP <90 mm Hg; 85.2% achieved
DBP <85 mm Hg; 83.2% achieved
DBP <80 mm Hg; 81.1% achieved
Felodipine 78%
ACEI   41%
BBs   28%
Diuretics   22%
ASA vs. placebo

HOT Trial 2 Results

- Lowest incidence of major CV events at DBP 82.6 mm Hg
- Optimal SBP at 138.5 mm Hg
- CV risk reduced by 30% and is lower than that observed in prospective trials using diuretics or BBs ($p < 0.05$)
- QOL improved in all groups, but most in DBP <80 mm Hg
- ASA reduced CV events by 15%, MI by 36%, but no change in CVA. Nonfatal bleeds greater, but no difference in fatal bleeds
- No increased risk of CV even down to DBP of 70 mm Hg
- CV risk reduction was even more significant in diabetic hypertensives ($p < 0.005$)

6. National Intervention Cooperative Study in Elderly Hypertensives (NICS-EH)
   CCB vs. Diuretic
   - 414 patients, age >60, started 1989
   - SBP 160–220 mm Hg
   - DBP <115 mm Hg
   - Treatment: nicardipine SR 20 mg bid vs. trichlormethiazide 2 mg qd
   - 5-year follow-up in Japan

CCB: 172/94–147/81 mm Hg
Diuretic: 173/93–147/79 mm Hg

Results

CV endpoints
CCB, 10.3%; Diuretic, 8.6%; p-value, NS
CV morbidity
CCB, 27.8%; diuretic, 26.8%; p-value, NS
Rates per 1000 persons per year

Modified from National Intervention Cooperative Study in Elderly Hypertensives Study Group: Randomized, double-blind comparison of a calcium antagonist and a diuretic in elderly hypertensives. (Hypertension 1999; 34:1129–1133.)

INSIGHT [168]

1. Double-blind, prospective, randomized; 703 centers; 8 countries
2. Men and women, 55–80 years of age with hypertension and one additional risk factor
3. Nifedipine GITS vs. HCTZ/amiloride + atenolol/enalapril
4. Endpoints: fatal or nonfatal stroke, MI, or CHF
5. 4.5-year follow-up. intention-to-treat (ITT) analysis
6. 6321 patients
7. BP >150/95 mm Hg or SBP >160 mm Hg (mean 173%)
8. Results

Adverse effects

	Nifedipine (n = 3157)		Co-amilozide (n = 3164)		p-Value
	n (%)	Number of patients withdrawn	n (%)	Number of patients withdrawn	
Adverse events					
All adverse events	1546 (49)	539	1327(42)	304	<0.0001
Serious adverse events	796 (25)	198	880 (28)	245	0.02
Symptomatic adverse events					
Peripheral edema	896 (28)	267	137 (4–3)	14	<0.0001
Syncope	47 (1.5)	9	89 (2.8)	6	0.0004
Headache	384 (12)	63	292 (9.2)	32	0.0002
Palpitation	81 (2.5)	4	86 (2.7)	8	0.71
Peripheral vascular disorder	95 (3–0)	3	168 (5.3)	13	<0.0001
Impotence	50 (1.6)	5	60 (1.9)	6	0.34
Rushing	135 (4.3)	40	74 (2.3)	18	<0.001
Diabetes	96(3.0)	1	137 (4.3)	8	0.01
Dizziness	254 (8.0)	21	318 (10.0)	17	0.006
Gout	41 (1.3%)	67 (2.1%)	1	0–01	
Accidental injury	41 (1.2)	4	69 (2.2)	4	0.007
Depression	124 (3.9)	6	182 (5.7)	13	0.0009
Metabolic adverse events					
Hypokalemia	61 (1.9)	0	195 (6.2)	8	<0.0001
Hyponatremia	8	0	61 (1.9)	12	<0.0001
Hyperlipidemia	127 (4.0)	0	202 (6.3)	0	<0.0001
Hyperglycemia	178 (5.6)	0	244 (7.7)	4	0.001
Hyperuricemia	40 (1.3)	3	201 (6.4)	1	<0.001
Impaired renal function	58 (1.8)	3	144 (4.6)	18	<0.0001

CV Endpoints

	Nifedipine	Co-amilozide	Odds ratio (95% CI)	p-Value
Primary outcomes				
Composite	200 (6.3%)	182 (5.8%)	1.11 (0.90–1.36)	0.34*
MI				
Nonfatal	61 (1.9)	56 (1.8)	1.09 (0.76–1.58)	0.52
Fatal	16 (0.5)	5 (0.2)	3.22 (1.18–8.80)	0.017
Sudden death	17 (0.5)	23 (0.7)	0.74 (0.39–1.39)	0.43
Stroke				
Nonfatal	55 (1.7)	63 (2.0)	0.87 (0.61–1.26)	0.52
Fatal	12 (0.3)	11 (0.3)	1.09 (0.48–2.48)	0.84
Heart failure				
Nonfatal	24 (0.8)	11 (0.3)	2.20 (1.07–4.49)	0.028
Fatal	2 (0.1)	1 (<0.1)	2.01(0.18–2213)	0.63
Other CV death	13 (0.4)	12 (0.4)	1.09 (0.50–2.38)	0.85
Secondary outcomes				
Composite[†]	383 (12.1)	397 (12.5)	0.96 (0.83–1.12)	0.62
Deaths				
All (first event)*	153 (4.8)	152 (4.8)	1.01 (0.80–1.27)	0.95
Non-CV	71 (2.2)	66 (2.1)	1.08 (0.77–1.52)	0.67
Unknown cause	22 (0.7)	34 (1.1)	0.65 (0.38–1.11)	0.14
CV	60 (1.9)	52 (1.6)	1.16(0.80–1.69)	0.4
Nonfatal CV events	230 (7.3)	245 (7.7)	0.94 (0.78–1.13)	0.50
Primary events	140 (4.4)	130 (4.1)	1.08 (0.85–1.38)	0.53
Angina (worsening or new)	57 (1.8)	77 (0.4)	0.74 (0.52–1.04)	0.10
TIA	25 (0.8)	25 (0.8)	1.00 (0.57–1.75)	1.0
Renal failure	8 (0.3)	13 (0.4)	0.62 (0.26–1.49)	0.38

*MI, stroke, heart failure, and CV death.
[†]Primary outcomes plus non-CV deaths, renal failure, angina, and transient 23 additional in nifedipine group and 20 in co-amilozide group occurred after a previous endpoint.

9. Conclusions
  a. More metabolic disorders on co-amilozide than on nifedipine including hypokalemia, hyponatremia, hyperuricemia, hyperglycemia, and renal impairment.
  b. Fewer serious adverse effects with nifedipine than co-amilozide.
  c. Equal BP reduction by 22/17–138/82 mm Hg.
  d. More new onset DM with co-amilozide (p = 0.02).
  e. Nifedipine and co-amilozide were equally effective in preventing overall CV and cerebrovascular morbidity and mortality.
  f. Wide CI and number of patients do not allow for definitive statistical analysis of some of the 10 and 20 endpoints with presumed significant p-values such as fatal MI and nonfatal CHF.
  g. More decline in GFR with co-amilozide (reduced GFR by 2.3 mL/min/year more than nifedipine [p = 0.001]).
  h. Incidence of impaired renal function with co-amilozide group was 4.6 vs. 1.8% in the nifedipine group (p = 0.001).
  i. Nifedipine slowed cardiac calcification by EBT better than co-amilozide. At year 3, progression of coronary calcification was 77.85% with co-amilozide and only 40% with nifedipine.

CLINICAL TRIALS

NORDIL [169]

1. Open-blinded endpoint (probe) design
2. Men and women, 50–69 years (mean age, 60) of age with primary hypertension
3. Treatment: diltiazem retard vs. Diuretic and/or BB
4. Endpoints: fatal and nonfatal MI, stroke, or sudden death
5. Follow-up: 5 years (mean 4.5) ITT analysis
6. Sample size: 10881 in 1032 in centers in Norway and Sweden
7. BP: DBP >100 mm Hg mean study BP was
  diuretic = 151.7/88.7 mm Hg
  diltiazem = 154.9/88.6 mm Hg
8. Results
The results are illustrarted in Tables 34 and 35.
9. Conclusions
  a. BP reduction
    SBP: diuretic <23.3 vs. diltiazem <20.3 mm Hg (p < 0.001)
    DBP: diuretic = diltiazem (18.7 mm Hg)
  b. Fatal and nonfatal stroke were more common in diuretic than in diltiazem group despite lower BP (p = 0.04), a 20% reduction with diltiazem (corrected 32% for difference in SBP).
  c. Fatal and nonfatal MI were equal between groups (p = 0.1), but the wide CI and lack of power make this conclusion more difficult to interpret.
  d. Significantly more adverse effects with diuretics related to fatigue, dyspnea, and impotence (p < 0.001) and with diltiazem related to headaches.
  e. CV endpoints in DM were equal between the two treatment groups.

Table 34 RR and Occurrence of Endpoints

	Number of patients with events		Event rate per 1000 patient-years		RR (95% CI)*	p
	Diltiazem group	Diuretics and BB group	Diltiazem group	Diuretics and BB group		
Primary endpoint	403	400	16.6	16.2	1.00 (0.87–1.15)	0.97
All stroke	159	196	6.4	7.9	0.80 (0.65–0.99)	0.04
Fatal stroke	21	22	0.8	0.9	0.96 (0.52–1.74)	0.89
All stroke plus TIA	200	236	8.1	9.5	0.84 (070–1.01)	0.07
All MI	183	157	7.4	6.3	1.16 (0.94–1.44)	0.17
Fatal MI	28	25	1.1	1.0	1.10 (0.64–1.88)	0.74
CV death	131	115	5.2	4.5	1.11 (0.87–1.43)	0.41
Total mortality	231	228	9.2	9.0	1.00 (0.83–1.20)	0.99
All cardiac events	487	470	20.2	19.2	1.04 (0.91–1.18)	0 57
DM	216	251	9.4	10.8	0.87 (0.73–1.04)	0.14
All cardiac events	105	128	4.2	5.1	0.82 (0.64–1.07)	0.14
CHF	63	53	2.5	2.1	1.16 (0.81–1.67)	0.42

TIA = transient ischemic attack; CHF = congestive heart failure.
*Cox's regression model adjusted for age, sex, systolic pressure, and baseline: status of DM and smoking.

Table 35 RR and Occurrence of Endpoints with DM at Baseline

	Number of patients with events		Event rate per 1000 patient-years		RR (95%CI)*	p
	Diltiazem group	Diuretics and BB	Diltiazem group	Diuretics and BB		
Primary endpoint	44	44	29.8	27.7	1.01 (0.66–1.53)	0.98
All stroke	20	20	13.3	12.3	0.97 (0.52–1.81)	0.92
Fatal stroke	1	3	0.6	1.8	0.29 (0.03–2.86)	0.29
All stroke plus TIA	20	23	13.3	14.2	0.85 (0.46–1.55)	0.6
All MI	17	18	11.2	11.1	0.99 (0.51–1.94)	0.99
Fatal MI	5	2	3.2	1.2	2.45 (0.47–12.8)	0.29
CV death	15	13	5.7	7.8	1.16 (0.55–2.44)	0.71
Total mortality	28	26	18.1	15.6	1.07 (0.63–1.84)	0.80
All cardiac events	54	52	37.2	33.3	1.04 (0.71–1.53)	0.82
Atrial fibrillation	9	14	5.9	85	0.63 (0.27–1.46)	0.28
CHF	13	7	8.5	4.2	1.46 (0.57–3.72)	0.43

*Cox's regression model adjusted for age, sex, systolic pressure, and baseline: status of DM and smoking.

CONVINCE [170, 210]

1. Double blind
2. Men and women, 55 years or older with hypertension and one additional risk factor
3. Treatment: COER-verapamil vs. HCTZ or atenolol
4. Endpoints: first occurrence of nonfatal stroke, nonfatal MI, or any CV disease–related death
5. Follow-up: 6 years terminated early at 3 years
6. 16602 patients in 661 sites worldwide
7. Mean initial BP 157/87 mm Hg was reduced equally among the two groups
8. All-cause and CV mortality were equal between treatment groups, but due to premature termination of the study, only 729 events were reached (2200 events were projected for significance; Table 36 and Figure 50)

Table 36 Convince Trial [210] Primary and Secondary Events by Treatment Assignment

	Number (%) of participants with events			p-Value
	COER Verapamil	Atenolol or HCTZ	Hazard ratio (95% CI)	
Primary (composite) outcome*	364 (4.5)	365 (4.4)	1.02 (0.88–1.18)	0.77
Fatal or nonfatal MI	133 (1.6)	166 (2.0)	0.82 (0.65–1.03)	0.09
Fatal or nonfatal stroke	133 (1.6)	118 (1.4)	1.15 (0.90–1.48)	0.26
CVD-related death	152 (1.9)	143 (1.7)	1.09 (0.87–1.37)	0.47
Primary event or CV hospitalization	793 (9.7)	775 (9.3)	1.05 (0.95–1.16)	0.31
Angina pectoris	202 (2.5)	190 (2.3)	1.09 (0.89–1.33)	0.39
Cardiac revascularization/ cardiac transplant	163 (2.0)	166 (2.0)	1.01 (0.82–1.26)	0.91
Heart failure	126 (1.5)	100 (1.2)	1.30 (1.00–1.69)	0.05
TIA and/or carotid endarterectomy	89 (1.1)	105 (1.3)	0.87 (0.66–1.15)	0.33
Accelerated/malignant hypertension	22 (0.3)	18 (0.2)	1.26 (0.67–2.34)	0.47
Renal failure (acute/ chronic)	27 (0.3)	34 (0.4)	0.81 (0.49–1.35)	0.43
Death	337 (4.1)	319 (3.8)	1.08 (0.93–1.26)	0.32
New cancer (excluding nonmelanoma skin cancer)	310 (3.8)	299 (3.6)	1.06 (0.91–1.24)	0.46
Death	95 (1.2)	93 (1.1)	1.04 (0.79–1.39)	0.76
Death or hospitalization due to bleeding	118 (1.4)	79 (1.0)	1.54 (1.15–2.04)	0.003
Deaths from bleeding	6 (0.1)	6 (0.1)	1.02 (0.33–3.17)	0.97
Death or hospitalization due to serious adverse event	1381 (16.9)	1363 (16.4)	1.04 (0.97–1.12)	0.29
Hospitalization for serious adverse event	1150 (14.1)	1143 (13.8)	1.03 (0.95–1.12)	0.44

COER = controlled onset extended-release.
*First occurrence of stroke, MI, or CVD-related death.

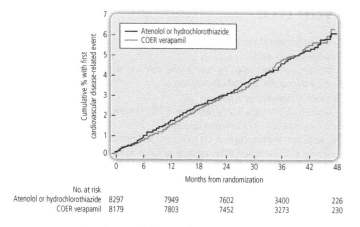

No. at risk					
Atenolol or hydrochlorothiazide	8297	7949	7602	3400	226
COER verapamil	8179	7803	7452	3273	230

COER indicates controlled-onset extended-release. The COER verapamil group experienced 364 cardiovascular disease-related events and the atenolol or hydrochlorothiazide group experienced 365 (hazard ration, 1.02; 95% CI, 0.88–1.18).

Figure 50 Incidence of Primary Outcome Measure Over Time.

PREVENT [171]

- 3 years, 825 patients with CHD
- Amlodipine vs. placebo
- No difference in CHD lesion by quantitative coronary angiography
- Significantly reduced carotid atherosclerosis
  1. B-mode ultrasound ($p < 0.009$)
  2. Carotid wall thickness (CWT) decreases 0.0024 mm/year (amlodipine)
  3. CWT increased 0.0121 mm/year (placebo)
- 31% reduction in composite of CV morbidity and mortality
  1. Nonfatal vascular events (CHF, unstable angina) 35% ($p = 0.02$)
  2. Revascularization (CABG, PTCA) reduced by 46% ($p = 0.001$)
- Amlodipine is effective in promoting regression of CWT, which parallels a lower CV morbidity and mortality.

VHAS [172]

- 498 hypertensive patients, 4 years
- Verapamil SR 240 mm Hg vs. chlorthalidone 25 mm Hg
- Mean thickness of carotid artery by B-mode ultrasound
    Verapamil—0.082 mm/year/mm
    Chlorthalidone—0.037 mm/year/mm ($p < 0.02$)
- Total fatal and nonfatal CV events
    Verapamil—19
    Chlorthalidone—35 ($p < 0.01$)
- More metabolic abnormalities with chlorthalidone (glucose, K^+, uric acid)
- BP reduction equal between groups
- Verapamil was more effective than the diuretic chlorthalidone in promoting regression of thicker carotid lesions that paralleled a lower CV event rate with verapamil.

PATE [173]

1. Patients age 60 years and older with essential hypertension (mean BP 150/83 mm Hg)
2. Treatment: ACEI (delapril) vs. CCB (manidipine)
3. 3-year study in 699 patients
4. Results
   a. Total mortality was equal
   b. Total CV morbidity and mortality was equal
   c. Possible "J curve" with SBP below 120 mm Hg related to cardiac events but not CVA
   d. BP reductions equal
   e. No difference in metabolic changes
   f. No difference in cancer morbidity and mortality.

Incidence of Fatal and Nonfatal CV Events [173]

	ACEI (n = 699)			Calcium antagonist (n = 1049)		
	Event	Fatal	Ratio*	Event	Fatal	Ratio*
CV events Fatal and nonfatal	34	7	22.5 X^2test	50 $p = 0.78$ (event) $p = 0.92$ (fatal)	10	19.7
Cerebrovascular events	14	3	9.3 X^2test	23 $p = 0.79$ (event) $p = 0.68$ (fatal)	6	9.1
Cerebral hemorrhage	3	2	2.0	4	4	1.6
Cerebral infarction	9	1	6.0	16	2	6.3
TIA	2	1.3	3			1.2
Cardiac events	20	4	13.3 X^2test	25 $p = p.54$ (event) $p = 0.35$ (fatal)	3	9.9
Angina pectoris	12	8.0	16	1		6.3
MI	3	2	2.0	6	1	2.4
Heart failure	3	2	2.0	1	1	0.4
Severe arrhythmia	2	1.3		2		0.8
Other CV events						
Aortic aneurysm				2	1	0.8

*Number of events/1000 patient-years.

ALLHAT [150]

On December 17, 2002, the National Heart, Lung and Blood Institute (NHLBI) released the ALLHAT study (Tables 37–43 and Figures 51–56). This is the largest

Table 37 ALLHAT Biochemical Results

	Chlorthalidone	Amlodipine	Lisinopril
Serum cholesterol (mg/dL)			
Baseline	216.1 (43.8)	216.5 (44.1)	215.6 (42.4)
4 years	197.2 (42.1)	195.6 (41.0)*	195.0 (40.6)*
Serum potassium (mmol/L)			
Baseline	4.3 (0.7)	4.3 (0.7)	4.4 (0.7)*
4 years	4.1 (0.7)	4.4 (0.7)*	4.5 (0.7)*
Estimated GFR[†] (mL/min/1.73 m^2)			
Baseline	77.6 (19.7)	78.0 (19.7)	77.7 (19.9)*
4 years	70.0 (19.7)	75.1 (20.7)*	70.7 (20.1)*

*p < 0.05 compared to chlorthalidone.

Table 38 ALLHAT Biochemical Results Fasting Glucose (mg/dL)

	Chlorthalidone	Amlodipine	Lisinopril
Total			
Baseline	123.5 (58.3)	123.1 (57.0)	122.9 (56.1)
4 years	126.3 (55.6)	123.7 (52.0)	121.5 (51.3)*
Among baseline nondiabetics with baseline <126 mg/dL			
Baseline	93.1 (11.7)	93.0 (11.4)	93.3 (11.8)
4 years	104.4 (28.5)	103.1 (27.7)	100.5 (19.5)*
Diabetes incidence (follow-up fasting glucose ≥ 126 mg/dL)			
4 years	11.6%	9.8%*	8.1%*

*p < 0.05 compared to chlorthalidone.

Table 39 ALLHAT non-fatal MI + CHD Death—Subgroup Comparisons—RR (95% CI)

Total 0.98 (0.90, 1.07)	Total 0.99 (0.91, 1.08)
Age < 65 0.99 (0.85, 1.16)	Age < 65 0.95 (0.81, 1.12)
Age ≥ 65 0.97 (0.88, 1.08)	Age ≥ 65 1.01 (0.91, 1.12)
Men 0.98 (0.87, 1.09)	Men 0.94 (0.85, 1.05)
Women 0.99 (0.85, 1.15)	Women 1.08 (0.92, 1.23)
Black 1.01 (0.86, 1.18)	Black 1.10 (0.94, 1.28)
Non-black 0.97 (0.87, 1.08)	Non-black 0.94 (0.85, 1.05)
Diabetic 0.99 (0.87, 1.13)	Diabetic 1.00 (0.87, 1.14)
Nondiabetic 0.97 (0.86, 1.09)	Nondiabetic 0.99 (0.88, 1.11)
0.50 1 2	0.50 1 2
Amlodipine better — Chlorthalidone better	Lisinopril better — Chlorthalidone better

Table 40 ALLHAT Stroke—Comparisons RR (95% CI)

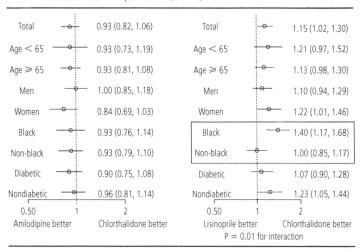

Total		0.93 (0.82, 1.06)
Age < 65		0.93 (0.73, 1.19)
Age ≥ 65		0.93 (0.81, 1.08)
Men		1.00 (0.85, 1.18)
Women		0.84 (0.69, 1.03)
Black		0.93 (0.76, 1.14)
Non-black		0.93 (0.79, 1.10)
Diabetic		0.90 (0.75, 1.08)
Nondiabetic		0.96 (0.81, 1.14)

0.50   1   2
Amlodipine better   Chlorthalidone better

Total		1.15 (1.02, 1.30)
Age < 65		1.21 (0.97, 1.52)
Age ≥ 65		1.13 (0.98, 1.30)
Men		1.10 (0.94, 1.29)
Women		1.22 (1.01, 1.46)
Black		1.40 (1.17, 1.68)
Non-black		1.00 (0.85, 1.17)
Diabetic		1.07 (0.90, 1.28)
Nondiabetic		1.23 (1.05, 1.44)

0.50   1   2
Lisinoprile better   Chlorthalidone better
P = 0.01 for interaction

Table 41 ALLHAT All-Cause Mortality—Subgroups Comparison—RR (95% CI)

Total		0.96 (0.89, 1.02)
Age < 65		0.96 (0.83, 1.10)
Age ≥ 65		0.96 (0.88, 1.03)
Men		0.95 (0.87, 1.04)
Women		0.96 (0.86, 1.07)
Black		0.97 (0.87, 1.09)
Non-black		0.94 (0.87, 1.03)
Diabetic		0.96 (0.87, 1.07)
Nondiabetic		0.95 (0.87, 1.04)

0.50   1   2
Amlodipine better   Chlorthalidone better

Total		1.00 (0.94, 1.08)
Age < 65		0.93 (1.81, 1.08)
Age ≥ 65		1.03 (0.95, 1.12)
Men		0.99 (0.91, 1.08)
Women		1.02 (1.91, 1.13)
Black		1.06 (0.95, 1.18)
Non-black		0.97 (0.89, 1.06)
Diabetic		1.02 (0.91, 1.13)
Nondiabetic		1.00 (0.91, 1.09)

0.50   1   2
Lisinopril better   Chlorthalidone better

CLINICAL TRIALS

Table 42 ALLHAT Combined CVD—Subgroup Comparisons RR (95% CI)

Subgroup	Amlodipine better / Chlorthalidone better	Subgroup	Lisinoprile better / Chlorthalidone better
Total	1.04 (0.99, 1.09)	Total	1.10 (1.05, 1.16)
Age < 65	1.03 (0.94, 1.12)	Age < 65	1.05 (0.97, 1.15)
Age ≥ 65	1.05 (0.99, 1.12)	Age ≥ 65	1.13 (1.06, 1.20)
Men	1.04 (0.98, 1.11)	Men	1.08 (1.02, 1.15)
Women	1.04 (0.96, 1.13)	Women	1.12 (1.03, 1.21)
Black	1.06 (0.96, 1.16)	Black	1.19 (1.09, 1.30)
Non-black	1.04 (0.97, 1.10)	Non-black	1.06 (1.00, 1.13)
Diabetic	1.06 (0.98, 1.15)	Diabetic	1.08 (1.00, 1.17)
Nondiabetic	1.02 (0.96, 1.09)	Nondiabetic	1.12 (1.05, 1.19)

Scale: 0.50 — 1 — 2; Amlodipine better / Chlorthalidone better; Lisinoprile better / Chlorthalidone better

P = 0.04 for interaction

Table 43 ALLHAT Heart Failure—Subgroup Comparisons–RR (95% CI)

Subgroup	Amlodipine better / Chlorthalidone better	Subgroup	Lisinopril better / Chlorthalidone better
Total	1.38 (1.25, 1.52)	Total	1.20 (1.09, 1.34)
Age < 65	1.51 (1.25, 1.82)	Age < 65	1.23 (1.01, 1.50)
Age ≥ 65	1.33 (1.18, 1.49)	Age ≥ 65	1.20 (1.06, 1.35)
Men	1.41 (1.24, 1.61)	Men	1.19 (1.03, 1.36)
Women	1.33 (1.14, 1.55)	Women	1.23 (1.05, 1.43)
Black	1.47 (1.24, 1.74)	Black	1.32 (1.11, 1.58)
Non-black	1.33 (1.18, 1.51)	Non-black	1.15 (1.01, 1.30)
Diabetic	1.42 (1.23, 1.64)	Diabetic	1.22 (1.05, 1.42)
Nondiabetic	1.33 (1.16, 1.52)	Nondiabetic	1.20 (1.04, 1.38)

Scale: 0.50 — 1 — 2; Amlodipine better / Chlorthalidone better; Lisinopril better / Chlorthalidone better

prospective clinical hypertension study to date with 42 418 patients randomized for 4–8 years (mean follow-up 4.9) in 623 clinical sites. This was a double-blind, randomized, multicenter, clinical trial with a primary endpoint of fatal CHD or nonfatal MI and secondary endpoints of all-cause mortality, stroke, combined CHD (nonfatal MI, CHD, death, coronary artery bypass graft [CABG], and hospitalization for angina), combined CVD (combined CHD, stroke, lower extremity revascularization, treated angina, fatal, hospitalized or treated CHF, and hospitalized or outpatient PAD), and finally other events such as renal outcomes (reciprocal serum creatinine, ESRD, and estimated GFR) and cancer. Metabolic parameters such as cholesterol, potassium, glucose, and new onset DM were also measured.

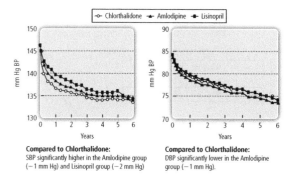

Compared to Chlorthalidone:
SBP significantly higher in the Amlodipine group
(−1 mm Hg) and Lisinopril group (−2 mm Hg)

Compared to Chlorthalidone:
DBP significantly lower in the Amlodipine
group (−1 mm Hg).

Figure 51 ALLAHAT BP Result by Treatment Group.

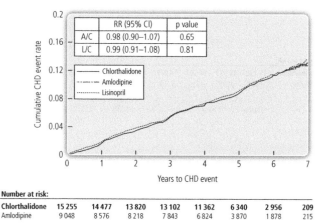

	RR (95% CI)	p value
A/C	0.98 (0.90–1.07)	0.65
L/C	0.99 (0.91–1.08)	0.81

Number at risk:

Chlorthalidone	15 255	14 477	13 820	13 102	11 362	6 340	2 956	209
Amlodipine	9 048	8 576	8 218	7 843	6 824	3 870	1 878	215

Figure 52 ALLHAT Cumulative Event Rates for the Primary Outcome (Fatal CHD or Non-fatal MI) by ALLHAT Treatment Group.

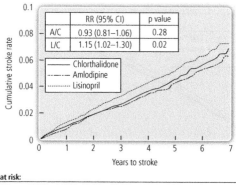

	RR (95% CI)	p value
A/C	0.93 (0.81–1.06)	0.28
L/C	1.15 (1.02–1.30)	0.02

Number at risk:

Chlorthalidone	15 255	14 515	13 934	13 309	11 570	6 385	3 217	567
Amlodipine	9 048	8 617	8 271	7 949	6 937	3 845	1 813	506

Figure 53 ALLHAT Cumulative Event Rates for Stroke by ALLHAT Treatment Group.

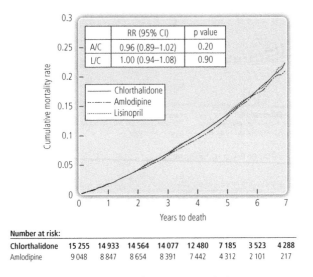

	RR (95% CI)	p value
A/C	0.96 (0.89–1.02)	0.20
L/C	1.00 (0.94–1.08)	0.90

Number at risk:

Chlorthalidone	15 255	14 933	14 564	14 077	12 480	7 185	3 523	4 288
Amlodipine	9 048	8 847	8 654	8 391	7 442	4 312	2 101	217

Figure 54 ALLHAT Cumulative Event Rates for All Cause Mortality by ALLHAT Treatment Group.

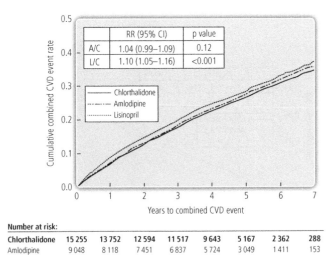

	RR (95% CI)	p value
A/C	1.04 (0.99–1.09)	0.12
L/C	1.10 (1.05–1.16)	<0.001

Number at risk:

Chlorthalidone	15 255	13 752	12 594	11 517	9 643	5 167	2 362	288
Amlodipine	9 048	8 118	7 451	6 837	5 724	3 049	1 411	153

Figure 55 ALLHAT Cumulative Event Rates for Combined CVD by ALLHAT Treatment Group.

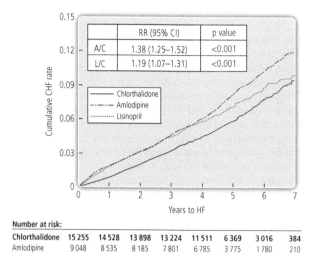

	RR (95% CI)	p value
A/C	1.38 (1.25–1.52)	<0.001
L/C	1.19 (1.07–1.31)	<0.001

Chlorthalidone
Amlodipine
Lisinopril

Number at risk:

Chlorthalidone	15 255	14 528	13 898	13 224	11 511	6 369	3 016	384
Amlodipine	9 048	8 535	8 185	7 801	6 785	3 775	1 780	210

Figure 56 ALLHAT Cumulative Event Rates for Combined CVD by ALLHAT Treatment Group.

The results of this study have been largely misinterpreted and misquoted by the media and in several medical journals. In fact, in the news release to the media, even the NHLBI had a misleading title with commissions and omissions that read as follows: "… NHLBI finds Traditional Diuretics Better Than Newer Medications for Treating Hypertension." Patients and physicians are once again confused about the data and what to do in the treatment of hypertension.

It is important to note that this study was performed in high-risk patients with vascular disease or CHD risk factors in an older age group over 55 years (average age was 67 years) and a large percentage of women (47%), African-Americans (35%), and type 2 diabetic patients (36%). The drugs compared were chlorthalidone, amlodipine, lisinopril, and doxazosin (dropped early in the trial). The drugs were given once a day in the AM as follows: chlorthalidone 12.5–25 mg, amlodipine 2.5–10 mg, and lisinopril 10–40 mg. Add-on therapy (tier 2 drugs) could be reserpine, clonidine, atenolol, and finally hydralazine as a tier 3 drug. The BP criteria for entry were untreated systolic or diastolic hypertension defined as ≥140/90 mm Hg, but ≤180/110 mm Hg at 2 visits or treated by hypertension defined as ≤160/100 mm Hg on one to two antihypertensive drugs at visit 1 or ≤180/110 mm Hg at visit 2 when medication may have been withdrawn partially. The mean BP at entry was 146/84 mm Hg. There were crossovers among the treatment groups of 7–9% at year 5, and about 40% of the patients in each group were on tier 2 medications with an average of at least two antihypertensive medications per patient.

What are the primary results?

1. BP

SBP: Amlodipine group was 1 mm Hg higher than the chlorthalidone group (p < 0.05). Lisinopril group was 2 mm Hg higher than the chlorthalidone group (p < 0.05). However, the SBP was 4 mm Hg higher in the black population treated with lisinopril than with chlorthalidone (p < 0.01).

DBP: Amlodipine group was 1 mm Hg lower than the chlorthalidone group (significant), and the lisinopril group was the same as chlorthalidone group. Therefore, amlodipine was equally effective as chlorthalidone in reducing mean arterial BP. As is evident, although these small differences reached statistical significance because of the larger group sizes, the absolute differences are quite small. If one compares chlorthalidone directly with amlodipine, since each had <1 mm Hg difference compared to the other with systolic and diastolic, respectively, there will be no real difference. It should also be pointed out that significantly more patients enrolled in the chlorthalidone arm than the other two (15255 for chlorthalidone vs. 9048 for amlodipine and 9054 for lisinopril) in design of the investigators. It was a "Heart Attack Trial" (HAT).

2. Primary endpoint of nonfatal MI and CHD death
Amlodipine (A) = chlorthalidone (C) = lisinopril (L). There was no significant difference among the three drugs ($p = 0.65$ for A/C and $p = 0.81$ for L/C). C = 11.5%; A = 11.3%; L = 11.4% (all 6-year rates).
The lack of difference in the primary endpoint in this study is a key and significant finding that was not clearly emphasized in the press (remember this is a high-risk, elderly, hypertensive population). It also points out that the small BP group differences had no clinical significance.

3. Secondary endpoints
   a. Stroke: There was a trend toward amlodipine being better than chlorthalidone with a 7% reduction in the amlodipine group, but this reduction was nonsignificant ($p = 0.28$). Chlorthalidone was better than lisinopril by 15% overall (6.3 vs. 5.6%; RR 1.15; 95% CI 1.02–1.30) ($p < 0.02$). This was 40% less in the black population only, but there was no difference in non-black population. This means lisinopril was as effective as chlorthalidone (NS) in the non-black population.
   b. CHF: Chlorthalidone was better than amlodipine by 38% (10.2 vs. 7.7%; RR 1.38; 95% CI 1.25–1.52 [6 years]) ($p < 0.001$) in preventing new onset nonfatal CHF. Chlorthalidone was better than lisinopril by 20% (8.7 vs. 7.7%; RR 1.19; 95% CI 1.07–1.31) ($p < 0.001$) in preventing new onset of nonfatal CHF.
   c. All-cause mortality: The three treatment groups were identical for mortality. For A/C $p = 0.20$ and for L/C $p = 0.90$.
   d. Combined CVD: Combined CHD, stroke, lower extremity revascularization, treated angina, fatal, hospitalized or treated CHF, hospitalized or outpatient PAD. Amlodipine equals chlorthalidone, and lisinopril had a 10% higher rate compared to chlorthalidone (33.3 vs. 30.9%; RR 1.10; 95% CI 1.05–1.16) ($p < 0.001$).
   e. Biochemical results: Chlorthalidone caused significantly more hypokalemia despite supplementation (0.3–0.4 mmol/L), which has been linked to sudden death, hyperglycemia, (3–5 mg%), hypercholesterolemia (1–2 mg%), and new onset DM (1.8–3.5%) than amlodipine or lisinopril ($p < 0.05$).
       Chlorthalidone also induced significantly more reduction in GFR (7–8 mL/min decrease) over 4.9 years and increased serum creatinine more than either amlodipine or lisinopril ($p < 0.05$). This demonstrates a potentially greater risk for CRI and ESRD and future need for renal replacement therapy such as dialysis or transplant in the chlorthalidone-treated patients. The expected decrease in GFR over 4.9 years is about 3–5 mL/min. Thus, chlorthalidone approximately doubled the expected decline in GFR.

There was no increased risk of cancer or gastrointestinal bleeding in the amlodipine or the lisinopril groups.

Conclusions

1. There is no difference in the primary endpoint of the study, fatal CHD, or nonfatal MI among the three treatment drug groups.
2. All-cause mortality was identical among the three treatment groups.
3. Chlorthalidone was superior to amlodipine and lisinopril in the prevention of new onset, nonfatal CHF. With lisinopril, this superiority was much more apparent in the black population.
4. Chlorthalidone was superior to lisinopril in stroke prevention in blacks but not in non-blacks. Chlorthalidone was not better than amlodipine in any subgroup of patients in stroke prevention.
5. Chlorthalidone induced more biochemical abnormalities such as hypokalemia, hyperglycemia, and hypercholesterolemia than amlodipine and lisinopril.
6. Chlorthalidone produced significantly more new onset DM than lisinopril and amlodipine.
7. Chlorthalidone produced significantly greater decline in GFR than amlodipine and lisinopril (7–8 mL/min). Expected rate is 3–5 mL/min. Thus, chlorthalidone approximately doubled the decline in GFR during the study period.
8. Amlodipine trended toward superiority compared to chlorthalidone in stroke prevention, but it did not reach statistical significance.
9. BP control was better with chlorthalidone than with lisinopril, but this control varied among the drugs, racial groups, and between SBP and DBP. Chlorthalidone reduced SBP more than amlodipine and lisinopril, but amlodipine reduced DBP more than chlorthalidone. Thus, amlodipine was equally effective as chlorthalidone in lowering mean arterial pressure.
10. In order to get BP from 146/86 to 134/75 mm Hg required an average of two drugs.

Interpretation and implications for treatment of hypertension

Most of the secondary outcome results in ALLHAT are driven by the reductions in CHF and in stroke in the black population. Some, but not all, of the differences can be explained by the differences in BP control as opposed to the specific drug class. For example, there was a 4-mm Hg difference in SBP in black patients in the lisinopril vs. the chlorthalidone groups. Based on meta-analysis studies, this difference could account for up to a 16% difference in stroke incidence. In the CHF patients, a 4-mm Hg difference in SBP could account for up to a 21% difference in CHF and 6% reduction in CHD and MI. Therefore, if one corrects for the SBP difference of 4 mm Hg in the lisinopril group, then the stroke reduction and the CHF reduction with chlorthalidone are not as impressive (i.e., 24% and 0%), respectively. In fact, lisinopril may have been better than chlorthalidone related to CHD and MI risk by 6%. In addition, both chlorthalidone and amlodipine are long-acting antihypertensive agents that control BP beyond 24 hours, whereas lisinopril loses its antihypertensive effect at about 16 hours. Would longer acting ACEIs, a twice per day regimen, or those with tissue selectivity have done better as was seen in HOPE and PROGRESS? In both these trials, a long-acting tissue-selective ACEI was administered resulting in significant reductions in CV and cerebrovascular morbidity and mortality. In the HOPE trial, the small reduction in BP did not account for the dramatic reductions in CV events, suggesting that the ACEI had nonhypotensive effects that were beneficial to the vascular system. However, the 24-hour ambulatory blood pressure monitor substudy did indicate significant reductions in BP with the ACEI. The final BP results could have been affected by the timing of the BP measurements. Also, the inaccuracy, observer bias or "rounding off effect" as well as the infrequency of cuff BP must be considered in ALLHAT.

The CHF differences may be explained by several theories:

1. Chlorthalidone is superior to other drugs.
2. Withdrawal of diuretics or other drugs at initiation of the study during randomization may have unmasked asymptomatic CHF and resulted in a greater frequency in the non-chlorthalidone-treated patients.
3. The improvement in other CVD endpoints may have shifted the CVD to CHF due to longer survival.
4. The definitions or clinical evaluation and diagnosis for CHF may not be accurate or consistent among the various clinical sites.
5. This is an elderly, high-risk population with possible unrecognized CHF and, thus, a different population subset than younger, lower risk hypertensives, or it may simply reflect the better follow-up and evaluation in study patients.
6. The chlorthalidone-treated patients may have masked mild or silent CHF symptoms prospectively, which would have biased clinical evaluation.
7. It should be remembered that in controlled clinical trials of patients with CHF, over 10 000 patients have been treated with ACEI vs. placebo and the ACEI (or ARBs), improvement in CHF was better. This result is difficult to explain in contrast to ALLHAT.

What should physicians do now to treat hypertension?

This study addresses only chlorthalidone, not other diuretics, and suggests that new onset nonfatal CHF is reduced more than with the other two drugs studied. It also suggests that strokes in blacks (but not non-blacks) are reduced more than with lisinopril, but not when compared to amlodipine. However, with respect to the caveats and the BP differences mentioned above, is chlorthalidone really better for CHF and strokes? How can these results be explained in view of the LIFE trial where an ARB was superior to a BB and in the HOPE and PROGRESS trials that showed superiority of ACEIs and in the ASCOT trial demonstrating superiority of combined amlodipine and perindopril over a thiazide diuretic and atenolol?

What are the long-term implications for the kidney and decline in GFR with chlorthalidone?

How can ALLHAT be explained in view of the data with RENAAL, IDNT, IRMA, AASK, INSIGHT, HOPE, and other studies? ESRD and dialysis are very expensive. Are there differences in specific drugs related to target organ protection? Recent reviews suggest that long-term use of thiazide diuretics may increase the incidences of ESRD.

What are the implications, long term, i.e., more than the 4–8 years of this study and the new onset diabetes and probable insulin resistance in the chlorthalidone group related to CVD and ESRD? Type 2 DM is the most common cause of kidney failure in the United States, but is not usually seen until more than a decade after onset. This increased risk of diabetes has enormous economic, morbidity, and mortality issues that are not addressed in ALLHAT. Many recent studies suggest that diuretics and BBs increase the incidence of type 2 DM as monotherapy or in combination and may also blunt the insulin sensitizing effects of ACEI and ARBs. Based on the ALLHAT trial, it is not recommended that chlorthalidone or diuretics should be used as first-line initial treatment of hypertension.

What are the long-term implications for the biochemical abnormalities with chlorthalidone?

Practically, most hypertensive patients will be on three to four hypertensive agents to reach new goal BP levels. These agents will need to be indapamide, chlorthalidone (or some other low-dose diuretic), amlodipine, or other CCB, ACEI, ARB, renin inhibitor, or possibly other medications. Control of BP and combination drugs must be paramount in the therapeutic regimen. Studies have suggested that the CCB, ACEI and ARB are actually the preferred agents when used in combination or as monotherapy.

One must weigh the results of ALLHAT with other studies (HOT, LIFE, HOPE, PROGRESS, SYST-EUR, INSIGHT, MRFIT, NORDIL, MRC, OSLO, RENAAL, IDNT, IRMA, AASK, ASCOT, and others). ALLHAT results do not support the results in all these other clinical trials.

One must also evaluate the patient demographics, underlying CVD, renal disease, and risk factors to select the most appropriate initial drug or drug combinations. Side effects, metabolic issues, and contraindications to chlorthalidone are important as well (sulfa allergy, pregnancy, metabolic, and renal problems, etc.).

ALLHAT will create guidance and some clarifications but also confusion and criticism as the data are analyzed more carefully and the later subset studies are published. In the meantime, it is not clear just how much new data have really been generated from ALLHAT and just how much it will change the practice of treating hypertension in practical terms. This story is unfolding and is far from over. All data are good if only to increase our questions and awareness of the complexity of treating hypertension. More studies are on the way with better and different designs and different population demographics that may challenge ALLHAT's ambiguous conclusions. It is known that elderly patients and those with concomitant CV risk factors, CV, or renal disease respond sooner and with more benefit at equal BP reductions compared to younger patients and those without concomitant CV or renal disease. After all, ALLHAT was really a study of high-risk, elderly hypertensives (average age = 67 years), and correlations to a younger population with different CV risks may not be accurate or appropriate.

STOP-2 [176]

- 6614 patients, age 70–84 years
- Study completed over 5 years
- Diuretic or BB vs. CCB or ACEI
- Equal BP reductions
- CV morbidity and mortality were equal
  Conventional: 19.8 events/1000
    New drugs: 19.8 events/1000
- Last visit 46% on two drugs and 61–66% on initial drugs
- Drug combinations: BB and diuretic or CCB and BB or ACEI and diuretic

All STOP-2 figures are reprinted with the permission from Ref. [14] (Figures 57–60).

Conclusions

1. CV morbidity and mortality were equal among the drug combination groups, but the CCB + ACEI combinations were not studied in STOP-2.
2. ACEI vs. CCB results in a significantly reduced rate of all MI (p = 0.018) and CHF (p = 0.025).
3. ACEI/CCB was significantly better (25%) than diuretic/BB in preventing stroke in elderly patients with ISH. (*Blood Pressure* 2004; 13: 137–143).

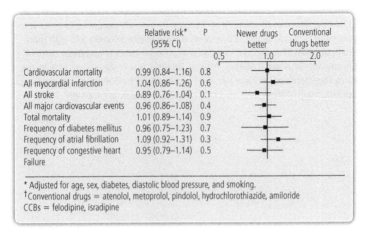

	Relative risk* (95% CI)	P	Newer drugs better	Conventional drugs better
Cardiovascular mortality	0.99 (0.84–1.16)	0.8		
All myocardial infarction	1.04 (0.86–1.26)	0.6		
All stroke	0.89 (0.76–1.04)	0.1		
All major cardiovascular events	0.96 (0.86–1.08)	0.4		
Total mortality	1.01 (0.89–1.14)	0.9		
Frequency of diabetes mellitus	0.96 (0.75–1.23)	0.7		
Frequency of atrial fibrillation	1.09 (0.92–1.31)	0.3		
Frequency of congestive heart Failure	0.95 (0.79–1.14)	0.5		

* Adjusted for age, sex, diabetes, diastolic blood pressure, and smoking.
†Conventional drugs = atenolol, metoprolol, pindolol, hydrochlorothiazide, amiloride
CCBs = felodipine, isradipine

Figure 57 STOP-2 Relative Risk of CV Mortality and Morbidity for All Newer Drugs vs. Conventional Drugs†.

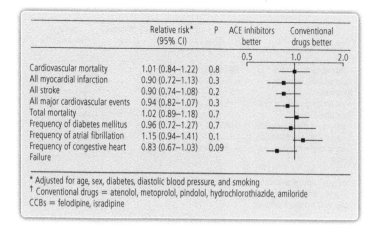

	Relative risk* (95% CI)	P	ACE inhibitors better	Conventional drugs better
Cardiovascular mortality	1.01 (0.84–1.22)	0.8		
All myocardial infarction	0.90 (0.72–1.13)	0.3		
All stroke	0.90 (0.74–1.08)	0.2		
All major cardiovascular events	0.94 (0.82–1.07)	0.3		
Total mortality	1.02 (0.89–1.18)	0.7		
Frequency of diabetes mellitus	0.96 (0.72–1.27)	0.7		
Frequency of atrial fibrillation	1.15 (0.94–1.41)	0.1		
Frequency of congestive heart Failure	0.83 (0.67–1.03)	0.09		

* Adjusted for age, sex, diabetes, diastolic blood pressure, and smoking
† Conventional drugs = atenolol, metoprolol, pindolol, hydrochlorothiazide, amiloride
CCBs = felodipine, isradipine

Figure 58 STOP-2 Relative Risk of CV Mortality and Morbidity for All ACE vs. Conventional Drugs[†].

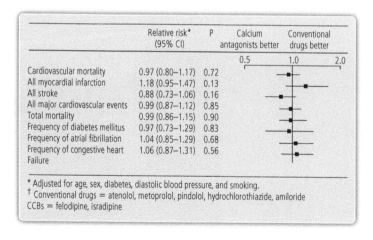

	Relative risk* (95% CI)	P	Calcium antagonists better	Conventional drugs better
Cardiovascular mortality	0.97 (0.80–1.17)	0.72		
All myocardial infarction	1.18 (0.95–1.47)	0.13		
All stroke	0.88 (0.73–1.06)	0.16		
All major cardiovascular events	0.99 (0.87–1.12)	0.85		
Total mortality	0.99 (0.86–1.15)	0.90		
Frequency of diabetes mellitus	0.97 (0.73–1.29)	0.83		
Frequency of atrial fibrillation	1.04 (0.85–1.29)	0.68		
Frequency of congestive heart Failure	1.06 (0.87–1.31)	0.56		

* Adjusted for age, sex, diabetes, diastolic blood pressure, and smoking.
† Conventional drugs = atenolol, metoprolol, pindolol, hydrochlorothiazide, amiloride
CCBs = felodipine, isradipine

Figure 59 STOP-2 Relative Risk of CV Mortality and Morbidity for Calcium Antagonists vs. Conventional Drugs[†].

	Relative risk* (95% CI)	P	ACE inhibitors better	Calcium antagonists better
Cardiovascular mortality	1.04 (0.86–1.26)	0.72		
All myocardial infarction	0.77 (0.61–0.96)	0.018		
All stroke	1.02 (0.84–1.24)	0.84		
All major cardiovascular events	0.95 (0.83–1.08)	0.42		
Total mortality	1.03 (0.89–1.19)	0.71		
Frequency of diabetes mellitus	0.98 (0.74–1.31)	0.91		
Frequency of atrial fibrillation	1.10 (0.90–1.34)	0.37		
Frequency of congestive heart Failure	0.78 (0.63–0.97)	0.025		

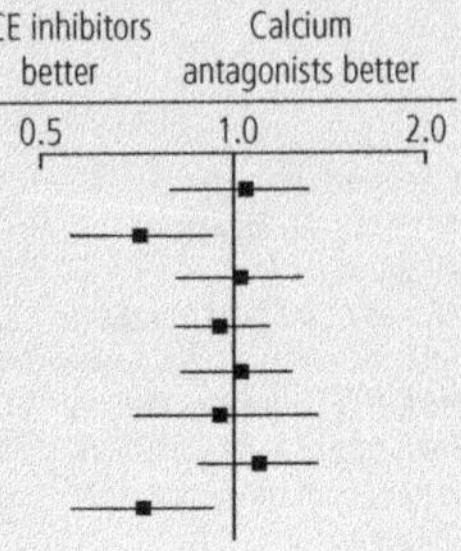

* Adjusted for age, sex, diabetes, diastolic blood pressure, and smoking
† Conventional drugs = atenolol, metoprolol, pindolol, hydrochlorothiazide, amiloride
CCBs = felodipine, isradipine

All five STOP-2 charts above are reprinted with the permission from Hansson L, Lindholm LH, Ekbom T, et al, for the STOP-Hypertension-2 Study Group: Randomized trial of old and new antihypertensive drugs in elderly patients: Cardiovascular mortality and morbidity the Swedish Trial in Old Patients with Hypertensive-2 Study. *Lancet* 1999; 354: 1751–1756.

Figure 60 STOP-2 Relative Risk of CV Mortality and Morbidity for ACE Inhibitors vs. Calcium Antagonists†.

IDNT [177]

1. 1715 hypertensive patients with nephropathy due to type 2 diabetes with severe proteinuria (mean >1 g/day)
2. Irbesartan vs. amlodipine vs. placebo
3. Mean treatment 2.6 years
Results

a. Irbesartan reduced risk of primary composite endpoint of doubling of creatinine ESRP or death by 20% vs. placebo ($p = 0.02$) and by 23% vs. amlodipine ($p = 0.006$).

  1) Risk of doubling of creatinine was 33% lower in irbesartan vs. placebo ($p = 0.0030$ and 37% lower in irbesartan vs. amlodipine ($p < 0.001$).
  2) ESRD risk was 23% lower with irbesartan vs. placebo or amlodipine ($p = 0.07$).
  3) Serum creatinine increased 24% more slowly in the irbesartan group than in the placebo group ($p = 0.008$) and 21% more slowly than in the amlodipine group ($p = 0.02$).
  4) Protection of renal function is independent of BP.

b. There were no significant differences in the rates of death from any cause or in the CV composite endpoint (CV mortality, nonfatal MI, CHF requiring hospitalization, CVA, or LE amputation).

AASK [178]

1. 1094 African-Americans age 18–70 years with nondiabetic hypertensive renal disease (GFR 20–65 mL/min/1.73 m)
2. Randomized, DB prospective, 3 × 2 factorial trial, 4 years
3. Compared two levels of BP and three antihypertensive drugs on GFR decline
4. BP levels: MAP = 102–107 mm Hg or MAP <92 mm Hg
5. Drugs: metoprolol vs. ramipril vs. amlodipine (open labels added drugs to BP control)
6. Outcomes measured
   a. Rate of change in GFR (GFR slope)
   b. Clinical composite outcome or reduction in GFR by 50% or more or >25 mL/min from baseline
   c. ESRD
   d. CVD events
   e. Death
7. Results
   a. Mean GFR slope did not differ between two BP groups.
   b. Clinical composite outcome did not differ between two BP groups.
   c. No difference in GFR slope among the three drugs.
   d. Ramipril reduced clinical composite outcomes by 22% vs. metoprolol (p = 0.04) and by 38% vs. amlodipine (p = 0.004). There was no difference between amlodipine and metoprolol.
   e. However, it was only in those patients with overt severe renal disease and 1 g protein/day (one-third of patients) that the ACEI or BB was better at slowing rate of GFR decline and delaying time to renal events than amlodipine.
   f. In the remaining two-third of patients with mild-to-moderate renal disease and <1 g of protein/day, amlodipine was as effective as ACEI in delaying or slowing the progression of renal disease (GFR).
   g. BP was similar in all three arms.
   h. No difference in CVD events among the three arms.
   i. Finally, if one evaluates the effects in those patients with <300 mg protein/day (urine protein/creatinine ratio <0.22), then there was no difference between amlodipine and ramipril related to decline in GFR.

Only in those patients with >1 g protein/day (urine protein/creatinine ratio >0.66) (one-sixth of total patients) was the overall change in GFR significantly less in the ACEI-treated group.

ABCD [179]

1. 470 patients with hypertension and type 2 diabetes
2. 5.3-year follow-up. Endpoint: GFR by 24-hour CRC1
3. Nisoldipine vs. enalapril
4. DBP >90 mm Hg at baseline to goal DBP <75 vs. DBP 80–89 mm Hg
5. Actual study mean BP

   Group I   132/78

   Group II   138/86
6. Results
   a. BP control in both groups with either nisoldipine- or enalapril-stabilized renal function in those without overt albuminuria.
   b. All-cause mortality decreased.
   c. Despite an increase in CV events in the CCB group, this study was not powered or designed to determine this outcome and is thus inconclusive.

ELSA [181, 207]

1. Prospective, randomized, double-blind, multinational trial
2. 2334 patients followed for 4 years. Ages 45–75 years
3. Treatment: lacidipine vs. atenolol (plus HCTZ)
4. BP levels at entry: 150–210/95–115 mm Hg
5. Endpoints: carotid atherosclerosis measured by maximal IMT with B-mode ultrasound.
6. Results
   a. Lacidipine IMT progression rate = 0.0087 mm/year, 40% reduction vs. atenolol (p = 0.0073).
   b. Atenolol IMT progression rate = 0.0145 mm/year.
   c. Lacidipine has less plaque progression and more plaque progression than atenolol.
   d. BP reductions were equal in clinical, but 24-hour arm showed atenolol to be more effective (–10/9 vs. –7/5 mm Hg).
   e. Trend toward relative reduction in CVA, major CV events, and mortality with lacidipine vs. atenolol (NS).
7. Conclusions

Lacidipine has anti-atherosclerotic actions independent of BP and is superior to atenolol despite the lacidipine group having higher 24-hour BM, more smokers, and less use of statins and anti-platelet drugs.

INVEST [182, 183]

1. 27000 CHD patients with hypertension in 1500 centers, mostly elderly (>60 years). Abnormal coronary angiogram or H/O or MI
2. Treatment: verapamil/trandolapril vs. atenolol/HCTZ-(V/T vs. A/H)
3. Outcomes: all-cause mortality, nonfatal MI, nonfatal CVA
4. Substudies on ABM, depression, QOL, genotyping
5. V/T treatment equals A/H treatment for BP control and all CV events
6. More D/M in A/H group. More CHF in V/T group (*JAMA* 2003; 290:2805–2816).

SHELL [184, 208]

1. Open, blinded endpoint (probe), 4800 patients
2. 1882 men and women, age 60 years and over with ISH
3. ISH with SBP >160 mm Hg and DBP <95 mm Hg
4. Treatment: lacidipine vs. chlorthalidone (L vs. C)
5. Endpoints: CV and cerebrovascular
6. Follow-up: 5 years in 115 centers in Italy
7. Substudies: 24 hours. ABM and ECHO
8. Equal BP reductions: chlorthalidone: 36.8/8.1 mm Hg; Lacidipine: 38.4/7.9 mm Hg
9. Total CV morbidity and mortality equal
10. L = C in reduction in SBP, CV events, and total mortality. (*Blood Pressure* 2003; 12:160–167).

MIDAS [185]

1. 883 patients with hypertension, 149.7 + 16.6/96.5 + 5.1 mm Hg
2. Average age 58 years, 3-year study
3. Randomized, double-blind trial in nine centers
4. Outcome: compare rate of progression of mean maximal IMT in carotid arteries with quantitative B-mode ultrasound
5. Treatment: isradipine vs. HCTZ
6. Results
   a. No difference in the rate of progression of mean maximum IMT between the two treatment groups
   b. HCTZ reduced BP more than isradipine, 19.5 vs. 16 mm Hg ($p = 0.002$)
   c. DBP was reduced equally in the two groups
   d. Higher incidence of vascular events CMI, CVD, CHF, angina, sudden death in isradipine vs. HCTZ group but it was not significant ($p = 0.07$)
   e. Higher increase in nonmajor vascular events and procedures, femoral-popliteal bypass graft in isradipine group ($p = 0.2$)
7. Conclusions

The lack of power, study design, and higher SBP in the isradipine group make the IMT and CV outcome data inconclusive.

GLANT [174, 175]

1. 1936 Japanese patients with mild-to-moderate essential hypertension, mean age of 60 years
2. ACEI (delapril) vs. CCB (various) such as short, intermediate, and long-acting CCB
3. 1-year study, prospective open trial
4. BP reduction greater in CCB vs. ACEI (p < 0.001)
5. CV and cerebrovascular morbidity and mortality were equal between groups.

FACET [180]

1. 380 patients with noninsulin-dependent diabetes mellitus (NIDDM) and hypertension
2. BP >140/90 mm Hg
3. Amlodipine vs. fosinopril
4. 3.5-year follow-up
5. Results
   a. BP control equal
   b. Metabolic parameters equal (lipids, Hg A1, C, glucose)
   c. Despite a lower combined CV outcome (MI, CVA, angina) with fosinopril, this study was not designed nor powered to evaluate clinical outcomes; thus, the CV outcome data are inconclusive.

PRESERVE [186]
- Nifedipine GITS vs. enalapril
- 303 men and women with essential hypertension and increased LV mass by echo
- 48-week study
- BP reductions equal 22/12 mm Hg in two groups
- LV mass index reduction equal in two groups

ACTION [160]

- 6000 patients with CHD over age 34 years
- Nifedipine GITS-DHP-CCB vs. placebo
- 5-year study

ASCOT Clinical Trials: LLA, BPLA, and LLA 2 × 2 [264–266]

- 19257 patients with hypertension and CVD risk, with at least three other CV risk factors
- Age 39–79 years
- BP >139/89 mm Hg
- Amlodipine ± perindopril (DHP-CCB ± ACEI) vs. BB ± diuretic (atenolol + bendroflumethiazide). Amlodipine 5–10 mg and perindopril 4–8 mg or atenolol 50–100 mg and bendroflumethiazide 1.25–2.5 mg

Cholesterol lowering with fixed dose atorvastatin 10 mg vs. placebo ARM

- 5-year study

Primary endpoint was nonfatal MI, including silent MI and fatal CHD. Analysis was by ITT.

- Lipid arm stopped at 3.3 years (prematurely), and the BP arm was stopped prematurely at 5.5 years with median follow-up and accumulated in total 106153 patient-years of observation (Figures 61–66 and Table 44).

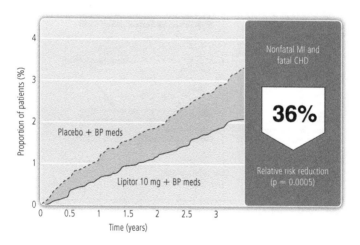

Figure 61 ASCOT LLA: Nonfatal MI and Fatal CAD.

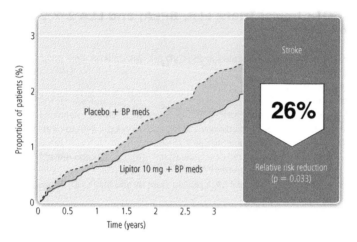

Figure 62 ASCOT LLA: Stroke.

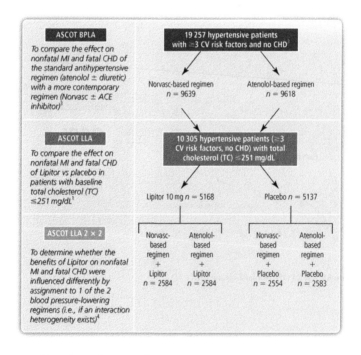

Figure 63 Anglo-Scandinavian Cardiac Outcomes Trial (ASCOT): Study Design.

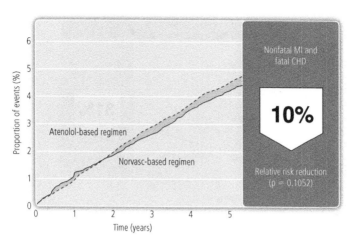

Figure 64 ASCOT BPLA Primary Endpoint: Nonfatal MI and Fatal CHD.

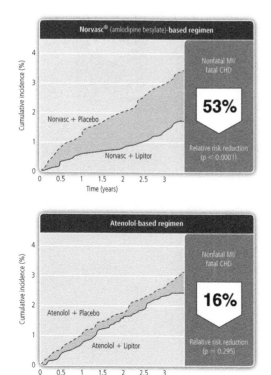

Figure 65 ASCOT LLA 2×2 Analysis.

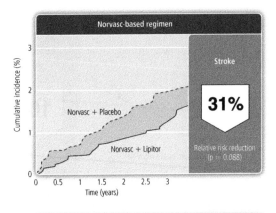

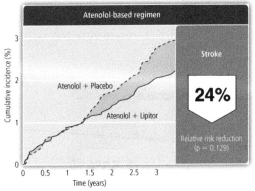

Figure 66 ASCOT LLA 2×2 Analysis.

Table 44 ASCOT: Baseline Patient Characteristics. Hypertensive patients with ≥3 risk factors and without CHD*

Baseline patient characteristics	ASCOT BPLA		ASCOT BPLA	
	Norvasc® (amlodipine besylate) arm $n = 9639$	Atenolol arm $n = 9618$	Lipitor® (atorvastatin calcium) arm $n = 5618$	Placebo arm $n = 5137$
Male	7381 (77%)	7361(77%)	4189 (81%)	4174 (81%)
Age (years)				
≤60	3558 (37%)	3534 (37%)	1882 (36%)	1853 (36%)
>60	6081 (63%)	6084 (63%)	3286 (64%)	3284 (64%)
Mean (SD)	63.0 (8.5)	63.0 (8.5)	63.1 (8.5)	63.2 (8.6)
White	9187 (95%)	9170 (95%)	4889 (94.6%)	4863 (94.7%)
Current smoker	3168 (33%)	3109 (32%)	1718 (33.3%)	1656 (32.2%)
Alcohol consumption (units/week)	8.0 (11.6)	7.9 (11.7)	8.0 (11.3)	8.2 (12.0)
SBP (mm Hg)	164.1 (18.1)	163.9 (18.0)	164.2 (17.7)	164.2 (18.0)
DBP (mm Hg)	94.8 (10.4)	94.5 (10.4)	95.0 (10.3)	95.0 (10.3)
Heart rate (beats/min)	71.9 (12.7)	71.8 (12.6)	71.3 (12.8)	71.8 (12.6)
BMI (kg/m^3)	28.7 (4.6)	28.7 (4.5)	28.6 (4.7)	28.7 (4.6)
Total cholesterol (mg/dL)	228 (43)	228 (43)	213 (31)	213 (31)
LDL-cholesterol (mg/dL)	147 (39)	147 (39)	132 (27)	132 (27)
HDL-cholesterol (mg/dL)	50 (15)	50 (15)	50 (15)	50 (15)
Triglycerides (mg/dL)	159 (89)	168 (89)	151 (80)	142 (80)
Glucose (mg/dL)	111 (37)	111 (37)	111 (37)	111 (37)
Creatinine (mg/dL)	1.1 (0.2)	1.1(0.2)	1.1(0.2)	1.1 (0.2)
Medical history				
Previous stroke or TIA	1050 (11%)	1063 (11%)	485 (9.4%)	516 (10%)
Diabetes	2567 (27%)	2578 (27%)	1258 (24.3%)	1274 (24.8%)
LVH	2091 (22%)	2076 (22%)	744 (14.4%)	729 (14.2%)
ECG abnormalities (other than LVH)	2206 (23%)	2249 (23%)	741 (14.3%)	729 (14.2%)
Peripheral vascular disease	586 (6%)	613 (6%)	261 (5.1%)	253 (4.9%)
Other relevant CVD	533 (6%)	486 (5%)	188 (3.6%)	207 (4.0%)

Values given are mean (SD) except for %.

LVH = left ventricular hypertrophy; TIA = transient ischemic attack.

*Hypertensive patients with no history of CHD but with three or more risk factors were eligible for study inclusion. These risk factors included a history of smoking, LVH or other specified ECG abnormalities, history of early CHD in a first degree relative, age ≥55 years, microalbuminuria or proteinuria, non-insulin-dependent diabetes, peripheral vascular disease, previous stroke or TIA, male sex, or ratio of plasma TC to HDL-C ≥6.

ASCOT LLA [264]

Atorvastatin-treated subjects had a 36% reduction in nonfatal MI and fatal CHD (p = 0.0005) and a 26% reduction in fatal and nonfatal CVA (p = 0.33) (Figures 61–63 and Table 44). These were hypertensive patients on a fixed dose of atorvastatin (10 mg) daily. The reduction in CV events was independent of the initial LDL-C baseline level. BP regimens and control were similar in the atorvastatin and the placebo groups throughout the trial and at study end.

ASCOT BPLA [265]

The primary endpoint of nonfatal MI and fatal CHD was lower in the amlodipine/perindopril group than in the atenolol/bendroflumethiazide group but did not reach clinical significance due to early termination of the study by the DBMB so that the specified number of events was not reached (Figures 63 and 64 and Table 44). However, all other event rates were significantly reduced more in the amlodipine/perindopril group as follows.

Results

Fatal and nonfatal stroke: decreased 23% (327 vs. 422; 0.77, 0.66–0.89, p = 0.0003)

Total CV events and procedures: decreased 16% (1362 vs. 1602; 0.84, 0.78–0.90, p < 0.0001)

All-cause mortality: reduced 11% (738 vs. 820; 0.89, 0.81–0.99, p = 0.025)

The incidence of developing diabetes was less on the amlodipine-based regimen by 30% (567 vs. 799; 0.63–0.78, p < 0.001).

Conclusion: The amlodipine-based regimen prevented more major CV events and induced less diabetes than that of the atenolol-based regimen. These effects appear to be independent of the BP effect and may be related to the specific drug regimens.

ASCOT LLA 2 × 2 [266]

The addition of atovorvastatin to an amlodipine-based regimen significantly reduced the indicence of the primary endpoint by 53% (p < 0.0001) vs. placebo (Figure 65). The RR reduction of 31% seen in fatal and nonfatal stroke when adding atorvastatin to an amlodipine-based regimen was not significant (p = 0.088) (Figure 66). In another secondary endpoint, the RR reduction of 27% seen in CV events and procedures when adding atorvastatin to an amlodipine-based regimen was significant (p = 0.001).

VALUE [267]

- 15245 patients with treated or untreated hypertension and high CVD risk
- Age over 50 years. Randomized, double-blind, parallel-group comparison
- Valsartan (ARB) vs. amlodipine (DHP-CCB)
- 6-year study with mean follow-up of 4.2 years. Primary endpoint was defined as a composite of cardiac mortality and morbidity.
- Amlodipine reduced BP more than valsartan, 4.0/2.1 mm Hg after 1 month and 1.5/1.3 mm Hg after 1 year (p < 0.0001) between groups. Reaching BP control of systolic <120 mm Hg by 6 months, independent of drug type, was associated with significant benefits for subsequent major outcomes. The BP response after just 1 month of treatment predicted events and survival.
- Primary composite of cardiac morbidity and mortality was equal with amlodipine and valsartan. However, secondary endpoints were different. The incidence of MI was significantly lower in the amlodipine groups than in the valsartan group (p = 0.02), and the incidence of stroke was also lower, but not significantly (p = 0.08). There was a positive trend for less heart failure with valsartan compared with amlopidine (p = 0.12) and a lower rate of new onset diabetes in the valsartan group compared with the amlodipine group (p < 0.0001).

BENEDICT [268]

The Bergamo Nephrologic Diabetes Complications Trial (BENEDICT) is a prospective, randomized, double-blind, parallel-group study primarily aimed at evaluating the possibility of preventing the progression to microalbuminuria (urinary albumin excretion [UAE] rate 20–200 mg/min, i.e., incipient nephropathy) in 1209 hypertensive, type 2 diabetic patients with a normal UAE rate (<20 mg/min). During phase A of the study, patients are randomized to a 3-year treatment with one of the following: (1) a nondihydropyridine CCB (verapamil SR 240 mg/day); (2) an ACEI (trandolapril 2 mg/day); (3) the combination of the above study drugs (verapamil SR 180 mg/day plus trandolapril 2 mg/day); or (4) placebo. Phase B of the study evaluates the progression to macroalbuminuria (UAE ≥200 mg/min) in patients who progress to microalbuminuria in phase A or are found with microalbuminuria during the screening phase; these patients are randomized to a 2-year treatment with either trandolapril (2 mg/day) alone or verapamil SR (180 mg/day) plus trandolapril (2 mg/day).

Compared to placebo, trandolapril alone or in combination with verapamil decreased the risks of developing microalbuminuria by 50%, whereas the effects of verapamil alone was similar to that of placebo.

Summary of published hypertension clinical trials involving primarily CCBs

1. The CCBs lower SBP and DBP as monotherapy equal to or better than all the other antihypertensive agents. This reduction is especially true in black and elderly hypertensive patients.

2. Both dihydropyridine and nondihydropyridine CCB significantly reduce total mortality, CV, cerebrovascular, and renal morbidity and mortality equal to or better than traditional conventional therapy with diuretics and BBs. However, the DHP-CCB is superior in the reduction of ischemic CVA compared to non–DHP-CCB. The combination of DHP-CCB and ACEI reduces CV events significantly better than a diuretic/BB combination (ASCOT trial).

3. CHD and fatal and nonfatal MI are reduced significantly with CCB (amlodipine), and this reduction is equal to that of diuretics (ALLHAT) and better than BBs (ASCOT). However, in the post-MI patient, the non–DHP-CCB may confer a survival advantage. The DHP-CCBs and diuretics are relatively contraindicated in the acute MI patient.

4. CVAs including ischemic stroke and intracranial hemorrhage are reduced significantly more with CCBs (10–15% better) in most studies, and there is a consistent trend in most other studies compared to diuretics, BBs, ACEIs, and ARBs. The DHP-CCB is superior to the non–DHP-CCB in reducing ischemic CVA. Amlodipine is equal to valsartan in reducing total cardiac events and mortality. Dementia may be prevented more with CCBs, particularly the DHP-CCB (SYST-EUR study), in the treatment of hypertension than with other antihypertensive agents. The CCBs reduce local cerebral resistance and correct the focal hypoperfusion without inducing a steal effect in patients with internal carotid artery (ICA) stenosis, thus preserving total cerebral perfusion.

5. Congestive heart failure may not be prevented as well with DHP-CCB as it is with diuretics and BBs, but study design, definitions of CHF, unmasking of

asymptomatic CHF, or masking of CHF in a prospective fashion may confound the interpretation of the true incidence of CHF, thus making the literature inconclusive on this point (ALLHAT, VALUE). Non–DHP-CCB should not be used in systolic CHF. However, CCBs improve diastolic relaxation and are excellent choice in the treatment of diastolic dysfunction and diastolic CHF.

6. Renal insufficiency (mild to moderate) with 24-hour urine protein <300 mg is prevented and treated as well with dihydropyridine or nondihydropyridine CCB compared to diuretics, BBs, ACEIs, and ARBs. However, in severe renal insufficiency, if the 24-hour urine excretion is over 1000 mg/day, then an ACEI or ARB is the preferred agent. Adding a CCB to an ACEI or ARB is very effective in reducing proteinuria and improving renal function. The combination of an ARB and a CCB appears to be as effective as the ACEI and CCB combination. The non–DHP-CCB would be the second preference agents. With mild-to-moderate renal insufficiency with 24-hour urine protein excretion between 300 and 1000 mg/day, either CCB, ACEI, ARB, or BB may result in equivalent renoprotection, although the data with BBs are less convincing and prospective clinical studies are fewer in number with lesser number of subjects.

   It should be noted, however, that certain diuretics, such as HCTZ, chlorthalidone, and other thiazide-like diuretics, may promote nephrotoxicity and increase the development of microalbuminuria, proteinuria, and progression of renal insufficiency to ESRD. This nephrotoxicity does not appear to be the case with the diuretic indapamide, which is renoprotective.

7. The CCBs are metabolically neutral or favorable on all biochemical parameters including serum glucose, lipids, potassium, magnesium, sodium, homocysteine, uric acid, and other blood tests. In addition, compared to diuretics, there is signficantly less new onset type 2 diabetes with the CCBs. CCBs improve insulin sensitivity, similar to ACEIs and ARBs.

8. The CCBs have anti-atherosclerotic effects in which they reduce progression and improve the regression of IMT in carotid arteries and plaques in both carotid and coronary atereries that are independent of their antihypertensive effects. This includes the coronary arteries and the carotid arteries in studies to date as evaluated by EBT, coronary arteriography, and B-mode ultrasound with the measurement of maximum mean IMT. This is especially true when compared to thiazide and thiazide-like diuretics and BBs.

9. There is no increased incidence of gastrointestinal bleeding or cancer with CCBs in any of the long-term comparative clinical trials. There is no increased risk of CHD or MI with the long-acting CCB in any of the recent, randomized, prospective clinical hypertension or CV trials.

10. CCBs are very effective in reducing LV mass and are equivalent to ACEIs and ARBs but significantly better than diuretics or BBs. In addition, they improve arterial compliance, C-I (large arteries) and C-2 (small resistance and oscillitory arterioles) compliances, vascular structure and function, and endothelial dysfunction.

Clinical hypertension trials with ARBs: Published trials (total 27 trials) and trials in progress [160]

1. Captopril Prevention Project (CAPPP)
2. Heart Outcomes Prevention Evaluation Study (HOPE)
3. Swedish Trial in Old Patients with Hypertension (STOP-2)
4. Perindopril Protection Against Recurrent Stroke Study (PROGRESS)

5. African-American Study of Kidney Disease and Hypertension (AASK)
6. Appropriate Blood Pressure Control in Diabetes Trial (ABCD)
7. Antihypertensive Therapy and Lipid-Lowering Heart Attack Prevention Trial (ALLHAT)
8. Australian National Blood Pressure Study 2 (ANBP-2)
9. Anglo-Scandinavian Cardiac Outcomes Trial (ASCOT)
10. BENEDICT
11. DIAB-HYCAR
12. EUROPA
13. HDS
14. HYVET
15. IDNT
16. PART-2
17. PEACE
18. Plaque Hypertension Lipid-Lowering Italian Study (PHYLLIS)
19. QUIET
20. SCAT
21. ADVANCE
22. PRESERVE
23. PROTECT
24. FACET
25. GLANT
26. PATE
27. ON-TARGET

CLINICAL TRIALS

PHYLLIS [160, 271]

Plaque Hypertension Lipid-Lowering Italian Study (PHYLLIS)

PHYLLIS was the first large hypertension trial to conduct office ABPM yearly in all patients. The main study—a multicenter, prospective, double-blind, randomized, controlled trial conducted over a period of 3 years—randomized 508 mildly hypertensive patients to a 2 × 2 factorial design treatment protocol. Patients were assigned to one of four treatments: an ACEI (fosinopril 20 mg once daily), a diuretic (HCTZ 12.5 mg once daily), diet plus a statin (pravastatin 40 mg once daily), or diet plus placebo (approximately 120 patients on each of the four treatment arms). At baseline, office BP was around 160/100 mm Hg, whereas ABPM was (as expected) lower, at around 122/72 mm Hg. Both these values were reduced to 140/82 and 135/70 mm Hg, respectively, on treatment.

There were essentially no differences in the BP reduction (about 8/6 mm Hg) between the ACEI and the diuretic; the addition of a statin did not further reduce BP in any group (mean changes in SBP were −8.7 and −7.1 mm Hg without and with statin, respectively, and mean changes in DBP were −6.2 and −5.5 mm Hg without and with statin, respectively). This replicates the finding in the much larger Heart Protection Study [4], where there was similarly no fall in BP with simvastatin, despite other reports to the contrary. The ABPM reduction of BP was similar on diuretic or ACEI. The diuretic group showed the most progression in bifurcation carotid IMT compared to all other groups.

QUIET [160, 270]

The Quinapril Ischemic Event Trial was designed to test the hypothesis that quinapril 20 mg/day would reduce ischemic events (the occurrence of cardiac death, resuscitated cardiac arrest, nonfatal MI, coronary artery bypass grafting, coronary angioplasty, or hospitalization for angina pectoris) and the angiographic progression of coronary artery disease in patients without systolic LV dysfunction. A total of 1750 patients were randomized to quinapril 20 mg/day or placebo and followed a mean of 27 ± 0.3 months. The 38% incidence of ischemic events was similar for both groups (RR 1.04; 95% CI 0.89–1.22; $p = 0.6$). There was also no significant difference in the incidence of patients having angiographic progression of coronary disease ($p = 0.71$). The rate of development of new coronary lesions was also similar in both groups ($p = 0.35$). However, there was a difference in the incidence of angioplasty for new (previously unintervened) vessels ($p = 0.018$). Quinapril was well tolerated in patients after angioplasty with normal LV function. Quinapril (20 mg) did not significantly affect the overall frequency of clinical outcomes or the progression of coronary atherosclerosis. However, the absence of the demonstrable effect of quinapril may be due to several limitations in study design.

SCAT [160, 274]

This long-term, multicenter, randomized, double-blind, placebo-controlled, 2 × 2 factorial, angiographic trial evaluated the effects of cholesterol lowering and ACE inhibition on coronary atherosclerosis in normocholesterolemic patients.

Methods and results: There were a total of 460 patients: 230 received simvastatin and 230 a simvastatin placebo and 229 received enalapril and 231 an enalapril placebo (some subjects received both drugs and some received a double placebo). Mean baseline measurements were as follows: cholesterol level, 5.20 mmol/L; triglyceride level, 1.82 mmol/L; HDL, 0.99 mmol/L; and LDL, 3.36 mmol/L. Average follow-up was 47.8 months. Changes in quantitative coronary angiographic measures between simvastatin and placebo, respectively, were as follows: mean diameters, –0.07 vs. –0.14 mm (p = 0.004); minimum diameters, –0.09 vs. –0.16 mm (p = 0. 0001); and percent diameter stenosis, 1.67 vs. 3.83% (p = 0.0003). These benefits were not observed in patients on enalapril when compared with placebo. No additional benefits were seen in the group receiving both drugs. Simvastatin patients had less need for percutaneous transluminal coronary angioplasty (8 vs. 21 events; p = 0.020), and fewer enalapril patients experienced the combined endpoint of death/MI/stroke (16 vs. 30; p = 0.043) than their respective placebo patients.

Conclusions: This trial extends the observation of the beneficial angiographic effects of lipid-lowering therapy to normocholesterolemic patients. The implications of the neutral angiographic effects of ACE inhibition are uncertain, but they deserve further investigation in light of the positive clinical benefits suggested here and seen elsewhere.

CLINICAL TRIALS

ADVANCE [160, 272]

The trial was done by 215 collaborating centers in 20 countries. After a 6-week active run-in period, 11 140 patients with type 2 diabetes were randomized to treatment with a fixed combination of perindopril and indapamide or matching placebo, in addition to current therapy. The primary endpoints were composites of major macrovascular and microvascular events, defined as death from CVD, nonfatal stroke or nonfatal MI, and new or worsening renal or diabetic eye disease, and analysis was by ITT. The macrovascular and microvascular composites were analyzed jointly and separately.

Findings: After a mean follow-up of 4.3 years, 73% of those assigned active treatment and 74% of those assigned control remained on randomized treatment. Compared with patients assigned placebo, those assigned active therapy had a mean reduction in SBP of 5.6 mm Hg and DBP of 2.2 mm Hg. The RR of a major macrovascular or microvascular event was reduced by 9% (861 [15.5%] active vs. 938 [16.8%] placebo; hazard ratio 0.91, 95% CI 0.83–1.00, p = 0.04). The separate reductions in macrovascular and microvascular events were similar but were not independently significant (macrovascular 0.92; CI 0.81–1.04, p = 0.16; microvascular 0.91; CI 0.80–1.04, p = 0.16). The RR of death from CVD was reduced by 18% (211 [3.8%] active vs. 257 [4.6%] placebo; 0.82, 0.68–0.98, p = 0.03) and death from any cause was reduced by 14% (408 [7.3%] active vs. 471 [8.5%] placebo; 0.86, CI 0.75–0.98, p = 0.03). There was no evidence that the effects of the study treatment differed by initial BP level or concomitant use of other treatments at baseline.

Interpretation: Routine administration of a fixed combination of perindopril and indapamide to patients with type 2 diabetes was well tolerated and reduced the risks of major vascular events, including death. Although the confidence limits were wide, the results suggest that over 5 years, one death due to any cause would be averted among every 79 patients assigned active therapy.

PROTECT [160, 275]

A high prevalence of increased IMT of the arterial wall has been documented in hypertension. These alterations in vascular wall structure may be the potent determinants for the promotion of the development of atherosclerosis. Direct histologic data from animal models of hypertension and indirect data from hypertensive patients have demonstrated a marked regression of increased IMT by ACE inhibition. Long-term effects of ACE inhibition on structural wall changes in humans have not been examined. Therefore, a multicenter, randomized, double-blind, European trial was designed to compare the effects of the ACEI perindopril and the diuretic HCTZ in slowing or reversing progression of increased IMT of carotid and femoral arteries in hypertensive patients. A total of 800 patients at 17 clinical centers in 7 European countries, aged 35–65 years, with hypertension and ultrasonographically proven IMT ≥ 0.8 mm of the common carotid artery will be randomly assigned to receive in a double-blind fashion either perindopril or HCTZ and will be followed for 24 months. High-resolution duplex sonography will be used to quantify IMT at baseline and twice a year during follow-up. A change of 0.1 mm of IMT from baseline is considered to be detectable, and the standard deviations of the changes from baseline are expected not to be higher than 0.2 mm. The primary endpoint of the study is the comparison of changes in IMT of the common carotid artery.

ANBP-2 [160, 209]

- 6083 elderly hypertensive patients
- PROBE design, community based
- Ages 65–84 years
- BP >159/89 mm Hg.
- ACEI vs. diuretic. ACEI reduced all CV events in males at significant levels compared to the diuretics. ACEI reduced MI better than diuretic by 17% in male subjects despite equal BP control ($p < 0.02$). There was no significant difference in the female subjects with any CV endpoint between the two treatment groups.
- 4.1-year median follow-up

DIAB-HYCAR [160]

Objective: To investigate whether a low dose of the ACEI ramipril lowers CV and renal events in patients with type 2 diabetes who have microalbuminuria or proteinuria. Design: Randomized, double-blind, parallel-group trial comparing ramipril (1.25 mg/day) with placebo (on top of usual treatment) for CV and renal outcomes for at least 3 years. Setting: Multicenter, primary care study conducted mostly by general practitioners in 16 European and North African countries. Participants: 4912 patients with type 2 diabetes aged >50 years who use oral antidiabetic drugs and have persistent microalbuminuria or proteinuria (urinary albumin excretion ≥20 mg/L in two consecutive samples) and serum creatinine ≤150 μmol/L.

Main Outcome Measures: The primary outcome measure was the combined incidence of CV death, nonfatal MI, stroke, heart failure leading to hospital admission, and end-stage renal failure. Results: Participants were followed for 3–6 (median 4) years. There were 362 primary events among the 2443 participants taking ramipril (37.8/1000 patient-years) and 377 events among the 2469 participants taking placebo (38.8/1000 patient-years; hazard ratio 1.03 [95% CI 0.89–1.20, p = 0.65]). None of the components of the primary outcome was reduced. Ramipril lowered SBP and DBP (by 2.43 and 1.06 mm Hg, respectively, after 2 years) and favored regression from microalbuminuria (20–200 mg/L) or proteinuria (>200 mg/L) to normal level (<20 mg/L) or microalbuminuria (p < 0.07) in 1868 participants who completed the study.

Conclusions: Low-dose (1.25 mg) ramipril once daily has no effect on CV and renal outcomes of patients with type 2 diabetes and albuminuria, despite a slight decrease in BP and urinary albumin. The CV benefits of a daily higher dose (10 mg) ramipril observed elsewhere are not found with an eightfold lower daily dose.

CLINICAL TRIALS

EUROPA [160, 273]

About 13655 patients were registered with previous MI (64%), angiographic evidence of coronary artery disease (61%), coronary revascularization (55%), or a positive stress test only (5%). After a run-in period of 4 weeks, in which all patients received perindopril, 12218 patients were randomly assigned perindopril 8mg once daily (n = 6110) or matching placebo (n = 6108). The mean follow-up was 4.2 years, and the primary endpoint was CV death, MI, or cardiac arrest. Analysis was by ITT.

Findings: Mean age of patients was 60 years (SD 9), 85% were male, 92% were taking platelet inhibitors, 62% BBs, and 58% lipid-lowering therapy. About 603 (10%) placebo and 488 (8%) perindopril patients experienced the primary endpoint, which yields a 20% RR reduction (95% CI 9–29, p = 0.0003) with perindopril. These benefits were consistent in all predefined subgroups and secondary endpoints. Perindopril was well tolerated.

Interpretation: Among patients with stable CHD without apparent heart failure, perindopril can significantly improve outcome. About 50 patients need to be treated for 4 years to prevent one major CV event. Treatment with perindopril, on top of other preventive medications, should be considered in all patients with CHD.

HDS [160, 276]

The Hypertension Diabetes Study is a 5-year follow-up in 758 NIDDM patients in a prospective, randomized, controlled study of therapy of mild hypertension. Patients were recruited who on antihypertensive therapy had SBP over 150 mm Hg or DBP over 85 mm Hg, or if not on therapy had SBP over 160 mm Hg or DBP over 90 mm Hg. Their mean BP at entry to the study was 160/94 mm Hg at a mean age of 57 years. They were allocated to tight control (aiming for SBP <150/SBP <85 mm Hg) or to less tight control (aiming for systolic <180/diastolic <105 mm Hg). The tight control group was allocated to primary therapy either with a BB (atenolol) or with an antiotensin converting enzyme inhibitor (captopril), with the addition of other agents as required. Over 5 years, the mean BP in the tight control group was significantly lower (143/82 vs. 154/88 mm Hg, p < 0.001). No difference was seen between those allocated to atenolol or captopril. The proportion of patients requiring three or more antihypertensive therapies to maintain tight control in those allocated to atenolol or captopril increased from 16 and 15%, respectively, at 2 years to 25 and 26%, respectively, at 5 years, whereas in the less tight control group at 2 and 5 years only 5 and 7%, respectively, required three or more therapies. There was no difference in the incidence of side effects or hypoglycemic episodes between those allocated to atenolol or captopril, but those allocated to atenolol increased their body weight by a mean of 2.3 kg compared with 0.5 kg in those allocated to captopril (p < 0.01). Allocation to atenolol was also associated with small increases in triglyceride and decreases in LDL and HDL cholesterol, which are of uncertain clinical relevance. The study is continuing to determine whether the improved BP control, which was obtained, will be beneficial in maintaining the health of patients by decreasing the incidence of major clinical complications, principally MI and strokes, and microvascular complications such as severe retinopathy requiring photocoagulation and deterioration of renal function.

CLINICAL TRIALS

HYVET [160]

- 2100 patients with hypertension
- Age >80 years
- BP 159–220/89–110 mm Hg
- Perindopril ACEI vs. diuretic (indapamide) vs. placebo
- 5-year follow-up. Expected completion in 2009

PART-2 [160, 277]

Objectives: The primary objective of this study was to investigate the effects of the ACEI, ramipril, on carotid atherosclerosis in patients with coronary, cerebrovascular, or peripheral vascular diseases. Background: ACEIs have been shown to reduce the risk of coronary events in various patient groups and to prevent the development of atherosclerosis in animal models. It has been hypothesized that the clinical benefits of ACEIs may, therefore, be mediated by effects on atherosclerosis.

Methods: Six hundred seventeen patients were randomized in equal proportions to ramipril (5–10 mg daily) or placebo. At baseline, 2 years and 4 years, carotid atherosclerosis was assessed by B-mode ultrasound, and LV mass was assessed by M-mode echocardiography.

Results: BP was reduced by a mean of 6 mm Hg systolic and 4 mm Hg diastolic in the ramipril group compared with the placebo group ($p < 0.001$). There was no difference between groups in the changes in common carotid artery wall thickness ($p = 0.58$) or in carotid plaque ($p = 0.93$). LV mass index decreased by 3.8g/m^2 (4%) in the ramipril group compared with the placebo group ($2p = 0.04$).

Conclusions: The results provide no support for the hypothesis that reduced atherosclerosis is responsible for the beneficial effects of ACEIs on major coronary events. It is more likely that the benefits are due to lower BP, reduced LV mass, or other factors such as reversal of endothelial dysfunction.

PEACE [269]

In the Prevention of Events with an ACEI (PEACE) trial, patients with chronic stable coronary disease and preserved systolic function were randomized to trandolapril or placebo and followed up for a median of 4.8 years. The urinary albumin-to-creatinine ratio (ACR) assessed in a core laboratory in 2977 patients at baseline and in 1339 patients at follow-up (mean 34 months) was related to estimated glomerular filtration rate and outcomes. The majority of patients (73%) had a baseline ACR within the normal range (<17 µg/mg for men and <25 µg/mg for women). Independent of the estimated glomerular filtration rate and other baseline covariates, a higher ACR, even within the normal range, was associated with increased risks for all-cause mortality ($p < 0.001$) and CV death ($p = 0.01$). The effect of trandolapril therapy on outcomes was not modified significantly by the level of albuminuria. Nevertheless, trandolapril therapy was associated with a significantly lower mean follow-up ACR (12.5 vs. 14.6 µg/mg, $p = 0.0002$), after adjustment for baseline ACR, time between collections, and other covariates. An increase in ACR over time was associated with increased risk of CV death (hazard ratio per log ACR 1.74, 95% CI 1.08–2.82).

Conclusions: Albuminuria, even in low levels within the normal range, is an independent predictor of CV and all-cause mortality.

On target and transcend (The ONTARGET Investigators, Telmisartan, Ramipril, or Both in Patients at High Risk for Vascular Events, NEJM 2008; 358: 1547–1559)

- 28 400 patients, men and women, high-risk CVD
- Randomized, double-blind, multicentered trial
- Telimisartan vs. ramipril vs. combination of both
- Primary endpoints:
  Composite CV death, MI, CVA, or hospitalization for CHF
- Secondary endpoints
  New CHF, revascularization, new DM, cognitive decline, dementia, and atrial fibrillation
- Other endpoints
  All-cause mortality
  Non-CV death
  LVH
  BP changes
  Acute ischemic syndrome
  TIA
  Nephropathy
  Microvascular DM complications
- Follow-up: 3.5–5.5 years, completion in 2008

CAPPP [133, 188]

- Prospective, randomized, open trial with blinded endpoint evaluation
- 10985 patients in 536 centers in Scandinavia
- Ages 25–66 years
- DBP .100 mm Hg
- Treatment: captopril vs. diuretics, BBs (conventional therapy). Note that only 50 mg qd or bid captopril was given.
- Primary endpoint: composite of fatal and nonfatal MI CVA and other CV events.
- Mean follow-up: 6.1 years. Only 0.25% lost follow-up.

Results
1. Primary endpoint composite was equal
2. Captopril 363 patients (11.1/1000 patient-years)
3. Conventional treatment (10.2/1000 patient-years)
   RR = 1.05 (95% CI 0.90–1.22), p = 0.52
- CV mortality was lower with captopril than with conventional treatment (76 vs. 95 events), RR = 0.77 (0.57–1.04) p = 0.092 (23% reduction).
- Rate of fatal and nonfatal MI was simple in both groups (0.96, p = 0.68).
- Total mortality was equal (0.93, p = 0.49).
- Fatal and nonfatal CVA were equal in DM patients.
- Fatal and nonfatal CVA were more common with captopril (189 vs. 148) in nondiabetic patients only, RR = 1.25 (1.01–1.55), p = 0.044 (25% increase).
- Rates of all other cardiac events were equal (0.94; p = 0.30)
- Initial SBP, DBP, creatinine, cholesterol, DM, and glucose were significantly higher in the captopril vs. conventional therapy. This indicates an overall higher baseline CV risk in the captopril patients.

SBP/DBP differences

	p-Value	Captopril	Conventional
Untreated	<0.0001	166.6/103.6	163.3/101.2
Treated	0.025	157.4/96.2	156.2/95.4

This initial BP was 3.3/2.4 mm Hg higher in the captopril previously untreated group and 1.2/0.8 mm Hg higher in the captopril previously treated patients.
- Reduced incidence for new onset DM in captopril group (0.86, p = 0.039).
- BP remained significantly higher in the captopril-treated patients compared to conventional therapy.
- Target BP was achieved more rapidly with conventional therapy in the first 6–12 months.
- Captopril was superior to conventional therapy in patients with DM in all CV endpoints (22% reduction).
  (0.78; p = 0.041).

Conclusions

- Captopril is superior to conventional BB and diuretic therapy in reducing the following:
  1. Fatal CV events
  2. Prevention of new onset DM
- Captopril is equal to diuretics and BBs in CVA reduction when BP levels are corrected between groups. A difference of 3.3/2.4 mm Hg accounts for about a 21% difference in CVA incidence.
- Captopril is superior to conventional therapy in hypertensive diabetic patients in reducing all CV events.
- Captopril decreases the incidence of new onset DM.
- Captopril has fewer adverse effects and higher compliance rate than conventional therapy.

HOPE (Heart Outcomes Prevention Evaluation Study) [278]

Objective
Primary endpoint of the study was composite of MI, stroke, or death from CV causes.

Inclusion criteria
Patients aged >55 years at high risk for CV events because of any evidence of vascular disease (CHD, stroke, PVD) or diabetes plus another coronary risk factor.

Exclusion criteria
Patients having heart failure or low-ejection fraction, already on ACEI therapy or vitamin E.

Study design
A total of 9297 patients were randomly assigned to receive ramipril (10 mg/day) or placebo for a mean of 5 years. In addition, all patients were randomly assigned to receive vitamin E, 400 IU/day, or placebo.

Patient characteristics
Mean age was 66 years, with just over 25% female; 80.6% had evidence of coronary artery disease, 52.8% a previous MI, 43.4% peripheral vascular disease, 38.3% diabetes, 46.5% hypertension, 65.8% an elevated cholesterol. Antiplatelet therapy (aspirin or other) was being taken by 76% at the time of enrollment, BBs by 40%, and lipid-lowering agents by 28.9%.

Results
The data safety monitoring board recommended termination of the study in early March 1999 owing to an overwhelming benefit of ramipril.

Vitamin E vs. Placebo: There were no significant differences in the primary outcome of death, MI, and stroke (16.2% in vitamin E group vs. 15.5% in placebo; $p = 0.35$). All-cause mortality was not different between the two groups either.

Ramipril vs. Placebo: In the ramipril group, there was a significant reduction in the primary endpoint from 17.7% in placebo to 14.1% in the treatment group (RR reduction of 22%; $p = 0.000002$). There was also a significant reduction in MI, stroke, and CV death. In addition, all-cause mortality was significantly reduced by 16% in the ramipril group ($p = 0.0058$).

Regarding BP reduction, there was an average reduction in SBP of 3.3 mm Hg in patients taking ramipril. The benefits on stroke and MI reduction achieved in the HOPE trial (31 and 20%, respectively) appear to be far greater than what would be expected from BP reduction alone. Moreover, the benefits were sustained across various quartiles of SBP and DBP, including those in the normal range.

Conclusions

There is overwhelming evidence that, in a broad range of high-risk patients, ramipril prevents CV death, stroke, and MI heart failure, development of diabetes diabetic microvascular complications including nephropathy. The benefits of ramipril are incremental to existing therapy. The beneficial effects of ramipril are independent of BP lowering. Vitamin E does not have any significant protective effect.

PROGRESS [187]

- 6105 subjects from 172 centers
- Hypertensive and nonhypertensive subjects with a history of CVA or TIA (1 month to 5 years)
- Treatment with perindopril or perindopril with indapamide vs. placebo against a background of standard care
- Mean BP 147/86 mm Hg (hypertensive group 159/94 mm Hg; nonhypertensive group 136/79 mm Hg)
- 4-year follow-up
- Average age 64 years, 11% were DM
- Primary outcome: total stroke (fatal or nonfatal)
- Secondary outcomes:
  - Fatal or disabling stroke
  - Total major vascular events comprising the composite of nonfatal stroke, nonfatal MI, or death from any vascular cause
  - Total and cause-specific deaths and hospital admissions
  - Dementia and cognitive function

Results
1. BP reduction
  - Overall: 9/4 mm Hg active vs. placebo
  - Combination therapy: 12.3/5 mm Hg
  - Single-drug therapy: 4.9/2.8 mm Hg
  - Hypertensive group: 9.5/3.9 mm Hg
  - Nonhypertensive group: 8.8/4.2 mm Hg
2. CVA reduction in all CVA subtypes
  - Combination therapy (perindopril plus indapamide): reduced 43%
  - Active treatment vs. placebo: reduced 28% (95% CI 17–38, $p < 0.0001$)
  - Single-drug treatment: NS (perindopril)
  - Active treatment group CVA had fewer fatal disabling or severe CVA vs. placebo
  - Similar reductions in risk of stroke in hypertensive and nonhypertensive patients ($p < 0.01$)
  - Cumulative CVA risk curves diverged early
  - Annual rate of new CVA 2.7% in treatment group vs. 3.8% in control group
3. Total major vascular events
  - Active treatment reduced 26% ($p < 0.0001$)
  - Decreased nonfatal CVA by 42% ($p < 0.0001$)
  - Decreased nonfatal MI by 38–42% ($p = 0.001$)
  - Vascular death was same in active and placebo groups
  - Decreased total major coronary events (nonfatal MI or death from CHD) by 26% (95% CI 6–42) ($p < 0.0001$)
4. Total deaths or deaths from vascular or nonvascular causes: NS
5. Hospital admissions reduced 9%
6. Dementia reduced 34% ($p < 0.0001$) and severe cognitive decline reduced 45% ($p < 0.0001$) in those with CVA.

Conclusions

- Perindopril (ACEI) + indapamide reduce all CVA in both hypertensive and nonhypertensive patients.
- Major coronary events are reduced twice as much compared to previous diuretic/BB-based trials.
- Dementia is reduced and cognitive decline is reduced.
- The reduction in nonfatal MI is greater than expected from the BP reduction suggesting an independent ACEI or indapamide effect.
- BP reductions (mean BP) down to 124/74 mm Hg showed continued benefit without any "J-shaped" curve.
- Very low adverse effects and withdrawal rate.

Summary of the clinical hypertension trials using primarily ACEIs

1. ACEIs are effective in reducing BP when administered at correct doses and dosing intervals in all patients regardless of age, gender, or race. Reductions in BP are equal to diuretics, BBs, CCBs, and angiotensin receptor antagonists as well as other classes of antihypertensive agents.
2. The role of tissue selectivity in clinical outcome studies remains to be proven, although surrogate endpoints suggest possible advantages of the tissue-selective ACEIs.
3. ACEIs should be administered in higher doses to achieve BP control. There is evidence that they have beneficial vascular effects that are due to both the antihypertensive effect and the nonantihypertensive effect, especially in reducing proteinuria.
4. CHD and MI morbidity and mortality have been significantly reduced. They are equal to (ALLHAT, STOP-2, CAPPP) or better than diuretic ANBP-2 and BBs (PROGRESS) and equal to CCB (ALLHAT) and superior to diuretics with BBs when used in combination with amoldipine (ASCOT) and superior to BBs as monotherapy, especially in the elderly hypertensive. In addition, they are effective in reducing recurrent MI in patients who have already had MI (HOPE and others).
5. CVAs are significantly reduced with ACEIs in all clinical trials (STOP-2, CAPPP, PROGRESS, HOPE, SCAT, ASCOT), with the possible exception of ALLHAT. However, the ALLHAT results are controversial due to the higher BP in the ACEI group, improper dosing, as was done in CAPPP, and the unfavorable results were limited to black hypertensive patients. Corrections for these factors indicate that ACEIs in ALLHAT were almost as effective as diuretics.
6. Congestive heart failure is significantly reduced. Systolic and diastolic dysfunction is improved. CHF is reduced equal to or better than diuretics (STOP-2, CAPPP, PROGRESS, HOPE). The ALLHAT data on CHF is controversial related to ACEI vs. diuretic due to higher BP levels on the ACEI, study design, potential masking of CHF symptoms on diuretics, and many other factors (see ALLHAT section).
7. Renal insufficiency, ESRD, microalbuminuria, and proteinuria are signficantly reduced compared to diuretics and BBs. They are preferred drugs, as are the ARBs in CRI and proteinuric states.

8. New onset DM is reduced significantly (HOPE, CAPPP, ALLHAT, STOP-2, ASCOT). They are preferred initial agents in hypertensive diabetes along with ARBs and CCBs. They are superior to diuretics and BBs in reducing CV events in the diabetic hypertensive (SYST-EUR, CAPPP).

9. Adverse effects are low and compliance with continuation of therapy is high. Initial rise in serum creatinine up to 20% above baseline is normal and expected in patients with any renal impairment and does not require treatment cessation.

10. Anti-atherogenic effects on the coronary and carotid arteries have been demonstrated (QUIET, SCAT, PART-2).

11. Improvement of vascular biology related to endothelial function and arterial compliance (both function and structure).

12. Reduce dementia and cognitive dysfunction (PROGRESS).

13. Neutral metabolic and biochemical changes, improvement in insulin sensitivity.

14. Reduce LVMI{expansion?} and LVH.

Clinical trials in hypertension with ARBs (eight trials) [160, 189, 190]

1. LIFE: Losartan Intervention For Endpoint reduction in hypertension (discussed in detail in following sections)

2. IDNT: Irbesartan Diabetes Nephropathy Trial (see renal and diabetes sections)

3. RENAAL: Randomized Evaluation of NIDDM with the Ang-II antagonist Losartan

4. SCOPE: Study of cognition and prognosis in elderly patients with hypertension (in progress)

5. VALUE: Valsartan Antihypertensive Long-Term Use Evaluation

6. On-Target and Transcend: see clinical trials section on ACEIs

7. MARVAL: see renal section

8. MOSES: eprosartan.

SCOPE
- 4000 patients with hypertension
- Age 70–89 with 2.5-year follow-up
- BP 160–179/90–99 mm Hg
- Endpoints of CVA, CHD, dementia
- ARB vs. placebo
- In progress

VALUE
- 15 313 patients
- Age >49 years with 6-year follow-up
- BP <210/115 mm Hg
  - Endpoints of CHD, CVA, CV death
  - ARB = DHP-CCB

LIFE [190]
- Double-blind, randomized, parallel-group trial
- 9193 subjects aged 55–80 years
- BP: 160–200/95–115 mm Hg
- LVH by ECG
- Follow-up: 4 years

Results:
- BP fell by 30.2/16.6 mm Hg in losartan group
    29.1/16.8 mm Hg in atenolol group
  - Primary composite endpoint of CV death, CVA, or MI
  Losartan 23.8/1000 patient-years
  Atenolol 27.9/1000 patient-years
  RR 0.87, 95% CI 0.77–0.98
  $p = 0.021$
  13% reduction favoring losartan
- CVD deaths were equal
  RR 0.89, 95% CI 0.73–1.07
  $p = 0.206$
- Fatal and nonfatal CVA reduced by losartan
  RR 0.75, 95% CI 0.63–0.89
  $p = 0.001$
  25% reductions favoring losartan
- MI (nonfatal and fatal): equal
  RR 1.07; 0.88–1.31
  $p = 0.491$
- New onset DM less frequent with losartan
- Losartan is better tolerated, has fewer adverse effects, and a better compliance rate.
- Losartan reduced composite CV endpoints significantly more than atenolol in the diabetic subgroup (24.5%; $p = 0.031$).
- Losartan reduced total mortality by 39% ($p = 0.002$) compared to atenolol.

Conclusion

1. Losartan prevents more CV morbidity and mortality than atenolol, for a similar reduction in BP.
2. Losartan prevents more CVA morbidity and mortality than atenolol, for a similar reduction in BP.
3. Losartan confers benefits in vascular disease independent of, and beyond, BP reduction. These benefits may be related to complete blockade of the renin-angiotensin system (RAS), improvement in endothelial function, arterial compliance, vascular function and structure, or other factors.
4. Losartan prevents more new onset DM than atenolol.
5. In the hypertensive diabetic patients, losartan is superior to atenolol in reductions.
   - CV death
   - CVA
   - MI
   - Total mortality.

LIFE Study: ISH Substudy [189]
- Double-blind, randomized, parallel-group study
- 1326 men and women, age 55–80 years (mean 70)
- SBP >160–200 mm Hg
  DBP <90 mm Hg (mean 174/83 mm Hg)
- ECG-LVH present
- Treatment: lorsartan vs. atenolol + HCTZ in either group
- Main outcome measure: composite endpoint of CV death, CVA, or MI
- Mean follow-up: 4.7 years.

Results

1. BP reduction equal in both groups 28/9 mm Hg but previously BP was 146/75 mm Hg in losartan group and 146/74 mm Hg in atenolol group (p = 0.04 for DBP)
2. Main outcome reduced by 25% with losartan vs. atenolol, 25.1 vs. 35.4 events/1000 patient-years
R = 0.75, 95% CI 0.56–1.01; (p = 0.06 adjusted risk and LVH degree unadjusted RR 0.71, 95% CI 0.53–0.95, p = 0.02)
3. MI: no difference
4. CV mortality: 8.7 vs. 16.9 events/1000 patient-years
RR 0.54, 95% CI 0.34–0.87
p = 0.01 46% reduction
5. Nonfatal and fatal CVA: 10.6 vs. 18.9 events/1000 patient-years
RR 0.60, 95% CI 0.38–0.92
p = 0.02, 40% reduction
6. New onset DM 12.6 vs. 16.9 events/1000 patient-years
RR 0.62, 95% CI 0.40–0.97
p = 0.04, 38% reduction
7. Total mortality: 21.2 vs. 30.2 events/1000 patient-years
RR 0.72, 95% CI 0.53–1.00
p = 0.046
8. LVH reduction: losartan better than atenolol p < 0.001
9. Curves for CV mortality and CVH separated early in favor of losartan
10. Losartan was better tolerated.

Conclusion

1. Losartan is superior to atenolol for treatment of patients with isolated systolic hypertension in reducing CVA, CV mortality, composite of CV morbidity and mortality, total mortality, new onset DM, and LVH.
2. The reduction in these events was independent of BP levels suggesting other beneficial effects of losartan on vascular events, possibly related to blockade of the RAS and favorable effects on vascular biology.

LIFE: Public health implications

- Based on NHANES III, 3.9 million people in the United States are over age 55 with high BP, LVH, and without CHF (2.7 million without diabetes).
- Assuming these patients experience events similar to LIFE participants randomized to atenolol, then over 4.8 years use of losartan would lead to:
  - 70 000 avoided CV morbidity/mortality clinical endpoints and 66 000 fewer first strokes
  - 54 000 less new onset diabetes cases.

LIFE: Summary 1

- Compared with atenolol-based therapy, losartan-based antihypertensive therapy was associated with:
  - Less CV morbidity and mortality (13%)
  - Less stroke (25%)
  - Less onset of diabetes (25%)

- Better regression in LVH
- Better tolerability with significantly fewer discontinuations for adverse events for similar BP reduction.

LIFE: Summary 2
- Following adjustment for effects on BP and LVH, the primary outcome seemed to be explained only partially by the effect on these parameters.
- In the diabetic subgroup:
  - Losartan provided better protection against CV morbidity and mortality, a reduction of 24%.
  - Losartan reduced total mortality by 39%.

LIFE: Conclusions
- Losartan offers better protection against CV morbidity and death (including stroke) compared to atenolol with benefits beyond BP reduction.
- Losartan was protective in the higher (e.g., DM) as well as the lower (e.g., nonvascular) risk group.
- Losartan reduces the rate of new onset of diabetes compared to atenolol.
- Losartan is significantly better tolerated than atenolol.
- These results are directly applicable in clinical practice.

Morbidity and mortality after stroke—eprosartan compared with nitrendipine for secondary prevention (MOSES study) [279]
Overview
- First study that compared two antihypertensive drugs
- Investigator created, initatied, and performed study
- Blinded endpoint committee
- 100% monitoring of all centers and all patients
- Well-defined hypertensive stroke patients
- Previous and study medication well balanced
- Very tight clinical control
- Early and comparable BP control
  Objective: To compare efficacy of eprosartan and nitrendipine in secondary stroke prevention and the reduction of CV and cerebrovascular morbidity and mortality.

MOSES: rationale
1. Why eprosartan?
   - Effectively reduces BP and is well tolerated
   - Reduces SNS activity
   - Increases poststroke survival in animal models
2. **Why nitrendipine?**
   - In the SYST-EUR study, nitrendipine reduced the frequency of stroke and dementia

MOSES: study design
1. PROBE design: Prospective, randomized, open-label, blinded endpoint
2. Primary endpoints: Total mortality + total number of CV and cerebrovascular events

3. Secondary endpoints: Functional status (Barthel's index, Rankin scale, and cognitive function)
4. Mean follow-up: 2.5 years
5. Before randomization: qualifying event documented by CCT or MRI and diagnosis of hypertension
6. Randomization: at entry—office BP, ABPM, MMS, Rankin, Barthel with pretreated patients—rolled over directly to study medication
7. Initital treatment dosage
   - Eprosartan 600 mg
   - Nitrendipine 10 mg
   - During the study, dosage was increased or combination with one of the following:
   a. Diuretics
   b. BBs
   c. ABs/other

MOSES: assessments

1. Procedures regularly performed
   - Sitting and ambulatory blood pressure measurements (ABPM)
   - Mini Mental Status Examination (MMSE) score
   - Documentation of all drugs taken
   - Barthel Index and Rankin scale
   - Electrocardiogram
   - Adverse event reporting

MOSES: trial profile

1. 1405 patients eligible for randomization
2. 710 assigned to eprosartan-based regimen; 685 assigned to the nitrendipine-based regimen
3. 29 patients withdrew consent before first intake of study drug (eprosartan)
4. 24 withdrew consent before first intake of study drug (nitrendipine)

MOSES: inclusion criteria

1. Hypertension (confirmed by ABPM) + cerebral ischemia (TIA, PRIND, complete stroke)
2. Cerebral hemorrhage during the last 24 months before study commencement (cerebral scan or MRI was necessary to confirm)

MOSES: baseline characteristics of patients

	Eprosartan	Nitrendipine
Total number of eligible patients	681	671
Sex		
Male: number (%)	365 (53.6%)	368 (54.8%)
Female: number (%)	316 (46.4%)	303 (45.2%)
Age (years)	67.7	68.1
BMI	27.7	27.4
Time between qualifying event and allocation	347.6	349.8

MOSES: baseline characteristics of patients with antihypertensive pretreatment—84%

	Eprosartan	Nitrendipine
Systolic office BP (mm Hg)	139.7	140.0
Diastolic office BP (mm Hg)	87.0	87.2
Heart rate	74.7	75.7

Qualifying Disease

	Eprosartan	Nitrendipine
Stroke	418 (61.4%)	407 (60.7%)
TIA	186 (27.3%)	184 (27.4%)
PRIND	36 (5.3%)	47 (7%)
Intracerebral hemorrhage	41 (6.0%)	33 (4.9%)

MOSES: Mini Mental Status Score; Rankin Scale Barthel Index

	Eprosartan	Nitrendipine
MMSE mean score	25.6	25.5
Modified Rankin Scale (score)	1.4	1.5
Barthel Index (score)	88.8	88.1

MOSES: conclusion 1
1. First comparison of two antihypertensive drugs in stroke patients
2. Well-defined hypertensive poststroke patients
3. Previous and study medications well balanced
4. Early and comparable BP control
5. High number of normotensive patients at study end
6. BP values confirmed by ABPM

MOSES: conclusion 2
1. Advantages for eprosartan with regard to:
- 20% fewer primary endpoints including recurrent events
- 25% fewer cerebrovascular events including recrurrent events
- 30% fewer first CV events

2. No difference between the groups with regard to:
- First primary endoints in each category
- First cerebrovascular events
- CV events including recurrent events
- Dementia

Valsartan Antihypertension Long-Term Use Evaluation Trial (VALUE) [280]

VALUE trial design
Objective
VALUE was designed to test the hypothesis that, for the same BP control, valsartan would reduce cardiac morbidity and mortality more than amlodipine in hypertensive patients at high CV risk.

Design
VALUE was a prospective, multinational, multicenter trial utilizing a double-blind, randomized, active-controlled, two-arm, parallel-group comparison. Patients were randomized to either valsartan- or amlodipine-based therapy. Additional antihypertensive medications were added in a five-step, response-dependent dose titration scheme to achieve a target BP goal of <140/90 mm Hg.

- Step 1: Patients were randomized to receive either valsartan (80 mg qd) or amlodipine (5 mg qd).
- Step 2: Doses were up-titrated to valsartan 160 mg or amlodipine 10 mg, depending on BP response.
- Steps 3 and 4: Addition of HCTZ 12.5 and 25 mg, respectively, based on achieved BP response.
- Step 5: Free add-on of antihypertensive agents other than ACEs, CCBs, ARBs, or diuretics other than HCTZ. The only exception was replacement of loop diuretics in patients with impaired renal function or CHF.

Study population
15 313 patients aged 50 years with treated or untreated hypertension who were at high CV risk. BP entry criteria were 160–210/95–115 mm Hg for untreated patients and 210/115 mm Hg for those already receiving antihypertensive therapy.

Study endpoints
Primary: Time to first cardiac event (composite of morbidity and/or mortality events):
- Cardiac morbidity: new or chronic CHF requiring hospital management, nonfatal acute MI, emergency procedures performed to prevent MI
- Cardiac mortality: sudden cardiac death, fatal MI, death during or after percutaneous transluminal coronary angioplasty (PTCA) or coronary artery bypass graft (CABG), death due to CHF, death associated with evidence of recent acute MI on autopsy

Secondary endpoints
- Fatal and nonfatal MI, fatal and nonfatal CHF, fatal and nonfatal stroke.
- Worsening of chronic stable angina or unstable angina, routine interventional procedures, potentially lethal arrhythmias, syncope or near-syncope, silent MI, and ESRD

Prescribed analysis
- New onset DM
- All-cause mortality—previously specified as a secondary endpoint

CLINICAL TRIALS

BP results

The most consistent and statistically significant difference between the two groups was in BP control. BP was substantially lower (4.0/2.1 mm Hg) in the amlodipine group in the early months starting from the end of month 1, when the patients were predominantly treated with monotherapy. The BP decrease observed favored amlodipine throughout the trial: on average, the BP difference between the two groups remained at least 2.0/1.5 mm Hg. At the end of the study, BP reductions from baseline were 17.3/9.9 mm Hg for the amlodipine group and 15.2/8.2 mm Hg for the valsartan group ($p < 0.0001$). The target BP ($<140/90$ mm Hg) was achieved in 56% of patients in the valsartan group and 62% in the amlodipine group. Fewer patients required add-on therapy with amlodipine (41%) than with valsartan (48%).

Endpoint results

The endpoint results and other results are illustrated in Table 45.

Conclusions

The primary composite endpoint occurred in 810 patients in the valsartan group (10.6%, 25.5/1000 patient-years) and 789 in the amlodipine group (10.4%, 24.7/1000 patient-years; hazard ratio 1.04, 95% CI 0.94–1.15, $p = 0.49$).

The main outcome of cardiac disease did not differ between the treatment groups. Unequal reductions in BP might account for differences between the groups in cause-specific outcomes. The findings emphasize the importance of prompt BP control in hypertensive patients at high CV risk.

Table 45 Value Trial: Endpoint Results

Endpoint results (value trial)

Primary endpoint results	Time to first cardiac morbidity or mortality: No significant difference between treatment groups, HR for valsartan 1.04 (0.94–1.15), p = 0.49
Results for components of primary endpoint	Cardiac morbidity: No significant difference between treatment groups, HR 1.02 (0.91–1.15), p = 0.71 Cardiac mortality: No significant difference between treatment groups, HR 1.01 (0.86–1.18), p = 0.90
Secondary endpoint results	Fatal and nonfatal MI: Significant difference between treatment groups favoring amlodipine, HR 1.19 (1.02–1.38), p = 0.02 Fatal and nonfatal stroke: No significant difference between treatment groups, HR 1.15 (0.98–1.35), p = 0.08 Fatal and nonfatal CHF: No significant difference between treatment groups, HR 0.89 (0.77–1.03), p =0. 12 All-cause mortality: No significant difference between treatment groups, HR 1.04 (0.94–1.14), p = 0.45
Other analyses	New onset diabetes: Significant difference between treatment groups favoring valsartan, OR 0.77 (0.69–0.86), p < 0.0001

Other results (value trial)

Serum creatine	Baseline: valsartan = 101.2; amlodipine = 100.9 End of study: valsartan = 108.1; amlodipine = 103.2
Safety and tolerability	Both treatment strategies were well tolerated with few severe adverse events. The discontinuation rates due to AEs were 11.9% for valsartan and 12.9% for amlodipine. Peripheral edema and hypokalemia were more common on valsartan: dizziness, headache, diarrhea, fatigue, serious angina, and syncope

CLINICAL TRIALS

Clinical Hypertension Trials in Hypertension with ARBs: Summary

1. Only one large clinical trial has compared an ARB (losartan) with a BB (atenolol) in hypertensive patients in regard to total CV endpoints. This is the LIFE trial. The results indicated significant superiority of losartan over atenolol in all of the following endpoints:
   a. Reduction in composite of CV morbidity and mortality including CV death, CVA, MI, and total mortality.
   b. Reduction in fatal and nonfatal CVA
   c. Reduction in new onset DM
   d. In the diabetic hypertensive, losartan significantly reduced (more than atenolol)
      1. CV death
      2. MI
      3. CVA
      4. Total mortality
2. VALUE demonstrated equal reduction in primary endpoints of composite cardiac morbidity and mortality with an ARB and DHP-CCB. Secondary endpoints for CVA were better with a CCB, but new onset DM was better with ARB. The MOSES trial showed superior results with an ARB in secondary prevention of CV events and CVA in patients with a previous CVA.
3. Renal endpoint clinical trials such as RENAAL, IDNT, and IRMA indicate reductions in progression to ESRD and decreased proteinuria with ARBs (lorsartan, irbesartan, telemasartan), in patients with DM and proteinuria.
4. ARBs reduce LVH signficantly and better than BBs.
5. ARBs improve endothelial dysfunction and arterial compliance and vascular biologic parameters of function and structure.
6. The side effect profile is low and they are well tolerated with high compliance rate.
7. The metabolic and biochemical profile is neutral or favorable.

CLINICAL TRIALS

222

SCOPE [281]

The Study on Cognition and Prognosis in the Elderly (SCOPE) assessed the effect of candesartan on CV and cognitive outcomes in elderly patients (aged 70–89 years) with mild-to-moderate hypertension. Patients were randomized to treatment with candesartan 8–16 mg daily (n = 2477) or placebo (n = 2460) and followed for 3.7 years on average. In agreement with the study protocol, other antihypertensive drugs were added if BP remained 160 mm Hg systolic and/or 90 mm Hg diastolic. Due to extensive add-on therapy, particularly in patients randomized to placebo, the between-treatment difference in BP was only 3.2/1.6 mm Hg. Nevertheless, the main analysis showed that nonfatal stroke was reduced by 28% (p = 0.04) in the candesartan group compared with the control group, and there was a nonsignificant 11% reduction in the primary endpoint, major CV events (p = 0.19). Of particular interest are significant risk reductions with candesartan in major CV events (32%, p = 0.013), CV mortality (29%, p = 0.049), and total mortality (27%, p = 0.018) in patients who did not receive add-on therapy after randomization and in whom the difference in BP was 4.7/2.6 mm Hg. Other analyses suggest positive effects of candesartan-based treatment on cognitive function, QOL and new onset diabetes. In conclusion, SCOPE strongly suggests that candesartan treatment reduces CV morbidity and mortality in old and very old patients with mild-to-moderate hypertension. Candesartan-based antihypertensive treatment may also have positive effects on cognitive function and QOL.

CLINICAL TRIALS

Part 6
Special Considerations in the Management of Hypertension Based on the Hypertension Clinical Trials

Handbook of Hypertension. By M.C. Houston. Published 2009 by Blackwell Publishing, ISBN: 978-1-4051-8250-8

CHD Risk Factor and Effects of Antihypertensive Drug Therapy

CHD: risk factors [53–55]

1. Hypertension—SBP and DBP[1]
2. Hyperlipoproteinemia:[1]
    (a) Hypercholesterolemia: increased LDL cholesterol (especially oxidized, acetylated, glycosylated, and other modified forms of LDL, small dense LDL-type B) and increased number of LDL particles.
    (b) Decreased HDL cholesterol and abnormal paraoxanase activity.
        (i) High HDL2 subfraction is associated with low incidence of CHD.
        (ii) HDL3 subfraction: less CHD association.
    (c) Hypertriglyceridemia: very low-density lipoprotein (VLDL) elevation and increased number of VLDL particles and large VLDL particles (often seen with low HDL) (especially those with increased total cholesterol). Remnant particles increase CHD risk.
    (d) Apolipoprotein A-I and A-II: low levels.
    (e) Apolipoprotein B: high levels.
    (f) Lipoprotein a (Lp(a)): high levels.
    (g) Increased APO-CII.
    (h) Serum free fatty acids (FFA).
3. Smoking[1]
4. Hyperglycemia (FBS over 75 mg%) (2 hour GTT over 110 mg%), DM, metabolic syndrome elevated hemoglobin A1C and AGEs (advanced glycosylation end products)
5. Insulin resistance[1]
6. Family history of premature CVD
7. Physical inactivity (lack of aerobic exercise)[1]
8. LVH1
9. Stress, anxiety, and depression
10. Type A personality (aggressive subtype)
11. Obesity (central),[1] BMI > 25, increased waist size, increased neck circumference, waist-to-hip ratio (WHR), % body fat
12. Male gender
13. Hyperuricemia1
14. Caffeine abuse
15. Age
16. Elevated HS-CRP.

SPECIAL CONSIDERATIONS

---

[1]Factors modified by antihypertensive therapy.

CHD: More Potential Risk Factors [55–67]

1. Excessive intake of alcohol may increase risk; however, small quantities of alcohol increase HDL3 subfraction and have anti-inflammatory effects that are associated with decreased risk of CHD [55, 58]. Low levels of carbohydrate-deficient transferrin (CDT) and high levels of gamma-glutamyl transpeptidase (GGTP) increase CHD risk
2. Increased platelet adhesion or aggregation (or both) and abnormal thrombogenic potential (TPA/PAI-1 ratio)[1] [59, 60]
3. Hemodynamic effects that alter arterial flow disturbances and induce endothelial damage, which enhances atherosclerosis (blood velocity, surfaces)[1] [61]
4. Renin, Ang-II, and endothelin: vasculotoxic and induce LVH[1] [62, 63]
5. Sympathetic nervous system overactivity, elevated catecholamines (NE and epinephrine [EPI] levels): induces LVH,[1] ED, vasoconstriction, platelet aggregation and is vasculotoxic [64]
6. Elevated blood viscosity[1] [65]
7. Hyperinsulinemia and insulin resistance[1] [66, 67] and increased proinsulin
8. Hyperfibrinogenemia[1] increased VWF and increased clotting factors (factors V, VII, IX, X, XII), deficiency of proteins C and S
9. Elevated homocysteine levels
10. Low vitamin C, E, lycopene, and reduced fruits and vegetables in diet (antioxidants)
11. Leukocytosis
12. Corneal arcus, diagonal earlobe crease, and hairy earlobes
13. Linoleic acid deficiency and reduced intake of omega-3 fatty acids
14. Short stature
15. Low levels of dehydroepiandrosterone sulfate (DHEAS)
16. Nonspecific ST–T wave changes on ECG
17. Lower socioeconomic status
18. Increased plasma levels of PAI-1
19. Elevated serum estradiol in men
20. Chromium deficiency
21. Lean hypertensive men (bottom 20% of IBW)
22. Polycythemia
23. Hypomagnesemia
24. Male pattern baldness
25. Elevated serum creatinine
26. Microalbuminuria and proteinuria
27. Chronic tachycardia and slow heart rate recovery after treadmill test
28. Elevated serum iron
29. Chronic infections (HSV, CMV, EBV, H. Flu, Chlamydia pneumoniae, H. pylori) (mycoplasma)
30. Chronic periodontal infection
31. Osteoporosis at menopause
32. Chronic cough or chronic inflammatory lung disease
33. Hypochloremia
34. Elevated intracellular adhesion molecules (ICAM-1) (V-CAM, P-selectin, etc.)

35. Low vitamin K levels
36. Increased myeloperoxidase levels (MPO)
37. Increased APO-E4
38. Low serum folate and MTHFR 677C T Æ polymorphism
39. Increased CD-14 monocytes and NK T cells
40. Low serum copper
41. Increased phospholipase A2
42. Increased serum leptin
43. Increased desaturated lecithin
44. Increased IL-6, IL-B, TNF-a, LPA (lipoprotein A)
45. Genetic increase in certain SNPs (single nucleotide polymorphisms) such as TSP-1 and TSP-4 (thrombospondins)
46. Hostility
47. Aortic calcifications
48. Elevated serum TNF-a
49. Elevated HSP (heated shock protein) in serum
50. Low serum calcitonin gene-related peptide (CGRP)
51. Low sex hormone binding globulin (SHBG)
52. Increased serum amyloid A (SAA)
53. Low levels of serum coenzyme Q-10
54. Low glutathione and glutathione peroxidase activity
55. Low intravascular superoxide dismutase (SOD)
56. High intake of refined carbohydrates, trans fats and saturated fats.

CHD Risk Factors: Influence of Diuretic and BB Therapy

	Diuretics Thiazide and thiazide-like	BBs (without ISA)
Hypokalemia	Yes	No
Hypomagnesemia	Yes	No
Dyslipidemia	Yes	Yes
Hypercholesterolemia	Yes	Yes
Hypertriglyceridemia	Yes	Yes
Increase LDL cholesterol	Yes	Yes
Lowered HDL cholesterol	Yes or no change	Yes
Elevated apolipoprotein B	Yes	Yes
Lowered apolipoprotein A	Yes	Yes
Elevated Lp(a)	Yes	Yes
Glucose intolerance and new onset DM	Yes	Yes
Insulin resistance	Yes	Yes
Hyperuricemia	Yes	Yes
Impaired aerobic exercise	Yes (minimal)	Yes
LVH regression	Yes (minimal)	Yes (minimal)
Improved diastolic dysfunction	No	Inconsistent
Increased blood viscosity	Yes	No
Increased catecholamines	Yes	Yes
Increased Ang-II	Yes	No
Potentiated arrhythmias	Yes	No
Acid–base abnormalities and other electrolyte disorders	Yes	No (rare hyperkalemia)
Blood velocity and arterial turbulence abnormalities	Yes	No
Hyperfibrinogenemia	Yes	No
Abnormal platelet function (aggregation and adhesion)	Yes	No
Increased thrombogenic potential increased PAI-1 and PAI-1/TPA ratio	Yes	No
Homocysteinemia	Yes	No
Proteinuria/microalbuminuria	Yes	No
Increased creatinine	Yes	No
Reduced GFR	Yes	No

Antihypertensive drugs and serum lipids [5, 68 ,77]

Antihypertensive drugs with known unfavorable effects on serum lipids

1. Diuretics: thiazides, chlorthalidone, loop diuretics, thiazide-like diuretics, metolazone (but not indapamide)
2. Beta-blockers (without ISA):
   (a) Atenolol (Tenormin)
   (b) Betaxolol (Kerlone)
   (c) Metoprolol (Lopressor, Toprol XL)
   (d) Nadolol (Corgard)
   (e) Propranolol (Inderal)

(f) Timolol (Blocadren)

(g) Bisoprolol (Zebeta).

3. Methyldopa (Aldomet)

4. Reserpine.

Antihypertensive drugs with potentially favorable effects on serum lipids

1. Alpha-blockers:

(a) Doxazosin (Cardura)

(b) Prazosin (Minipress)

(c) Terazosin (Hytrin).

2. Calcium channel blockers:

(a) Amlodipine (Norvasc)

(b) Diltiazem (Cardizem SR, CD, LA, Dilacor XR, Tiazac, and others)

(c) Felodipine (Plendil)

(d) Isradipine (DynaCirc)

(e) Nicardipine (Cardene, Cardene SR)

(f) Nifedipine (Adalat CC, Adalat Oros, Procardia XL)

(g) Verapamil (Calan SR, Isoptin SR, Verelan, Covera HS)

(h) Nisoldipine (Sular).

3. Central alpha-agonists:

(a) Clonidine (Catapres and Catapres-TTS)

(b) Guanabenz (Wytensin)

(c) Guanfacine (Tenex).

Antihypertensive drugs with neutral effects on serum lipids

1. Angiotensin-converting enzyme inhibitors:

(a) Benazepril (Lotensin)

(b) Captopril (Capoten)

(c) Enalapril (Vasotec)

(d) Fosinopril (Monopril)

(e) Lisinopril (Prinivil, Zestril)

(f) Quinapril (Accupril)

(g) Ramipril (Altace)

(h) Moexipril (Univasc)

(i) Trandolapril (Mavik)

(j) Perindopril (Aceon).

2. Direct vasodilators:

(a) Hydralazine (Apresoline)

(b) Minoxidil (Loniten).

3. BBs with ISA:

(a) Acebutolol (Sectral)

(b) Penbutolol (Levatol)

(c) Pindolol (Visken)

(d) Carteolol (Cartrol).

4. BBs with vasodilating and/or alpha-blocking activity:

(a) Labetalol (Trandate, Normodyne)

(b) Carvedilol (Coreg)

(c) Nebivolol.
5. Indapamide (Lozol) and SARAs
6. Ang-II inhibitors:
    (a) Losartan (Cozaar)
    (b) Valsartan (Diovan)
    (c) Irbesartan (Avapro)
    (d) Telmisartan (Micardis)
    (e) Candesartan cilexetil (Atacand)
    (f) Eprosartan (Teveten)
    (g) Olmesartan (Benicar).

Serum lipids and antihypertensive therapy with diuretics and BBs: summary

1. The effects are dose related: higher doses of BBs have more adverse effects, but even low doses of thiazide and thiazide-like diuretics (HCTZ 12.5 mg, chlorthalidone 12.5 mg) have adverse effects. However, indapamide does not adversely affect glucose or lipids, and SARAs are neutral.
2. Elevations blunted but not prevented by:
    (a) nutritional restriction of fats, carbohydrates, and weight loss;
    (b) exercise and reduction of smoking.
3. Duration: adverse effects persist with long-term therapy well above initial serum lipid levels.
4. Diuretics plus nonselective BBs cause additive adverse effects.
5. Thiazide and thiazide-like diuretics have similar adverse lipid effects in equipotent doses except for indapamide, which has neutral effects on lipids.
6. BBs may differ depending on several factors:
    (a) Nonselective: greatest adverse alteration in serum lipids
    (b) Cardioselective: less adverse alteration in serum lipids
    (c) ISA, vasodilating, and alpha-/beta-blockers: least alteration in lipids (neutral effect).
7. Diuretic effects on serum lipids appear to be more pronounced in postmenopausal women, men, and obese patients.
8. Increase in lipids is more marked in patients with higher baseline values (average change is about 10–20%).
9. Abnormal lipid levels reverse to normal after cessation of therapy (takes 2–4 months).

Composite effects of antihypertensive drugs on CHD risk factors

The composite effects of antihypertensive drugs on CHD risk factors [5, 78–84] are illustrated in Table 46.

CCBs and atherosclerosis (CHD reduction) trials

Nifedipine vs. propranolol vs. isosorbide [85]	CHD/angina
Nifedipine vs. placebo (INTACT) [86]	Mild CHD/angina
Nifedipine vs. placebo (INTACT2) [125]	Mild CHD/angina
Verapamil vs. non-CCB [87]	CHD/angina
Verapamil vs. placebo (FIPS) [87]	CHD/angina
Isradipine vs. HCTZ (MIDAS) [88]	Carotid artery

Nicardipine vs. placebo [89]   CHD
Verapamil vs. chlorthalidone (VHAS)   CHD/CVD/carotid
Amlodipine vs. placebo (PREVENT)   CHD/CVD/carotid
Nifedipine vs. co-amilozide (INSIGHT)   CHD by EBT
Lacidipine vs. atenolol (ELSA)   Carotid IMT

Table 46 Effects of Antihypertensive Drugs on CHD Risk Factors

	Thiazide and thiazide-like diuretics	Indapamide	BBs without ISA	BBs with ISA	Labetalol	Guane-thidine, guanadrel
Hypertension	↓	↓	↓	↓	↓	↓
Dyslipidemia	↑	→	↑	→	→	→
Glucose intolerance	↑	→	↑	↑	↑	→
Insulin resistance	↑	→	↑	↑	?	?
LVH	→	↓	→/↓	↑	↓	↓
Exercise	→/↓	→	↓	↓	→/↓	↓
Potassium	↓	↓*	→/↑	→	→	→
Magnesium	↓	↓*	→	→	→	→
Uric acid	↑	↑*	↑	↑	↑	→
Blood viscosity	↑	→	→	→	→	→
Blood velocity	→/↑	→	↓	→	→	→
Catecholamines	↑	↓	↑	↑	→	↓
Ang-II	↑	→	↓	→	↓	↑
Arrhythmia potential	↑	→	↓	→/↑	→	↑
Fibrinogen	↑	→	?	?	?	?
Platelet function	↑	↓	→/↓	?	?	?
Thrombogenic potential	↑	↓	?	?	?	?
Antiatherogenic	→	→	↑†	?	?	↑
Homocysteinemia	↑	→	→	→	→	?
Renal dysfunction						
Proteinuria, MAU	↑	→/↑	→/↑	→/↑	→/↑	?
CHD RR ratio	17:20	3:20	6:20	7:20	3:20	3:20

BB = beta-blocker; CHD = coronary heart disease; ISA = intrinsic sympathomimetic activity; LVH = left ventricular hypertrophy; MAU = microalbuminuria.
*Minimal.
†Animal studies.
‡Animal and human studies.
↓ Reduced; ↑ increased; → no change; ? unknown.

Central alpha-agonists	Methyl-dopa	Direct vaso-dilators	Alpha-blocker	Angio-tensin-converting enzyme inhibitors	Ang-II inhibitors	Calcium blockers	Reserpine
↓	↓	↓	↓	↓	↓	↓	↓
↓	↑	→	↓	→	→	↓	↑
↓	→	→	↓	↓	↓	↓	→
↓	→	→	↓	↓	↓	→/↓	?
↓	↓	↑	↓	↓	↓	↓	↓
→	→	→	→	→	→	→	↓
→	→	→	→	↑	↑	→	→
→	→	→	→	→/↑	→/↑	→	→
→/↓	→/↓	→	→	↓	↓	→/↓	→
→	→	↓	↓	→	→	?	?
↓	↑	↑	↓	↓	↓	↓	↓
↓	↓	↑	→/↓	↓	↓	↓	↓
↓	↓	↑	→/↓	↓	↓	↓	↓
↓	↓	↑	→	↓	↓	↓	↑
?	?	?	↓	?	?	?	?
↓	→	?	?	↓	↓	↓	?
?	?	?	?	?	?	↓	?
?	?	?	?	↓[†]	↓[†]	↓[‡]	↑[†]
?	?	?	?	→	→	→	?
→/↑	→/↑	→/↑	→/↑	→/↑	↓	↓	→
0:20	2:20	5:20	0:20	0:20	0:20	0:20	3:20

Antihypertensive Drugs and CHD Risk Factors: Summary

Favorable effects (0:20 CHD RR ratio)
1. Calcium channel blockers:
   (a) Amlodipine (Norvasc)
   (b) Diltiazem (Cardizem SR, CD, LA, Dilacor XR, Tiazac, and others)
   (c) Felodipine (Plendil)
   (d) Isradipine (DynaCirc)
   (e) Nicardipine (Cardene, Cardene SR)
   (f) Nifedipine (Adalat CC, Adalat Oros, Procardia XL)
   (g) Verapamil (Calan SR, Isoptin SR, Verelan, Covera HS)
   (h) Nisoldipine (Sular).
2. Alpha-blockers:
   (a) Doxazosin (Cardura)
   (b) Prazosin (Minipress)
   (c) Terazosin (Hytrin).
3. Central alpha-agonists:
   (a) Clonidine (Catapres and Catapres-TTS)
   (b) G-uanabenz (Wytensin)
   (c) Guanfacine (Tenex).
4. Angiotensin-converting enzyme inhibitors:
   (a) Benazepril (Lotensin)
   (b) Captopril (Capoten)
   (c) Enalapril (Vasotec)
   (d) Fosinopril (Monopril)
   (e) Lisinopril (Prinivil, Zestril)
   (f) Quinapril (Accupril)
   (g) Ramipril (Altace)
   (h) Moexipril (Univasc)
   (i) Trandolapril (Mavik)
   (j) Perindopril (Aceon).
5. Ang-II blockers:
   (a) Losartan (Cozaar)
   (b) Valsartan (Diovan)
   (c) Irbesartan (Avapro)
   (d) Telmisartan (Micardis)
   (e) Candesartan cilexetil (Atacand)
   (f) Eprosartan (Teveten)
   (g) Olmesartan (Benicar).

Neutral effects (0–5:20 CHD RR ratio)
1. Diuretics (selected):
   (a) Amiloride (Midamor)
   (b) Indapamide (Lozol)
   (c) Spironolactone (Aldactone)
   (d) Eplerenone (INSPRA)
   (e) Triamterene (Dyrenium).

2. Direct vasodilators:
   (a) Hydralazine (Apresoline)
   (b) Minoxidil (Loniten).
3. Central alpha-agonist:
   (a) Methyldopa (Aldomet).
4. Alpha-/beta-blocker or vasodilating BB:
   (a) Labetalol (Trandate, Normodyne)
   (b) Carvedilol (Coreg)
   (c) Nebivolol.
5. Neuronal-inhibiting drugs:
   (a) Guanadrel (Hylorel)
   (b) Guanethidine (Ismelin)
   (c) Reserpine (Serpasil).

Unfavorable effects (over 5:20 CHD RR ratio)

1. Diuretics (selected):
   (a) Chlorthalidone (Hygroton, Thalitone)
   (b) Loop diuretics (furosemide, bumetanide, ethacrynic acid, torsemide)
   (c) Quinazolines (metolazone)
   (d) Thiazides: chlorothiazide, HCTZ, polythiazide, methyclothiazide.
2. BBs without ISA:
   (a) Atenolol (Tenormin)
   (b) Betaxolol (Kerlone)
   (c) Metoprolol (Lopressor, Toprol XL)
   (d) Nadolol (Corgard)
   (e) Propranolol (Inderal, Inderal LA)
   (f) Timolol (Blocadren)
   (g) Bisoprolol (Zebeta).
3. BBs with ISA:
   (a) Acebutolol (Sectral)
   (b) Penbutolol (Levatol)
   (c) Pindolol (Visken)
   (d) Carteolol (Cartrol).

Hypertension and Renal Disease

Classification of chronic kidney disease [1]

Stage	Description	GFR (mL/min/1.73 m²)
1	Kidney damage with normal or increased GFR	>90
2	Kidney damage with mild decreased GFR	60–89
3	Moderate decreased GFR	30–59
4	Severe decreased GFR	15–29
5	Kidney failure (ESRD)	<15 (or dialysis)

Classification of urinary protein excretion

Urinary protein excretion rate per day	Description/nomenclature
<30 mg albumin	Not identified as disease state
30–300 mg albumin	Microalbuminuria
>300 mg albumin	Macroalbuminuria
>330 mg total protein	Overt proteinuria
>1000 mg total protein	Macroproteinuria
>3500 mg total protein	Nephrotic range proteinuria

Hypertension and renal disease

Hypertensive nephrosclerosis accounts for 23% of the prevalent ESRD in the United States and 26% of incident new cases in 2000. In consideration of the critical role of BP control on renal disease progression, hypertensive nephrosclerosis and diabetic nephrosclerosis together accounted for 57.5% of prevalent ESRD and 69% of incident new cases of ESRD in 2000 [2].

It is estimated that 11% of the American adult population over age 20 have evidence of chronic kidney disease with at least Stage 1 nephropathy [3]. Furthermore, although 32% of the US adult population has hypertension, 58% of the hypertensive adult American population is estimated to have at least mild reduction of GFR (Stage 2). The proportion of patients with treated hypertension with impaired renal function is 64%, and the proportion of patients with untreated hypertension with impaired renal function is 52%. At least one study is supportive of the hypothesis that patients with primary hypertension are born with fewer functioning nephrons [4].

Although no data show a reduction in ESRD related to the treatment of stage I–II mild to moderate hypertension, elevations of BP have been shown to be a strong independent risk factor for ESRD [5].

Clinical trials, both prospective and retrospective, suggest that 15–35% of patients with mild to moderate hypertension progress to renal insufficiency on stepped-care therapy (diuretics and BBs) despite adequate BP control. This progression is particularly true for African-American hypertensive patients [6].

It is postulated that chronic elevations of intraglomerular capillary pressure (Pgc) accelerate the loss of glomeruli and nephron function seen with normal aging. The relative difference in the resistance to flow between the afferent (preglomerular) and efferent (postglomerular) arterioles determines the glomerular capillary pressure.

As BP increases, there is a progressive rise in RVR, decrease in effective renal blood flow (RBF) and renal plasma flow (RPF), and a later decrease in GFR. Decline in GFR is initially hemodynamic (reversible) but becomes irreversible because of accelerated glomerulosclerosis and nephron loss. Once the functioning global number of nephrons falls by more than 50%, autoregulation becomes impaired and afferent (preglomerular) arteriolar dilatation induces structural hypertrophy and functional hyperfiltration of each remaining intact "remnant" nephron. Hyperperfusion and hyperfiltration result in glomerular hypertension, which accelerates further global loss of remnant nephrons.

Antihypertensive therapy that normalizes both systemic BP and intraglomerular pressure while preserving the autoregulatory ability of the afferent arteriole would be expected to provide protection of glomerular filtration function.

Ang-II, catecholamines, and vasopressin regulate efferent (postglomerular) arteriolar vasoconstriction. Drugs that interfere with or attenuate Ang-II, catecholamines, or vasopressin actions (ACEIs, angiotensin receptor antagonists, and CCBs) may offer renal protection beyond BP reduction alone, whereas drugs that increase Ang-II, catecholamines, and vasopressin (diuretics) may promote glomerular injury despite systemic BP reduction. Drugs that cause regression of glomerular and renal vascular hypertrophy may improve renal function or prolong renal survival (ACEIs, angiotensin receptor antagonists, and CCBs).

Clinical trials have demonstrated that different drug categories have different abilities to prevent the decline of GFR in hypertensive patients. ACEIs have been demonstrated to be beneficial in kidney diseased patients with both diabetic [7] and nondiabetic nephropathy with both microalbuminuria and macroproteinuria [8, 9]. ARBs have been demonstrated to be beneficial in patients with type 2 DM, with microproteinuria or macroproteinuria. CCBs have been shown to be renoprotective in patients with nephropathy that is either diabetic or hypertensive, but CCB monotherapy has limited application for renal protection when macroproteinuria is present. Combining CCBs with either ACEIs or ARBs is very effective. Combination therapy of ACEIs with ARBs is also showing considerable benefit in nondiabetic primary nephropathies [10].

Both SBP and DBP correlate with the development and progression of renal insufficiency and end-stage renal failure, but SBP is more important than DBP as a risk factor. Any degree of hypertension can promote acceleration of renal disease progression.

Meta-analysis demonstrates that hypertensive nephrosclerosis is reduced proportionately with the reduction in BP. Target BP should be 110–120/70–75 mm Hg in hypertensive patients with renal impairment and macroproteinuria and in hypertensive diabetics. Target BP in the absence of macroproteinuria and diabetes is less clear; results of the MDRD trial show that there is benefit of aggressive BP reduction below 130/85, but the AASK trial did not demonstrate significant benefit in preventing adverse renal outcomes in a population of high-risk African-Americans with Stages 3 and 4 nephropathy without macroproteinuria or diabetes in lowering BP from group mean of 141/85 to a group mean of 128/78. Other investigators have demonstrated that while intensive BP lowering (MAP 92) does not slow the rate of GFR decline in type 1 diabetics compared to usual therapy (MAP 100 to 107), that intensive therapy does confer the benefit of significant proteinuria reduction compared to usual therapy [11].

Hypertension-related renal disease: postulated mechanisms

Figure 67 illustrates hypertension-related renal disease: postulated mechanisms [4, 5, 90–93].

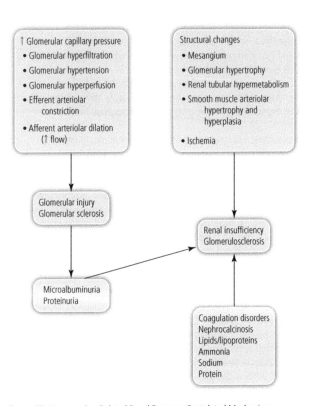

Figure 67 Hypertension-Related Renal Damage: Postulated Mechanisms.

Is thiazide diuretic-based antihypertensive therapy associated with increased risk of renal injury?

Although most antihypertensive trials in North America incorporating a diuretic arm in the study design have been designed to use the diuretic chlorthalidone, the thiazide diuretic HCTZ remains the most commonly prescribed diuretic for BP control in North America.

HCTZ has been shown in laboratory animals to increase RVR, intraglomerular pressure, and the production of vasotoxic cytokines including transforming growth factor beta (TGFb) and PAI-1 as well as stimulating production of renin, Ang-II, aldosterone, and homocysteine, all of which have been associated with increased vascular injury. HCTZ has been shown to accelerate glomerular injury in the L-NAME model of glomerulosclerosis, whereas ACEIs, ARBs, and CCBs have all been shown to retard renal injury in that model.

The NHANES III gave a valuable cross-section sampling of the presence of hypertension, the adequacy of hypertension therapy, and the use of various antihypertensive agents in the United States during data sampling from 1988 to 1994. An analysis of these data has shown that in patients with hypertension, the presence of elevated creatinine level was 1.7-fold increased (nearly doubled) with the prescription of diuretics (after adjusting for the number of medications prescribed, age, sex, race, and diabetes) [12].

A number of clinical trials lend evidence in support of the contention that thiazide-based antihypertensive therapy is either nephrotoxic or fails to exert discernible renoprotection. The European Working Party on High Blood Pressure in the Elderly (EWPHE) trial [13], the Hypertension in Elderly Patients in Primary Care (HEP) trial [14], and the Swedish Trial in Old Patients (STOP) with Hypertension [15] all demonstrated significant increases in serum creatinine level in the patients receiving step-care therapy with thiazide diuretics either alone or in combination with BBs (HEP, STOP) or with alpha methyldopa (EWPHE).

In the SHEP trial, after 3 years of follow-up, serum creatinine level had not changed in the placebo group but had significantly increased in the actively treated group (chlorthalidone) [16]. The incidence of mild renal insufficiency was similar in placebo and active treatment groups regardless of the absence or presence of diabetes. This suggests that chlorthalidone therapy does not offer the intended benefits in renal disease even while CV and stroke endpoints are significantly reduced.

Analysis [17] of the SYST-EUR trial studying changes in renal function in untreated and treated patients showed that serum creatinine levels did not change over 5 years in patients randomized to nitrendipine monotherapy, whereas patients receiving HCTZ either alone or in combination with study medication showed a significant increase in serum creatinine level.

The INSIGHT [18] demonstrated that when compared with CCB therapy the diuretic co-amiloride conferred ~2.5-fold increased risk of impaired renal function developing during 4 years of follow-up (4.6 vs. 1.8%).

The ALLHAT [19] found that therapy based on the diuretic chlorthalidone was associated with a significantly lower GFR at 2 and 4 years of follow-up compared to both therapies based on the CCB amlodipine or the ACEI lisinopril.

Analysis of diuretic prescribing practices in the United States showed that a direct relationship exists between total American spending for all diuretic therapy and the rate of increase in the incidence rate of ESRD 4 years later. Renal failure incidence attenuates following reductions of diuretic distribution in the United States. Given that the total Medicare spending for ESRD in 2000 approached $14 billion and is rising at ~6% annually, further study of the economic impact of expanded diuretic use in the United States is warranted.

Major clinical trials showing renoprotection

Table 47 summarizes the major clinical trials showing renoprotection.

Effects of antihypertensive drugs on renal function

Effects of antihypertensive drugs on renal function are summarized in Table 48 [4, 5].

Table 47 Major Clinical Trials Showing Renoprotection

Clinical trial	Primary renal disease	No. of participants	Design and therapy	Outcome description
REIN-1 [20]	Nondiabetic renal disease with macroproteinuria between 1 and 3 g daily	78 active treatment 88 placebo	Ramipril up to 5 mg daily vs. placebo	Ramipril reduced macroproteinuria and slowed GFR decline by 56%, greater than expected by BP control alone
REIN-2 [21]	Nondiabetic renal disease with nephrotic range proteinuria above 3 g daily	117 patients	Ramipril up to 5 mg daily vs. placebo	52% reduction in rate of GFR decline
IRMA-2 [22]	Hypertensive type 2 DM	590 patients	Double-blind placebo-controlled trial of irbesartan 150 mg daily, 300 mg daily and placebo	70% risk reduction of renal endpoints seen in 300 mg dose group; risk reduction for 150 mg group was not significant
IDNT [23]	Hypertensive type 2 DM	1715 patients	Double-blind placebo-controlled irbesartan vs. amlodipine vs. conventional BP therapy	Irbesartan reduced risk of renal endpoints by 20% compared to placebo and 23% compared to amlodipine
RENAAL [24]	Type 2 DM with nephropathy	1513 patients	Losartan vs. placebo	16% risk reduction in active treatment group

COOPERATE [25]	Nondiabetic adult patients with Stages 2–4 nephropathy, with or without hypertension	336 patients	Losartan vs. trandolapril vs. combination therapy of both drugs	Combination therapy reduced risk of doubling creatinine or ESRD by 62% compared to trandolapril monotherapy and 60% compared to losartan monotherapy
AASK [26]	Nondiabetic hypertensive African-Americans with mild to severe renal impairment (Stages 2–4 nephropathy)	1094 patients	Amlodipine vs. metoprolol vs. ramipril based therapy; BP goals assigned either 102–107 MAP "usual" goal or <92 MAP	ACEI reduced risk of achieving the composite endpoint by 22% compared to BB and 38% compared to CCB. No difference between BB and CCB; no added advantage of achieving aggressive BP target
MARVAL [27]	Type 2 DM with microalbuminuria, with or without hypertension	332 patients	Valsartan 80mg/day vs. amlodipine 5 mg/day for 24 weeks	Valsartan treated patients had significant 44% reduction in albumin excretion compared to baseline, amlodipine treated patients had nonsignificant 8% reduction

(Continued)

Table 47 (Continued)

Clinical trial	Primary renal disease	No. of participants	Design and therapy	Outcome description
CALM [28]	Type 2 DM with hypertension and microalbuminuria	199 patients	Randomized to receive candesartan or lisinopril monotherapy for the first 12 weeks; then half the patients were randomized to receive combination therapy of both drugs for the second 12-week period	At 12 weeks both candesartan and lisinopril monotherapy significantly reduced proteinuria; at 24 weeks the combination therapy achieved lower BP control than either monotherapy, but proteinuria was not significantly further reduced
MICROHOPE [29]	Diabetic patients with at least one other CV risk factor, no proteinuria	3577 patients (subset of HOPE trial)	Randomized to ramipril 10mg/day or placebo	24% risk reduction of overt nephropathy after 4.5 years independent of BP reduction
EUCLID [30]	Normotensive nonalbuminuric type 1 DM patients	530 patients	Placebo-controlled lisinopril therapy trial with 2-year follow-up	Lisinopril therapy in normotensive nonalbuminuric diabetics reduces the excretion of urinary albumin by 18% after 2 years of follow-up
AIPRI [31]	All chronic nephropathies but predominantly nondiabetic	583 patients	Benazepril vs. placebo	53% risk reduction

Study	Population	Patients	Design	Results
MDRD [32]	Study 1: Stage 3 nephropathy including diabetic and nondiabetic Study 2: Stage 4 nephropathy including diabetic and nondiabetic	Study 1: 585 patients Study 2: 255 patients	Study 1: Patients assigned usual or low dietary protein intake; BP randomized to "usual" 107 MAP or "low" 92 MAP using any medications Study 2: Patients assigned to low or very low dietary protein intake; BP randomized as in Study 1	Patients in Study 1 had no change in rate of GFR decline regardless of protein intake or BP control. Pooled results of both study arms showed that patients with proteinuria treated to lower BP target MAP 92 had slower decline in GFR.
UKPDS [33]	Type 2 DM and hypertension	758 patients	Captopril vs. atenolol	No significant difference between medications; all benefits were ascribed to magnitude of BP lowering
ABCD [34]	Hypertensive type 2 DM with various degrees of proteinuria	470 patients	Randomized to either CCB nisoldipine or ACEI enalapril; randomized to two levels of BP control "intensive (132/78)" or "moderate (138/86)"	No difference observed between levels of BP control for renal function decline. Both CCB and ACEI were equally protective of GFR and proteinuria

(Continued)

Table 47 (*Continued*)

Clinical trial	Primary renal disease	No. of participants	Design and therapy	Outcome description
Collaborative Study Group [35]	Type 1 DM with overt proteinuria	207 active treatment 202 placebo	Captopril 25 mg TID vs. placebo 3-year median follow-up	Captopril associated with 50% decline in death, dialysis and transplantation independent of BP difference

AASK = African American Study of Kidney Disease and Hypertension; ABCD = Appropriate Blood Pressure Control in Diabetes Trial; ACEI = angiotensin-converting enzyme inhibitors; BB = beta-blocker; BP = blood pressure; CCB = calcium channel blocker; CV = cardiovascular; DM = diabetes mellitus; ESRD = end-stage renal failure; GFR = glomerular filtration rate; HOPE = Heart Outcomes and Prevention Evaluation study; IDNT = Irbesartan Diabetic Nephropathy Trial; IRMA = Irbesartan in patients with type 2 diabetes and microalbuminuria; MAP = mean arterial pressure; RENAAL = Randomized Evaluation of NIDDM with the Ang-II antagonist Losartan; UKPDS = United Kingdom Prospective Diabetes Study.

Table 48 Effects of Antihypertensive Drugs on Renal Function

	Diuretics	Beta-blockers	BBs with ISA	Beta-blockers + alpha-blockers	Direct vasodilators	Neuronal inhibitors	Calcium channel blockers	Ang-II inhibitors + ACEIs	Central alpha-agonists	Alpha methyldopa	Alpha-blockers
GFR	→/↓	→/↓	↑	↑	→/↑	→	↑	→	↑/→	↑/→	→/↑
ERPF	→/↓	→/↓	↑	↑	→/↑	→	↑	↑	↑	↑	→/↑
GFR/ERPF	↑	↑	↑	↑	↑	→	↑	↑	↑	↑	↑
RBF	→/↓	→/↓	→/↑	→/↑	→/↑	→	↑/→	↓/→	↑/→	↑/→	→
RVR	↑	→/↑	↑	↑	↓	→	→/↓	→	→	→	?
IGCP	↑	?	?	?	↑	?	↓/↑	→	?	?	?
Urinary albumin	↑	?	?	?	↑	?	↓/↑	→	?	?	?
Urinary$_{Na+}$	↑	→/↓	→/↓	↑	→	→/↓	↑	↑	→/↑	↓	→/↓
Urinary$_{K+}$	↑	→/↓	↑	↑	↑	↑	↑/→	→/↓	↑	↑	↑
Urinary$_{Mg}{}^{2+}$	↑	→/↓	↑	↑	↑	↑	↑	→	↑	↑	↑
Plasma volume	↓	→/↑	→/↑	→/↑	↑	→/↓	↓	→/↓	→/↓	↓	→/↓

ACEI = angiotensin-converting enzyme inhibitors; BB = beta-blocker; ERPF = effective renal plasma flow; GFR = glomerular filtration rate; IGCP = intraglomerular capillary pressure; RBF = renal blood flow; RVR = renal vascular resistance.
↓ Reduced; ↑ increased; → no change; ? unknown.

References: hypertension and renal disease

1. National Kidney Foundation: K/DOQI Clinical Practice Guidelines for Chronic Kidney Disease: Evaluation, Classification and Stratification. *Am J Kidney Dis* 2002; 39(suppl 1): S1–S266.
2. US Renal Data System: USRDS 2002 Annual Data Report. The National Institutes of Health, National Institute of Diabetes and Digestive and Kidney Diseases, Bethesda, MD, 2002.
3. Coresh J, et al. Prevalence of chronic kidney disease and decreased kidney function in the adult US population: Third National Health and Nutrition Examination Survey. *Am J Kidney Dis* 2003; 41: 1–12.
4. Keller G, et al. Nephron number in patients with primary hypertension. *N Engl J Med* 2003; 348(2): 101–108.
5. Klag MJ, et al. Blood pressure and end-stage renal disease in men. *N Engl J Med* 1996; 334: 8–13.
6. Rostand SG, et al. Renal insufficiency in treated essential hypertension. *N Engl J Med* 1989; 320: 684–688.
7. Bakris GL, et al. Preserving renal function in adults with hypertension and diabetes: A consensus approach. *Am J Kidney Dis* 2000; 36(3): 646–661.
8. Jafar TH, et al. Angiotensin-converting enzyme inhibitors and progression of nondiabetic renal disease. *Ann Intern Med* 2001; 135: 73–87.
9. Kshirsagar AV, et al. Effect of ACE inhibitors in diabetic and nondiabetic chronic renal disease: A systematic overview of randomized placebo-controlled trials. *Am J Kidney Dis* 2000; 35(4): 695–707.
10. Russo D, et al. Coadministration of losartan and enalapril exerts additive antiproteinuric effect in IgA nephropathy. *Am J Kidney Dis* 2001; 38: 18–25.
11. Lewis JB, et al. Effect of intensive blood pressure control on the course of type I diabetic nephropathy. *Am J Kidney Dis* 1999; 34(5): 809–817.
12. Coresh J, et al. Prevalence of high blood pressure and elevated serum creatinine level in the United States. *Arch Intern Med* 2001; 161: 1207–1216.
13. Fletcher A, et al. Risks and benefits in the trial of the European Working Party on high blood pressure in the elderly. *J Hypertens* 1991; 9: 225–230.
14. Coope J, et al. Randomised trial of treatment of hypertension in elderly patients in primary care. *BMJ* 1986; 293: 1145–1151.
15. Ekbom T, et al. Antihypertensive efficacy and side effects of three beta-blockers and a diuretic in elderly hypertensives: A report from the STOP-hypertension study. *J Hypertens* 1992; 10: 1525–1530.
16. Savage PJ, et al. Influence of long-term low-dose diuretic-based antihypertensive therapy on glucose, lipid, uric acid and potassium levels in older men and women with isolated systolic hypertension. The Systolic Hypertension in the Elderly Program. *Arch Intern Med* 1999; 158: 741–751.
17. Voyaki SM, et al. Follow-up of renal function in treated and untreated older patients with isolated systolic hypertension. *J Hypertens* 2001; 19: 511–519.
18. Brown MJ, et al. Morbidity and mortality in patients randomized to double-blind treatment with a long-acting calcium-channel blocker or diuretic in the International Nifedipine GITS study: Intervention as a Goal in Hypertension Treatment (INSIGHT). *Lancet* 2000; 356: 366–372.
19. The ALLHAT Study Group. Major outcomes in high-risk hypertensive patients randomized to angiotensin-converting enzyme inhibitor or calcium-channel blocker vs. diuretic. *JAMA* 2002; 288: 2981–2997.

20. Ruggenenti P, et al. Renoprotective properties of ACE-inhibition in non-diabetic nephropathies with non-nephrotic proteinuria. *Lancet* 1999; 354: 359–364.

21. The GISEN Group. Randomised placebo-controlled trial of effect of ramipril on decline in glomerular filtration rate and risk of terminal renal failure in proteinuric, non-diabetic nephropathy. *Lancet* 1997; 349: 1857–1863.

22. Parving H, et al. The effect of irbesartan on the development of diabetic nephropathy in patients with type 2 diabetes. *N Engl J Med* 2001; 345(12): 870–878.

23. Lewis EJ, et al. Renoprotective effect of the angiotensin-receptor antagonist irbesartan in patients with nephropathy due to type 2 diabetes. *N Engl J Med* 2001; 345(12): 851–860.

24. Brenner BM, et al. Effects of losartan on renal and cardiovascular outcomes in patients with type 2 diabetes and nephropathy. *N Engl J Med* 2001; 345(12): 861–869.

25. Nakao N, et al. Combination treatment of angiotensin-II receptor blocker and angiotensin-converting-enzyme inhibitor in non-diabetic renal disease (COOPERATE): A randomized controlled trial. *Lancet* 2003; 361: 117–124.

26. Wright JT, et al. Effect of blood pressure lowering and antihypertensive drug class on progression of hypertensive kidney disease. *JAMA* 2002; 288: 2421–2431.

27. Viberti G, et al. Microalbuminuria reduction with valsartan in patients with type 2 diabetes mellitus. *Circulation* 2002; 106: 672–678.

28. Mogensen CE, et al. Randomised controlled trial of dual blockade of renin-angiotensin system in patients with hypertension, microalbuminuria and non-insulin dependent diabetes: The Candesartan and Lisinopril Microalbuminuria (CALM) study. *BMJ* 2000; 321(7274): 1440–1444.

29. Heart Outcomes Prevention Evaluation (HOPE) Study Investigators. Effects of ramipril on cardiovascular and microvascular outcomes in people with diabetes mellitus: Results of the HOPE study and MICRO-HOPE substudy. *Lancet* 2000; 355: 253–259.

30. The EURODIAB Controlled Trial of Lisinopril in Insulin-Dependent Diabetes Mellitus (EUCLID) Study Group. Randomised placebo-controlled trial of lisinopril in normotensive patients with insulin-dependent diabetes and normoalbuminuria or microalbuminuria. *Lancet* 1997; 349(9068): 1787–1792.

31. Maschio G, et al. Effect of the angiotensin-converting enzyme inhibitor benazepril on the progression of chronic renal insufficiency. The Angiotensin-Converting Enzyme Inhibition in Progressive Renal Insufficiency Study Group. *N Engl J Med* 1996; 334: 939–945.

32. Klahr S, et al. The effects of dietary protein restriction and blood pressure control on the progression of chronic renal disease. *N Engl J Med* 1994; 330(13): 877–884.

33. UK Prospective Diabetes Study Group. Efficacy of atenolol and captopril in reducing risk of macrovascular and microvascular complications in patients with hypertension and type 2 diabetes: UKPDS 39. *BMJ* 1998; 317: 713–720.

34. Estacio RO, et al. Effect of blood pressure control on diabetic microvascular complications in patients with hypertension and type 2 diabetes. *Diabetes Care* 2000; 23(suppl 2): B54–B64.

35. Lewis EJ, et al. The effect of angiotensin-converting enzyme inhibition on diabetic nephropathy. *N Engl J Med* 1993; 329: 1456–1462.

SPECIAL
CONSIDERATIONS

DM and Hypertension Summary [191, 192]

1. The aggregate of major CV, renal events, and total mortality was lowest in more actively treated patients with lower BP (Tables 49–65 and Figures 68–80). The recommended BP goal is 110/70 mm Hg. Thus, more intensive BP lowering is recommended.
2. Approximately four antihypertensive drugs will be required to reach these goal levels for BP.
3. ACEIs and ARBs with CCBs showed better reduction in CV events compared to conventional diuretic or BB therapy, especially in CHD, CHF, and CVA events.
4. ACEI + CCB is superior to diuretic and BB in combination treatment to reduce CV events (SYST-EUR vs. SHEP).
5. Renal insufficiency, microalbuminuria, and proteinuria are best prevented by ACEIs and ARBs as initial therapy. Selective use of CCBs depending on the level of proteinuria (i.e., <1 g/24 hours) [192] is also renoprotective and reduces proteinuria. ACEIs, ARBs, and CCBs are superior to diuretics and BBs (IDNT, IRMA, RENAAL, CAPPP, ABCD-HT, LIFE, AASK, HOPE, MICROHOPE, ASCOT, VALUE).
6. New onset type 2 DM is more common with diuretics and BBs than other drug classes (HOPE, CAPPP, STOP-II, LIFE, UKPDS, SHEP, MICROHOPE, INSIGHT, NORDIL, NICS-EH, ARICS, ALLHAT, ASCOT, VALUE).
7. The addition of a thiazide diuretic to an RAAS drug or CCB will partially negate the improved insulin sensitivity with the RAAS agent or CCB and result in a higher glucose and hemoglobin A1C than would occur with monotherapy without the diuretic.

Table 49 Hypertension and DM [191]

Causes of Death Among People with Diabetes

Cause	% of deaths
Ischemic heart disease	40
Other heart disease	15
Diabetes (acute complications)	13
Cancer	13
Cerebrovascular disease	10
Pneumonia/influenza	4
All other causes	5

From Geiss LS, et al. Mortality in non-insulin-dependent diabetes. In: *Diabetes in America*, 2nd edn., National Diabetes Data Group. Bethesda, MD, 1995: 233–257.

Table 50 JNC-7 Recommendations for Patients with DM

Combination of two or more drugs to achieve BP <130/80 mm Hg
ACEI and ARB slow progression and reduce albuminuria
ARBs reduce progression to macroalbuminuria

Table 51 UK Prospective Diabetes Study

Captopril vs. Atenolol

Endpoint	Relative risk	95% CI
Any endpoint	1.10	0.86–1.41
Diabetes death	1.27	0.82–1.97
Any death	1.14	0.81–1.61
MI	1.20	0.82–1.76
Stroke	1.12	0.59–2.12
PAD	1.48	0.35–6.19
Microvascular disease	1.29	0.80–2.10

MI = myocardial infarction; PAD = peripheral arterial disease.
$n = 400$ vs. 358.
From Ref. [19], with permission.

Table 52 SHEP and SYST-EUR in Diabetic and Nondiabetic Patients

	Diabetics		Nondiabetics	
	SHEP	SYST-EUR	SHEP	SYST-EUR
N (% of total)	590 (12.3)	492 (10.5)	4149 (87.7)	4203 (89.5)
Mean BP reduction corrected for placebo				
Systolic (mm Hg)	−9.8	−8.6	−12.5	−10.3
Diastolic (mm Hg)	−2.2	−3.9	−4.1	−4.6
Risk in placebo group (events/1000 patient-years)				
Total mortality	35.6	45.1	21.8	21.6
CV endpoints	63.0	55.0	36.8	28.9
Stroke	28.8	26.6	15.0	12.3
Coronary events	32.2	23.1	15.2	12.4
Percent change with active treatment (95% CI)				
Mortality	−26 (−54, 18)	−64 (−83, −25)	−15 (−32, 6)	−18 (−40, 13)
All CV endpoints	−34 (−54, −6)	−68 (−84, −35)	−34 (−45, −21)	−30 (−47, −8)
Stroke	−22 (55, 34)	−86 (−96, −58)	−38 (−54, −17)	−39 (−60, −7)
Coronary events	−56 (−75, −23)	−58 (−87, 37)	−19 (−38, 5)	−22 (−47, 17)

BP = blood pressure; CV = cardiovascular; SHEP = Systolic Hypertension in the Elderly Program; SYST-EUR = Systolic Hypertension in Europe.

Table 53 Trials Comparing More with Less Intensive or Active with Placebo Treatment: Effects on Renal Function [191]

Trial	Renal variable	Patients n	BP	A	Treatment Comparison	Years	BP difference (mm Hg)	More intensive or active	Less intensive or placebo	p-Value
SHEP [31]	SCr (Δ μmol/L)	583	HT	–	D vs. Pl	3	−9.8/−2.2	+4.8	+0.7	NS
UKPDS [15]	SCr (Δ)	1148	HT	–	More vs. less	9	−10/−5	–	–	NS
HOT [6]	SCr (Δ μmol/L)	1501	HT	–	More vs. less	3.8	−3/−3	+2.2	+2.7	NS
SYST-EUR [10]	SCr (Δ μmol/L)	492	HT	–	CA vs. Pl	2	−8.6/−3.9	+3.3	+4.4	NS
IDNT [12]	SCr (Δ μmol/L)	1148	HT	OA	AIIA vs. Pl	3	−4/−3	+40	+53	0.008
	SCr (Δ μmol/L/year)	1136	HT	OA	CA vs. Pl	3	−3/−3	+51	+52	NS
Ravid et al. [26]	100/SCr (Δ)	94	NT	MA	ACEI vs. Pl	5	−4	−0.01	−0.12	<0.05
Lebovitz et al. [27]	GFR (Δ mL/min/ 1.73 m²/month)	121	HT	–	ACEI vs. Pl	2	−2.2	−0.13	−0.47	0.012
Ahmad et al. [28]	GFR (Δ mL/min/ 1.73 m²/month)	103	NT	MA	ACEI vs. Pl	5	0/−3	−5	−5	NS
Ravid et al. [29]	CrCl (Δ mL/min/ year)	156	NT	NA	ACEI vs. Pl	6	−4	−1.5	−2.4	0.040
ABCD-HT [34]	CrCl (Δ mL/min/ 1.73 m²/year)	470	HT	–	More vs. less	5	−6/−8	−7	−11	NS
ABCD-NT [8]	CrCl (Δ mL/min/ 1.73 m²/year)	480	HT	–	More vs. less	5	−9/−6	−8	−8	NS

| IRMA [14] | CrCl (Δ mL/min/1.73 m²/year) | 590 | HT | MA | AIIA vs. PI | 2 | −2/0 | −8.5 | −4.8 | NS |
| RENAAL [13] | est CrCl (Δ mL/min/1.73 m²/year) | 1513 | HT | OA | AIIA vs. PI | 3.4 | −2.5/−0.5 | −4.4 | −5.2 | 0.01 |

A = albuminuria; ABCD = Appropriate Blood Pressure Control in Diabetes Trial; ACEI = angiotensin-converting enzyme inhibitors; AIIA = Ang-II receptor antagonists; BP = blood pressure; CA = calcium antagonists; CrCl = estimated creatinine clearance; D = diuretics; GFR = glomerular filtration rate; HOT = Hypertension Optimal Treatment; HT = hypertensives; IDNT = Irbesartan Diabetic Nephropathy Trial; IRMA = Irbesartan in patients with type 2 diabetes and microalbuminuria; MA = microalbuminuria; NA = no albuminuria; NS = nonsignificant; NT = normotensives; OA = overt albuminuria; PI = placebo; RENAAL = Randomized Evaluation of NIDDM with the Ang-II antagonist Losartan; SCr = Serum creatinine; SHEP = Systolic Hypertension in the Elderly Program; SYST-EUR = Systolic Hypertension in Europe; UKPDS = United Kingdom Prospective Diabetes Study.
The BP differences (diff) between treatment groups are expressed as SBP/DBP or (single figure) as mean BP.

254

Table 54 Trials Comparing More with Less Intensive or Active with Placebo Treatment: Effects on Renal Dysfunction or Failure [191]

Trial	Renal variable	Treatment Comparison	Years	More intensive or active	Less intensive or placebo	p-Value	Relative risk	95% CI
SHEP [31]	% Patients with SCr > 176.8 μmol	D vs. Pl	3	18	29	NS		
HOT [6]	% Patients with SCr > 176.8 μmol	More vs. less	3.8	9.8	12.2	NS		
UKPDS [15]	n renal failure per 1000 patient-years	More vs. less	9	1.4	2.3	NS		
SYST-EUR [10]	n renal failure per 1000 patient-years	CA vs. Pl	2	5.7	5.7	NS		
IDNT [12]	% Patients with 2× SCr + ESRD + death	AIIA vs. Pl	3	32.6	39.0	0.02	0.80	0.66–0.97
	% Patients with 2 × SCr	AIIA vs. Pl	3	16.9	23.7	0.003	0.67	0.52–0.87
	% Patients with ESRD	AIIA vs. Pl	3	14.2	17.8	0.07	0.77	0.57–1.03
	% Patients with 2 × SCr + ESRD + death	CA vs. Pl	3	41.1	39.0	NS	1.04	0.86–1.25
	% Patients with 2 × SCr	CA vs. Pl	3	25.4	23.7	NS	1.06	0.84–1.35
	% Patients with ESRD	CA vs. Pl	3	18.3	17.8	NS	1.00	0.76–1.32
RENAAL [13]	% Patients with 2× SCr + ESRD + death	AIIA vs. Pl	3.4	15.9	18.1	0.02	0.84	0.72–0.98
	% Patients with 2 × SCr	AIIA vs. Pl	3.4	7.9	10.0	0.006	0.75	0.61–0.92
	% Patients with ESRD	AIIA vs. Pl	3.4	6.9	9.1	0.002	0.72	0.58–0.89

AIIA = Ang-II receptor antagonists; CA = calcium antagonists; D = diuretics; ESRD = end-stage renal failure; HOT = Hypertension Optimal Treatment; IDNT = Irbesartan Diabetic Nephropathy Trial; NS = nonsignificant; Pl = placebo; RENAAL = Randomized Evaluation of NIDDM with the Ang-II antagonist Losartan; SCr = Serum creatinine; SHEP = Systolic Hypertension in the Elderly Program; SYST-EUR = Systolic Hypertension in Europe; UKPDS = United Kingdom Prospective Diabetes Study.

Table 55 Trials Comparing More with Less Intensive or Active with Placebo Treatment: Effects on UAE [191]

Trial	Renal variable	Treatment		More intensive or active	Less intensive or placebo	p-Value
		Comparison	Years			
Ravid et al. [26]	ΔUAE (mg/24 hour)	ACEI vs. Pl	5	−3	+187	<0.05
Lebovitz et al. [26]	ΔUAE (mg/24 hour)	ACEI vs. Pl	2	−310	+470	NR
Ahmad et al. [28]	ΔUAER (μg/min)	ACEI vs. Pl	5	−35	+32	<0.001
Ravid et al. [29]	ΔUAE (mg/24 hour)	ACEI vs. Pl	6	−4.2	−15.7	0.001
MICROHOPE [11]	ΔUA/Cr ratio	ACEI vs. Pl	4.5	+1.35	−1.9	0.02
ABCD-HT [34]	% ΔUAE	More vs. less	5	+0.1	+0.2	NS
ABCD-NT [8]	% ΔUAE	More vs. less	5	+0.36	+0.066	0.001
IDNT [12]	% ΔUAE	AIIA vs. Pl	3	−33	−10	NS
	% ΔUAE	CA vs. Pl	3	−6	−10	NS
RENAAL [13]	Δlog UAE	AIIA vs. Pl	3.4	−35	+5	0.0001
IRMA [14]	Δlog UAE	AIIA vs. Pl	2	−31	−2	<0.001

ABCD = Appropriate Blood Pressure Control in Diabetes Trial; ACEI = angiotensin-converting enzyme inhibitors; AIIA = Ang-II receptor antagonists; CA = calcium antagonists; Cr = creatinine; HT = hypertensives; IDNT = Irbesartan Diabetic Nephropathy Trial; IRMA = Irbesartan in patients with type 2 diabetes and microalbuminuria; NR = not reported; NS = nonsignificant; NT = normotensives; Pl = placebo; RENAAL = Randomized Evaluation of NIDDM with the Ang-II antagonist Losartan; UA = uric acid; UAE = urinary albumin excretion.

The data of Lebovitz et al. [26] are from the subgroup of patients with baseline overt albuminuria.

Table 56 Trials Comparing More with Less Intensive or Active with Placebo Treatment: New or Worsening Proteinuria [191]

Trial	Renal variable	Treatment Comparison	Years	More intensive or active	Less intensive or placebo	P-Value	RR or OR (95% CI)
Ravid et al. [26]	From MA to OA (%)	ACEI vs. PI	5	12	42	<0.001	
Lebovitz et al. [26]	From MA to OA (%)	ACEI vs. PI	3	7	21	NR	
Ahmad et al. [28]	From MA to OA (%)	ACEI vs. PI	5	7.7	23.5	<0.001	
Ravid et al. [29]	From MA to MA (%)	ACEI vs. PI	6	6.5	19.0	<0.042	
Gaede et al. [29]	From MA to OA (%)	More vs. less multi-management	3.8	10.4	24.4	0.01	0.27* (0.10–0.75)
UKPDS [15]	New MA (n/1000 patient-years)	More vs. less	6	20.3	28.5	0.009	0.76 (0.51–0.99)
	New OA (n/1000 patient-years)	More vs. less	6	5.3	8.6	NS	0.61 (0.31–1.21)
MICROHOPE [11]	New MA	ACEI vs. PI	4.5	–	–	NS	0.91 (0.80–1.04)
SYST-EUR [10]	New OA (n/1000 patient-years)	CA vs. PI	2	18.8	58.0	0.008	0.29 (0.12–0.69)
ABCD-HT [34]	From NA to MA (%)	More vs. less	5	25	18	NS	
	From MA to OA (%)	More vs. less	5	16	23	NS	
ABCD-NT [8]	From NA to MA (%)	More vs. less	5	Lower	Higher	0.012	
	From MA to OA (%)	More vs. less	5	Lower	Higher	0.028	
IRMA [14]	From MA to OA (%)	AIIA vs. PI	2	5.2	14.9	<0.001	0.30 (0.14–0.61)

ABCD = Appropriate Blood Pressure Control in Diabetes Trial; ACEI = angiotensin-converting enzyme inhibitors; AIIA = Ang-II receptor antagonists; CA = calcium antagonists; HT = hypertensives; IRMA = Irbesartan in patients with type 2 diabetes and microalbuminuria; MA = microalbuminuria; NA = no albuminuria; NR = not reported; NS = nonsignificant; NT = normotensives; OA = overt albuminuria; OR = odds ratio; PI = placebo; RR = relative risk; SYST-EUR = Systolic Hypertension in Europe; UKPDS = United Kingdom Prospective Diabetes Study.

Table 57 Trials Comparing Regimens Based on Different Drug Classes: Renal Effects [191]

Trial	Treatment		Patients			Change in CrCl mL/min/1.73 m²			Renal failure % patients			Change in UAE %			New MA % patients			New OA % patients		
	Comparison	Years	n	BP	A	1	2	p-Value	1	2	p-Value	1	2	p-Value	1	2	p-Value	1	2	p-Value
UKPDS [23]	ACEI vs. BB	9	758	HT	–				1.3	1.4	NS				31*	26*	NS	5*	10*	NS
INSIGHT [20]	CA vs. D	3.5	1302	HT	–				0.6	1.1	NS							19	20	NS
ABCD-HT [34]	ACEI vs. CA	5	470	HT	–	−10	−8	NS				−0.3	+0.2	<0.05†	20	23	NS			
ABCD-NT [8]	ACEI vs. CA	5	354	NT	–	−7	−7	NS						NS			NS			
IDNT [12]	AIIA vs. CA	3	1146	HT	OA	−5.5‡	−6.8‡	NR	32.6	41.1	0.006	−33	−6	NR						
LIFE [25]	AIIA vs. BB	5	1195	HT	–													7	13	0.002

ABCD = Appropriate Blood Pressure Control in Diabetes Trial; ACEI, angiotensin-converting enzyme inhibitors; AIIA = Ang-II receptor antagonists; BB = beta-blocker; CA = calcium antagonists; CrCl = creatinine clearance; D = diuretics; HT = hypertensives; IDNT = Irbesartan Diabetic Nephropathy Trial; INSIGHT = International Nifedipine GITS Study: Intervention as a Goal in Hypertension Treatment; LIFE = Losartan Intervention for Endpoint Reduction; MA = microalbuminuria; NR = not reported; NS = nonsignificant; NT = normotensives; OA = overt albuminuria; UAE = urinary albumin excretion; UKPDS = United Kingdom Prospective Diabetes Study.

*MA and OA at the end of the study, independently of baselines.

1 and 2 indicate the first and the second treatments, respectively, of the column treatment comparison.

†Significance lost after 3.5 years.

‡Changes in creatinine clearance per year.

Table 58 Trials Comparing Different Antihypertensive Regimens: Worsening of Diabetes [191]

Trial	n	Treatment Comparison	Years	Variable	Treatment 1	2	p-Value
UKPDS [15]	1148	More vs. less	4	Final HbA1c (%)	7.2	7.2	NS
			8	Final HbA1c (%)	8.3	8.3	NS
MICROHOPE [11]	3577	ACEI vs. PI	4.5	ΔHbA1c (%)	2.2	2.0	NS
ABCD-HT [34]	470	More vs. less	5	Final HbA1c (%)	10.2	9.9	NS
ABCD-NT [8]	480	More vs. less	5	Final HbA1c (%)	10.5	10.5	NS
IRMA [14]	590	AIIA vs. PI	2	ΔHbA1c (%)	0.4	0.3	NS
UKPDS [23]	758	ACEI vs. BB	4	Final HbA1c (%)	7.0	7.5	<0.01
			8	Final HbA1c (%)	8.3	8.4	NS
			4	Added antidiabetics (%)	53	66	<0.005
			8	Added antidiabetics (%)	71	81	<0.05
ABCD-HT [34]	470	ACEI vs. CA	5	Final HbA1c (%)	10.0	10.0	NS
ABCD-NT [8]	480	ACEI vs. CA	5	Final HbA1c (%)	10.8	10.2	NS

ABCD = Appropriate Blood Pressure Control in Diabetes Trial; ACEI = angiotensin-converting enzyme inhibitors; AIIA = Ang-II receptor antagonist; BB = beta-blocker; CA = calcium antagonists; HT = hypertensives; IRMA = Irbesartan in patients with type 2 diabetes and microalbuminuria; NS = nonsignificant; NT = normotensives; PI = placebo; UKPDS = United Kingdom Prospective Diabetes Study.

Table 59 Trials Comparing Different Antihypertensive Regimens: New Onset Diabetes [191]

Trial	n	Treatment		New onset diabetes					RR (95% CI)
		Comparison	Years	% Patients		n/1000 patient-years		p-Value	
				1	2	1	2		
SHEP [29]	3209	D vs. Pl	3	8.6	7.5			NS	
HOPE [4]	5720	ACEI vs. Pl	4.5	3.6	5.4			<0.001	0.66 (0.51–0.85)
NORDIL [21]	10881	CA vs. D/BB	4.5			9.4	10.8	NS	0.87 (0.73–1.04)
STOP-2 [45]	1409	CA vs. D/BB	5			9.9	10.0	NS	0.97 (0.73–1.29)
INSIGHT [29]	6321	CA vs. D	3.5	4.3	5.6			<0.05	
NICS-EH [46]	414	CA vs. D	5	0	1.9			NS	
CAPPP [47]	10985	ACEI vs. D/BB	6.1					0.039	0.86 (0.74–0.99)
STOP-2 [45]	4418	ACEI vs. D/BB	5			9.6	10.0	NS	0.96 (0.72–1.27)
STOP-2 [45]	4401	ACEI vs. CA	5			9.6	9.9	NS	0.98 (0.74–1.31)
LIFE [48]	7998	AIIA vs. BB	4.8	6	8	13.0	17.4	0.001	0.75 (0.63–0.88)

ACEI = angiotensin-converting enzyme inhibitors; AIIA = Ang-II receptor antagonists; BB = beta-blocker; CA = calcium antagonists; CAPPP = Captopril Prevention Project; D = diuretics; HOPE = Heart Outcomes and Prevention Evaluation study; LIFE = Losartan Intervention for Endpoint Reduction; INSIGHT = International Nifedipine GITS Study; Intervention as a Goal in Hypertension Treatment; NICS-EH = National Intervention Cooperative Study in Elderly Hypertensives; NORDIL = Nordic Diltiazem Study; NS = nonsignificant; Pl = placebo; RR = relative risk; SHEP = Systolic Hypertension in the Elderly Program; STOP-2 = Swedish Trial in Old Patients with Hypertension-2.

Table 60 Primary Trials of Hypertension Control in Diabetes

Trial	Intervention and primary agents	Primary subgroup analysis	Total CV events		Total mortality		Microvascular endpoints	
			Relative risk	Absolute risk	Relative risk	Absolute risk	Relative risk	Absolute risk
SHEP	Thiazide diuretic vs. usual care	Subgroup	0.66 (0.46 to 0.94)	0.08 (0.01 to 0.14)	0.74 (0.46 to 1.18)	0.02 (−0.04 to 0.08)	Not reported	Not reported
SYST-EUR	CCB vs. placebo	Subgroup	0.38 (0.20 to 0.81)	0.08 (0.03 to 0.13)	0.59 (0.31 to 1.09)	0.05 (−0.01 to 0.09)	Not reported	Not reported
HOPE	ACEI vs. placebo	Subgroup	0.75 (0.64 to 0.88)	0.05 (0.02 to 0.07)	0.76 (0.63 to 0.92)	0.03 (0.01 to 0.05)	0.84 (0.71 to 0.99)	0.03 (0.00 to 0.05)
RENAAL	ARB vs. placebo	Primary	0.90*	0.02 (−0.03 to 0.07)	1.02 (0.73 to 1.19)	−0.01 (−0.05 to 0.03)	0.79 (0.66 to 0.95)[a]	0.04 (0.00 to 0.09)[a]
IPDM	ARB vs. placebo	Primary	Not reported	Not reported	Not reported	Not reported	0.30 (0.14 to 0.61)[b]	0.10 (0.04 to 0.16)[b]
HOT	Target DBP <80mm Hg or <90mm Hg; agents = felodipine, then ACEI or BB	Subgroup	0.49 (0.14 to 0.78)	0.05 (0.02 to 0.08)	0.56 (0.31 to 1.02)	0.03 (0.00 to 0.05)	Not reported	Not reported
UKPDS	Target BP <180/105mm Hg vs. <150/85mm Hg; agents = captopril or atenolol	Primary	0.66**	Not reported	0.82 (0.63 to 1.08)	0.04 (−0.01 to 0.09)	0.63 (0.44 to 0.89)	0.05 (0.01 to 0.09)

| ABCD | Target DBP 75 mm Hg vs. 80–89 mm Hg; agent = nisoldipine or enalapril | Primary | No difference | Not reported | 0.51 (0.27 to 0.97) | 0.05 (0.00 to 0.10) | No difference[c] | No difference |

Adapted from Vijan S, Hayward RA. Treatment of hypertension in type 2 diabetes melitus: Blood pressure goals, choice of agents and setting priorities in diabetes care. *Ann Intern Med* 2003; 138: 593–602.

ABCD = Appropriate Blood Pressure Control in Diabetes Trial; ACE = angiotensin-converting enzyme; ACEI = ACE inhibitor; ARB = angiotensin receptor blocker; BB = beta-blocker; BP = blood pressure; CV = cardiovascular; CCB = calcium channel blocker; DBP = diastolic BP; HOPE = Heart Outcomes and Prevention Evaluation study; HOT = Hypertension Optimal Treatment; IPDM = Irbesartan in Patients with Type 1 Diabetes and Microalbuminuria; RENAAL = Randomized Evaluation of NIDDM with the Ang-II antagonist Losartan; SHEP = Systolic Hypertension in the Elderly Program; SYST-EUR = Systolic Hypertension in Europe; UKPDS = United Kingdom Prospective Diabetes Study. Values in parentheses are 95% cIs.

[a]Renal outcomes (doubling of serum creatinine concentration and risk for ESRD).

[b]Comparison for 300-mg dose of irbesartan; 150-mg dose did not significantly reduce risk, risk is for progression of nephropathy.

[c]No combined endpoint reported. RRs for individual endpoints comparing intensive with moderate BP control were as follows; progression from normoalbuminuria to microalbuminuria, 1.38 (CI, 0.84–2.27); progression from microalbuminuria to overt albuminuria, 0.70 (CI, 0.36–1.36); retinopathy progression, 0.88 (CI, 0.68–1.15); and neuropathy progression, 1.30 (CI, 1.01–1.66).

*p > 0.2.

**p = 0.019.

Table 61 Effects of Different Drug Classes in Treatment of Hypertension in Diabetes

Trial	Intervention and primary agents	Primary subgroup analysis	Total CV events		Total mortality		Microvascular endpoints	
			Relative risk	Absolute risk	Relative risk	Absolute risk	Relative risk	Absolute risk
ABCD	Enalapril vs. nisoldipine	Primary	0.43 (0.25 to 0.73)	0.09 (0.04 to 0.13)	0.77 (0.36 to 1.67)	0.02 (−0.03 to 0.06)	Not reported	Not reported
FACET	Fosinopril vs. amlodipine	Primary	0.49 (0.26 to 0.95)	0.07 (0.01 to 0.13)	0.81 (0.22 to 3.02)	0.01 (−0.03 to 0.04)	Not reported	Not reported
CAPPP	Captopril vs. thiazide diuretic or BB	Subgroup	0.59 (0.38 to 0.91)	Not reported	0.54 (0.31 to 0.96)	Not reported	Not reported	Not reported
UKPDS	Captopril vs. atenolol	Primary	1.29 (0.92 to 1.81)	Not reported	1.14 (0.81 to 1.61)	−0.02 (−0.08 to 0.03)	1.29 (0.80 to 2.10)	−0.02 (−0.06 to 0.02)
NORDIL	Diltiazem vs. BB or diuretics	Subgroup	1.01 (0.66 to 1.53)	−0.01 (−0.06 to 0.04)	1.07(0.63 to 1.84)	−0.01 (−0.05 to 0.03)	Not reported	Not reported
INSIGHT	Nifedipine GITS vs. co-amilozide	Subgroup	0.99 (0.69 to 1.42)	0.00 (−0.03 to 0.03)	0.75† (0.52 to 1.09)	Not reported	Not reported	Not reported
STOP-2 (3 groups)	CCB vs. diuretics or BB	Subgroup	0.91 (0.66 to 1.26)	0.03 (−0.06 to 0.11)	0.79 (0.54 to 1.14)	0.05 (−0.03 to 0.12)	Not reported	Not reported
	ACEI vs. diuretics or BB		0.85 (0.62 to 1.18)	0.04 (−0.04 to 0.12)	0.88 (0.62 to 1.26)	0.03 (−0.05 to 0.10)	Not reported	Not reported
	ACEI vs. calcium-channel		0.94 (0.67 to 1.32)‡	0.01 (−0.07 to 0.10)	1.14 (0.78 to 1.67)	20.02 (−0.10 to 0.05)	Not reported	Not reported
IDNT (3 groups)	Irbesartan vs. placebo	Primary	0.91 (0.72 to 1.14)	0.02 (−0.04 to 0.07)	0.92 (0.69 to 1.23)	0.01 (−0.03 to 0.06)	0.80 (0.66 to 0.97)§	0.06 (0.01 to 0.12)
	Amlodipine vs. placebo		0.88 (0.69 to 1.12)	0.03 (−0.02 to 0.08)	0.88 (0.66 to 1.19)	0.02 (−0.03 to 0.06)	1.04 (0.86 to 1.25)§	−0.02 (−0.08 to 0.04)

IDNT (3 groups)							
Irbesartan vs. placebo	Primary	0.91 (0.72 to 1.14)	0.02 (−0.04 to 0.07)	0.92 (0.69 to 1.23)	0.01 (−0.03 to 0.06)	0.80 (0.66 to 0.97)§	0.06 (0.01 to 0.12)
Amlodipine vs. placebo		0.88 (0.69 to 1.12)	0.03 (−0.02 to 0.08)	0.88 (0.66 to 1.19)	0.02 (−0.03 to 0.06)	1.04 (0.86 to 1.25)§	−0.02 (−0.08 to 0.04)
Irbesartan vs. amlodipine		1.03 (0.81 to 1.31)	20.01 (−0.06 to 0.04)	1.04 (0.77 to 1.40)	0.00 (−0.05 to 0.04)	0.77 (0.63 to 0.93)§	0.09 (0.03 to 0.14)
LIFE							
Losartan vs. atenolol	Secondary	0.76 (0.58 to 0.98)	0.05 (0.01 to 0.10)	0.61 (0.45 to 0.84)	0.06 (0.02 to 0.10)	‖	‖
ALLHAT (2 groups)							
Lisinopril vs. chlorthalidone	Secondary	1.08 (1.00 to 1.17)	Not reported	1.02 (0.91 to 1.13)	Not reported	Not reported	Not reported
Amlodipine vs. chlorthalidone		1.06 (0.98 to 1.15)	Not reported	0.96 (0.87 to 1.07)	Not reported	Not reported	Not reported

Adapted from Vijan S, Hayward RA. Treatment of hypertension in type 2 diabetes mellitus: Blood pressure goals, choice of agents and setting priorities in diabetes care. *Ann Intern Med* 2003; 138: 593–602.

ABCD = Appropriate Blood Pressure Control in Diabetes; ACE = angiotensin-converting enzyme; ACEI = ACE inhibitor; ALLHAT = Antihypertensive and Lipid-Lowering Treatment to Prevent Heart Attack Trial; BB = beta-blocker; CAPPP = Captopril Prevention Project; CCB = calcium channel blocker; CV = cardiovascular; FACET = Fosinopril vs. Amlodipine Cardiovascular Events Trial; GITS = gastrointestinal therapeutic system; IDNT = Irbesartan Diabetic Nephropathy Trial; INSIGHT = International Nifedipine GITS Study: Intervention as a Goal in Hypertension Treatment; LIFE = Losartan Intervention for Endpoint Reduction; NORDIL = Nordic Diltiazem; STOP-2 = Swedish Trial in Old Patients with Hypertension-2; UKPDS = United Kingdom Prospective Diabetes Study.

*Values in parentheses are 95% CIs.

Brown M. Personal communication.

†The risk for MI in the ACEI group was 0.51 (CI, 0.28 to 0.92) compared with the CCB group.

§Composite microvascular endpoint = doubling of serum creatinine concentration + development of ESRD 1 all-cause mortality; individually, only doubling of the serum creatinine concentration was statistically significantly lower with irbesartan compared with either placebo or amlodipine.

‖Risk for microalbuminuria was lower in the losartan group, although the risk/hazard ratio is not presented (p = 0.002).

Table 62 RENAAL: Impact of Losartan on Primary Composite Endpoint*

	Losarltan[†] group		Placebo[†] group		p-Value	% Relative risk reduction (95% CI)
	n	%	n	%		
Primary composite endpoint*	327	43.5	359	47.1	0.02	16 (2 to 28)
Doubling of serum creatinine	162	21.6	198	26.0	0.006	25 (8 to 39)
ESRD	147	19.6	194	25.5	0.002	28 (11 to 42)
Death	158	21.0	155	2.03	0.88	−2 (−27 to 19)
ESRD or death	255	34.0	300	39.4	0.01	20 (5 to 32)
Doubling of serum creatinine and ESRD	226	30.1	263	34.5	0.01	21 (5 to 34)

Adapted from Brenner et al. *N Engl J Med* 2001; 345: 861–869.
AB = alpha-blocker; BB = beta-blocker; CCB = calcium channel blocker; ESRD = end-stage renal disease; RR = relative risk; RENAAL = Randomized Evaluation of NIDDM with the Ang-II antagonist Losartan; SCr = serum creatinine.
*Composite of a doubling of SCr, ESRD, or death.
[†]In combination with open-label diuretic, CCB, BB, AB, and/or centrally acting agent.

Table 63 RENAAL: Concurrent Use of DHP-CCB with ARB

- 66% of patients in losartan group were using DHP-CCB
- Risk of primary outcome ↓ 16.1% with DHP-CCB + losartan vs. 16% with losartan alone*
- Concurrent DHP-CCB + ARB is safe in patients with diabetic nephropathy
  - Provides benefit of additional BP lowering and does not have negative renal effects

ARB = angiotensin receptor blockers; DHP-CCB = dihydropyridine calcium channel blocker; ESRD = end-stage renal disease; RENAAL = Randomized Evaluation of NIDDM with the Ang-II antagonist Losartan; SCr = serum creatinine.
*Doubling of baseline SCr, ESRD, or death [212].

Table 64 Diabetic Nephropathy Meta-Analysis [221]

Key points
- One study in type 1 DM (Lewis et al.) demonstrates albuminuria reduction and renal function protection with ACEI vs. placebo
- One study in type 2 DM demonstrates renal function protection with ACEI vs. placebo (Lebovitz et al.)
- Two studies in type 2 DM demonstrate renal function protection with ARB vs. placebo or CCB vs. placebo (RENAAL, IDNT, respectively)

ACEI = angiotensin-converting enzyme inhibitor; ARB = angiotensin receptor blockers; CCB = calcium channel blocker; DM = diabetes mellitus; IDNT = Irbesartan Diabetes Nephrology Trial; RENAAL = Randomized Evaluation of NIDDM with the Ang-II antagonist Losartan.

Table 65 Trials Comparing Intensive vs. Regular or Active vs. Placebo BP Control: Effect on Albuminuria and Renal Function [221]

Trial	n	Years	Condition*	BP treatment	p-Value difference	Value	p-Value albuminuria	Renal value	p-Value function	Value
Lewis et al. [19]	409	3	DM1 ON	ACEi vs. PI	-3/-1		-0.3/NR‖	<0.001	-43%§	<0.007
Lebovitz et al. [23]	121	3	DM2 ON	ACEi vs. PI	-4.9	<0.001	7%/21%¶	NR	0.20/-0.33*	0.004
Nielsen et al. [24]	43	3	DM2 ON	ACEi vs. 3B+D	-4/-1		-55%/-15%**	<0.01	-0.59/-0.54#	NS
UKPDS 38 [26]	1148	9	DM2	Tight vs. regular	-10/-5		7%/6.6%¶	NS	No difference	
UKPDS 39 [27]	1148	9	DM2	ACEi vs. OB	1/2		5%/9%¶	NS	No difference	
Gaede et al. [31]	149	3.8	DM2 MA	Intensive vs. regular	-7/-3		10.9%/25%¶	<0.01	-	
ABCD [32]	470	5	DM2 MA ON	Intensive vs. moderate	-6/-8		16%/23%¶	NS	No difference	
ABCD [32]	470	5	DM2 MA ON	ACEi vs. CCB	No difference		19%/20%¶	NS	No difference	
MICBOHOPE [33]	3577	4.5	DM2 MA	ACEi vs. PI	-2.5/-1		6%/7%¶	0.07	-	
IRMA [44]	590	2	DM2 MA	ARB 300 vs. 150 vs. PI	141/144/144‡‡		5.2%/9.7%/14.9%¶	<0.001		
IDNT [45]	1715	2.6	DM2 ON	ARB vs. CCB vs. PI	98.0/98.3/101.3‡‡	0.001	-33%/-6%/-10%**		23%/20%§§	0.006/0.02
RENAAL [46]	1513	3.4	DM2 ON	ARB vs. PI	98.6/99.9‡‡		-35%/No change**	<0.001	16%§§	0.02

Renal function deterioration was not an endpoint in these trials.

ABCD = Appropriate Blood Pressure Control in Diabetes Trial; BP = blood pressure; DBP = diastolic BP; IDNT = Irbesartan Diabetes Nephrology Trial; IRMA = Irbesartan in patients with type 2 diabetes and microalbuminuria(AQS1); MBP = mean BP; NR = not reported; NS = not significant; RENAAL = Randomized Evaluation of NIDDM with the Ang-II antagonist Losartan; SBP = systolic BP; UKPDS = United Kingdom Prospective Diabetes Study.

*DM1/DM2 = DM type 1 or 2; MA = microalbuminuria, subclinical nephropathy; ON = overt nephropathy.

†ACEi = angiotensin-converting enzyme inhibitors; ARB = angiotensin receptor blockers; BB = beta-blockers; CCB = calcium channel blockers; D = diuretics; PI = placebo plus nonstudy drugs if needed (for IRMA the two doses of 300 and 150mg are shown, for IDNT the groups of active drugs are two).

‡Difference of SBP/DBPmm Hg of the first treatment from the second is shown, (−) = less BP in the first treatment, if one number is shown it represents MBP.

§Percent reduction in risk of doubling of serum creatinine.

‖Absolute decrease in g/day during follow-up.

¶Percentage of patients progressing to overt nephropathy.

#Decrease in GFR mL/min/1.73 m²/month.

**Percentage reduction of proteinuria.

††Median SBP during follow-up.

‡‡Median MBP during follow-up.

§§Percent reduction in risk of approaching the composite endpoints of the first treatment vs. second or third.

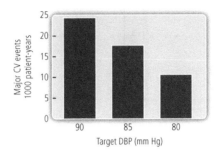

Figure 68 Major CV Events in Patients with Diabetes in Relation to TBP Groups.

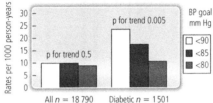

From Hanson L, Zanchelli A, Carruthers SG, et al. Effects of intensive blood-pressure lowering and low-dose aspirin in patients with hypertension: Principal results of the Hypertension Optimal Treatment (HOT) randomised trial. *Lancet* 1998; 351: 1755–1762, with permission.

BP = blood pressure; CV = cardiovascular; HOT = hypertension optimal treatment.

Figure 69 Large Clinical Trials in Hypertension and Type 2 Diabetes or Impaired Glucose Metabolism [191].

Tight vs. less tight BP control		
Endpoint	Relative risk	9–5% CI
Any endpoint	0.76	0.62–0.92
Diabetes death	0.68	0.49–0.94
Any death	0.82	0.63–1.08
MI	0.79	0.59–1.07
Stroke	0.56	0.35–0.89
PAD	0.51	0.19–1.37
Microvascular disease	0.63	0.44–0.89
n = 758 vs. 390.		

From Ref. [18], with permission.
MI = myocardial infarction; PAD = peripheral arterial disease.

Figure 70 UK Prospective Diabetes Study.

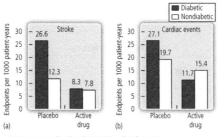

CCB treatment reduced stroke 69% (a) and cardiac events
57% (b) in diabetic hypertensives
Benefit of active treatment began soon after randomization, when
most patients were still on monotherapy with nitrendipine.
CCB = calcium channel blocker

Adapted from Prisant LM, Louard RJ: Controversies surrounding the treatment
of the hypertensive patient with diabetes. *Curr Hypertens Rep* 1999;
1: 512–520, with permission.

Figure 71 SYST-EUR: Effect of Active Treatment in Diabetic (*n* = 492) and Nondiabetic (*n* = 4203) Hypertensive Patients (n = 4695). Median Follow-up Was 2 Years.

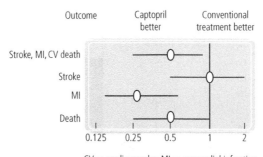

CV = cardiovascular; MI = myocardial infarction.

Figure 72 CAPPP: Patients with Diabetes [133].

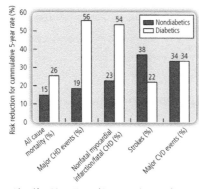

Adapted from Prisant LM, Louard RJ: Controversies surrounding
the treatment of the hypertensive patient with diabetes.
Curr Hypertens Rep 1999; 1: 512–520, with permission.

BB = beta blocker; CHD = coronary heart disease; CVA = cerebrovascular accidents;
CVD = cardiovascular disease.

Figure 73 SHEP: Relative Risk Reduction of Endpoints by Active Treatment vs. Placebo for Diabetic (*n* = 583) and Nondiabetic (*n* = 4149) Patients by Treatment Group. Mean Follow-up Was 4.5 Years.

267

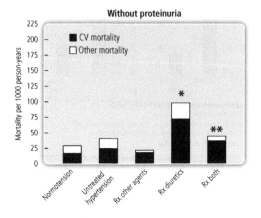

Without proteinuria

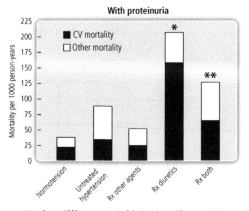

With proteinuria

Mortality per 1000 person-years in diabetic patients without proteinuria
and with proteinuria according to hypertension status and type of antihypertensive
treatment (Rx) during each year of follow-up. Diuretics increased
CV mortality and total mortality compared to other antihypertensive drugs
or no treatment.
*p<0.025; **p<0.025 vs. treatment with diuretics alone.
From Ref. [94].
CV = cardiovascular.

Figure 74 Hypertensive Diabetics: Mortality, CHD, and Antihypertensive Therapy [94].

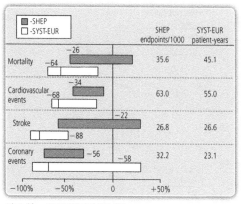

Adapted from *NEJM* 1999; 340: 677–684.

CV = cardiovascular; SHEP = Systolic Hypertension in the Elderly Program;
SYST-EUR = Systolic Hypertension in Europe.

Figure 75 Diabetic Patient.

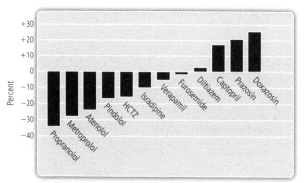

The effects on insulin sensitivity index of 3–6 months of antihypertensive monotherapy
given to groups of hypertensive patients.

Adapted from Lithell HO. Effect of antihypertensive drugs on insulin, glucose, and lipid
metabolism. *Diabetes Care* 1991; 14: 203–209.
HCTZ = hydrochlorothiazide.

Figure 76 Insulin Sensitivity and Antihypertensive Drugs.

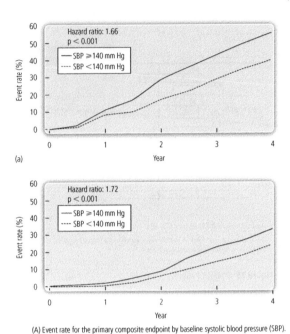

(a)

(b)

(A) Event rate for the primary composite endpoint by baseline systolic blood pressure (SBP).
(B) Event rate for end-stage renal disease (ESRD) alone by baseline SBP.

Figure 77 BP Level Effects on Type 2 DM Nephropathy [212].

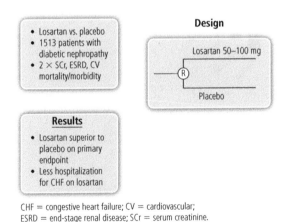

CHF = congestive heart failure; CV = cardiovascular;
ESRD = end-stage renal disease; SCr = serum creatinine.

Figure 78 RENAAL.

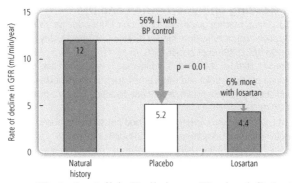

(a)

ARB = Ang-II receptor blocker; BP = blood pressure; GFR = glomerular filtration rate.
Adapted from Bakris et al. *Am J Kidney Dis* 2000; 36: 646–661; Brenner et al.
N Engl J Med 2001; 345: 861–869.

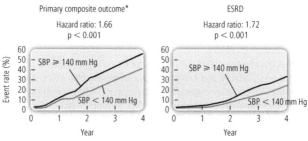

(b)

BP = blood pressure; ESRD = end-stage renal disease; SBP = systolic blood pressure.

Figure 79 (a) RENAAL: Effects of BP Control, ARB on GFR Decline. (b) RENAAL: Primary Composite Outcome and ESRD for Baseline SBP ⩾ 140 vs. < 140 mm Hg.

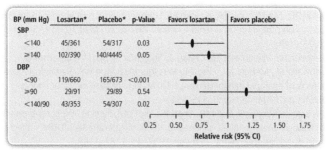

Comparison of ESRD outcomes in the groups randomized to losartan (given as losartan potassium) vs. placebo at different achieved mean BPs up until primary composite event.
*Data are number of events/total number of patients.
BP = blood pressure; DBP = diastolic BP; SBP = Systolic BP.

Figure 80 ESRD outcomes in RENAAL.

Further Reading on Hypertension and DM

1. K/DOQI clinical practice guidelines for chronic kidney disease: Evaluation, classification and stratification. Kidney Disease Outcome Quality Initiative. *Am J Kidney Dis* 2002; 39(suppl 2): S46–S75.
2. Miettinen H, Haffner SM, Lehto S, Ronnemaa T, Pyorala K, Laakso M. Proteinuria predicts stroke and other atherosclerotic vascular disease events in nondiabetic and non-insulin-dependent diabetic subjects. *Stroke* 1996; 27: 2033–2039.
3. Weir MR. Diabetes and hypertension: Blood pressure control and consequences. *Am J Hypertens* 1999; 12(suppl): 170S–178S.
4. Bidani AK, Schwartz MM, Lewis EJ. Renal autoregulation and vulnerability to hypertensive injury in remnant kidney. *Am J Physiol* 1987; 252: F1003–F1010.
5. Ritz E, Keller C, Bergis K, Strojek K. Pathogenesis and course of renal disease in IDDM/NIDDM: Differences and similarities. *Am J Hypertens* 1997; 10(suppl): 202S–207S.
6. Ismail N, Becker B, Strzelczyk P, Ritz E. Renal disease and hypertension in non-insulin-dependent diabetes mellitus. *Kidney Int* 1999; 55: 1–28.
7. Waeber B, Feihl F, Ruilope LM. Diabetes and hypertension. *Blood Press* 2001; 10: 311–321.
8. Parving HH. Hypertension and diabetes: The scope of the problem. *Blood Press* 2001; 10(suppl 2): 25–31.
9. US Renal Data System: USRDS 1999 Annual Data Report. National Institute of Diabetes and Digestive and Kidney Disease, Bethesda, MD, 1999: 25–38.
10. Bretzel RG. Effects of antihypertensive drugs on renal function in patients with diabetic nephropathy. *Am J Hypertens* 1997; 10(suppl): 208S–217S.
11. Lewis EJ, Hunsicker LG, Bain RP, Rohde RD. The effect of angiotensin-converting-enzyme inhibition on diabetic nephropathy. The Collaborative Study Group. *N Engl J Med* 1993; 329: 1456–1462.
12. Kasiske BL, Kalil RS, Ma JZ, Liao M, Keane WF. Effect of antihypertensive therapy on the kidney in patients with diabetes: A meta-regression analysis. *Ann Intern Med* 1993; 118: 129–138.
13. Weidmann P, Schneider M, Bohlen L. Therapeutic efficacy of different antihypertensive drugs in human diabetic nephropathy: An updated meta-analysis. *Nephrol Dial Transplant* 1995; 10: 39–45.
14. Maki DD, Ma JZ, Louis TA, Kasiske BL. Long-term effects of antihypertensive agents on proteinuria and renal function. *Arch Intern Med* 1995; 155: 1073–1080.
15. Lebovitz HE, Wiegmann TB, Cnaan A, Shahinfar S, Sica DA, Broadstone V, Schwartz SL, Mengel MC, Segal R, Versaggi JA, Bolton WK. Renal protective effects of enalapril in hypertensive NIDDM: Role of baseline albuminuria. *Kidney Int* 1994; 45(suppl): S150–S155.
16. Nielsen FS, Rossing P, Gall MA, Skott P, Smidt UM, Parving HH. Long-term effect of lisinopril and atenolol on kidney function in hypertensive NIDDM subjects with diabetic nephropathy. *Diabetes* 1997; 46: 1182–1188.
17. UK Prospective Diabetes Study (UKPDS) Group. Intensive blood-glucose control with sulphonylureas or insulin compared with conventional treatment and risk of complications in patients with type 2 diabetes (UKPDS 33). *Lancet* 1998; 352: 837–853.

18. UK Prospective Diabetes Study Group. Tight blood pressure control and risk of macrovascular and microvascular complications in type 2 diabetes: UKPDS 38. *BMJ* 1998; 317: 703–713.

19. UK Prospective Diabetes Study Group. Efficacy of atenolol and captopril in reducing risk of macrovascular and microvascular complications in type 2 diabetes. UKPDS 39. *BMJ* 1998; 317: 713–720.

20. Hansson L, Zanchetti A, Carruthers SG, Dahlof B, Elmfeldt D, Julius S, Menard I, Rahn KH, Wedel H, Westerling S. Effects of intensive blood pressure lowering and low-dose aspirin in patients with hypertension: Principal results of the Hypertension Optimal Treatment (HOT) randomized trial. *Lancet* 1998; 351: 1755–1762.

21. Guidelines Subcommittee: 1999 World Health Organization—International Society of Hypertension Guidelines for the Management of Hypertension. *J Hypertens* 1999; 17: 151–183.

22. Kjeldsen SE, Os I, Farsang C, Mallion JM, Hansson L, Sleight P. Treatment of hypertension in patients with type-2 diabetes mellitus. *J Hypertens* 2000; 18: 1345–1346.

23. Gaede P, Vedel P, Parving HH, Pedersen O. Intensified multifactorial intervention in patients with type 2 diabetes mellitus and microalbuminuria: The Steno type 2 randomized study. *Lancet* 1999; 353: 617–622.

24. Estacio RO, Jeffers BW, Gifford N, Schrier RW. Effect of blood pressure control on diabetic microvascular complications in patients with hypertension and type 2 diabetes. *Diabetes Care* 2000; 23(suppl 2): B54–B64.

25. Heart Outcomes Prevention Evaluation (HOPE) Study Investigators. Effects of ramipril on cardiovascular and microvascular outcomes in people with diabetes mellitus: Results of the HOPE study and MICRO-HOPE substudy. *Lancet* 2000; 355: 253–259.

26. Velussi M, Brocco E, Frigato F, Zolli M, Muollo B, Maioli M, Carraro A, Tonolo G, Fresu P, Cernigoi AM, Fioretto P, Nosadini R. Effects of cilazapril and amlodipine on kidney function in hypertensive NIDDM patients. *Diabetes* 1996; 45: 216–222.

27. Bakris GL, Copley JB, Vicknair N, Sadler R, Leurgans S. Calcium channel blockers versus other antihypertensive therapies on progression of NIDDM associated nephropathy. *Kidney Int* 1996; 50: 1641–1650.

28. Viberti G, Mogensen CE, Groop LC, Pauls JF. Effect of captopril on progression to clinical proteinuria in patients with insulin-dependent diabetes mellitus and microalbuminuria. European Microalbuminuria Captopril Study Group. *J Am Med Assoc* 1994; 271: 275–279.

29. EUCLID Study Group. Randomised placebo-controlled trial of lisinopril in normotensive patients with insulin-dependent diabetes and normoalbuminuria or microalbuminuria. *Lancet* 1997; 349: 1787–1792.

30. Ravid M, Brosh D, Levi Z, Bar-Dayan Y, Ravid D, Rachmani R. Use of enalapril to attenuate decline in renal function in normotensive, normoalbuminuric patients with type 2 diabetes mellitus. A randomised, controlled trial. *Ann Intern Med* 1998; 128: 982–988.

31. Kon V, Fogo A, Ichikava I. Bradykinin causes selective efferent arteriolar dilation during angiotensin I converting enzyme inhibition. *Kidney Int* 1993; 44: 545–550.

32. Price DA, De'Oliveira JM, Fisher ND, Hollenberg NK. Renal hemodynamic response to an angiotensin II antagonist, eprosartan, in healthy men. *Hypertension* 1997; 30: 240–246.

33. Pitt B, Poole-Wilson PA, Segal R, Martinez FA, Dickstein K, Camm AJ, Konstam MA, Riegger G, Klinger GH, Neaton J, Sharma D, Thiyagarajan B. Effect of losartan compared with captopril on mortality in patients with symptomatic heart failure: Randomized trial—the Losartan Heart Failure Survival Study ELITE II. *Lancet* 2000; 355: 1582–1587.

34. Muirhead N, Feagan BF, Mahon J, Lewanczuk RZ, Rodger NW, Botteri F, Oddou-Stock P, Pecher E, Cheung R. The effects of valsartan and captopril on reducing microalbuminuria in patients with type 2 diabetes mellitus: A placebo-controlled trial. *Curr Ther Res* 1999; 60: 650–660.

35. Lacourciere Y, Belanger A, Godin C, Halle JP, Ross S, Wright N, Marion J. Long-term comparison of losartan and enalapril on kidney function in hypertensive type 2 diabetics with early nephropathy. *Kidney Int* 2000; 58: 762–769.

36. Parving HH, Lehnert H, Brochner-Mortensen J, Gomis R, Andersen S, Arner P. The effect of irbesartan on the development of diabetic nephropathy in patients with type 2 diabetes. *N Engl J Med* 2001; 345: 870–878.

37. Lewis EJ, Hunsicker LG, Clarke WR, Berl T, Pohl MA, Lewis JB, Ritz E, Atkins RC, Rohde R, Raz I. Renoprotective effect of the angiotensin-receptor antagonist irbesartan in patients with nephropathy due to type 2 diabetes. *N Engl J Med* 2001; 345: 851–860.

Selection of Therapy Based on Subsets of Hypertension

Selection of antihypertensive therapy based on the subsets of hypertension approach allows for the categorization of drugs into three groups: drugs of choice, alternatives, and contraindicated drugs. The first column refers to the diseases that are often associated with hypertension. A drug should be selected considering all disease factors. Drugs are listed in alphabetical order, not by preference, in each column.

Key code:
AB = Alpha blocker
ABB = Alpha-/beta-blocker
ACEI = Angiotensin-converting enzyme inhibitor
ARB = Angiotensin receptor blocker
BB = Beta blocker
CAA = Central alpha-agonist
CCA = Common carotid artery
CCB = Calcium channel blocker
D = diuretic
DHP = Dihydropyridine
DV = Direct vasodilator
Non-DHP = Nondihydropyridine
SARA = Serum aldosterone receptor antagonist
RI = Renin inhibitor

Concomitant condition	Drug(s) of Choice	Alternatives	Relative or absolute contraindication
Abnormal vascular compliance	ACEI ARB CCB RI	D	Selective BB Nonselective BB
Addictive syndromes: withdrawal from opiates, tobacco, alcohol	CAA (clonidine)		Nonselective BB
Angina: mixed	BB without ISA CCB	AB ABB ACEI ARB CAA D RI	BB with ISA DV
Angina: obstructive	BB without ISA CCB	AB ABB ACEI ARB CAA D RI	BB with ISA DV

(Continued)

Concomitant condition	Drug(s) of Choice	Alternatives	Relative or absolute contraindication
Angina: vasospastic	CCB	AB ABB ACEI ARB CAA D RI	BB with ISA BB without ISA DV
Anxiety/stress	CCA BB without ISA		
Cerebrovascular disease, prevention of CVA and post-CVA	ACEI ARB CCB D RI	AB ABB CAA DV	BB without ISA BB with ISA
Chronic liver disease	AB BB CAA CCB	ABB ACEI ARB D RI	Methyldopa
CHF systolic	ABB ACEI ARB BB without ISA D SARA	CCA DHP-CCB RI	AB BB with ISA Non–DHP-CCB
Cognitive dysfunction and prevention of vascular dementia	ACEI ARB CCB (DHP) Indapamide	D RI	BB
CHD high-risk	ABB ACEI ARB BB CCB	AB CAA D RI	DV
Cyclosporine-induced hypertension	CCB		
Depression	AB ACEI ARB CCB	D DV	ABB BB CAA Reserpine
Diabetes mellitus	ACEI ARB CCB RI	ABB AB BB with ISA CAA DV Indapamide SARA	BB without ISA Thiazide diuretics
Diabetic diarrhea and gustatory sweating	Clonidine		

Concomitant condition	Drug(s) of Choice	Alternatives	Relative or absolute contraindication
Diastolic dysfunction	ABB ACEI ARB BB with ISA CCB	BB without ISA CAA D (caution with volume)* RI	AB DV
Dyslipidemia	ABB AB ACEI ARB CAA CCB RI	BB with ISA DV Indapamide	BB without ISA D (thiazides)
Essential tremor	BB without ISA CAA		
Exercise	ACEI ARB CAA CCB-DHP RI	AB ABB BB with ISA D DV	BB w?ithout ISA
GERD	ACEI ARB RI	AB ABB BB CCA D	CCB (lower LES tone)
Glaucoma	ABB BB CAA D	BB with ISA	
Homocysteinemia	ACEI ARB CCB RI	ABB CAA DV	BB D
Hyperuricemia	ARB	AB ACEI CAA CCB DV RI	ABB BB D
Hyperthyroidism	BB	CAA	
LVH	ACEI ARB CAA CCB Indapamide RI	AB ABB BB without ISA D	BB with ISA DV
Menopausal symptoms	CAA	BB without ISA	DV
Metabolic syndrome	ACEI ARB CCB RI	AB ABB CAA Indapamide SARA	BB† D‡

(Continued)

Concomitant condition	Drug(s) of Choice	Alternatives	Relative or absolute contraindication
Microvascular angina	CCB	AB ACEI ARB CAA RI	ABB BB
Migraine headache (prophylactic)	ACEI ARB BB without ISA CCB CAA	AB A BB RI	DV
Mitral valve prolapse	BB without ISA CCB-non-DHP CAA	ABB ACEI ARB RI	AB D DV
Obesity	ACEI ARB CAA CCB RI	ABB AB D DV	BB
Obstructive airway disease	AB ACEI ARB CAA CCB RI	D DV	ABB BB
Peptic ulcer disease	CCB CAA	AB ABB ACEI ARB BB D DV	Reserpine
Peripheral vascular disease	CCB (DHP)	AB ACEI ARB CAA D DV RI	ABB BB
Post-MI: non-Q-wave	ACEI ARB BB without ISA CCB (non-DHP)	AB ABB CAA CCB (DHP) D RI	BB with ISA DV
Post-MI: Q-wave normal LV function	ABB ACEI ARB BB SARA	CAA CCB RI	BB with ISA D DV

Concomitant condition	Drug(s) of Choice	Alternatives	Relative or absolute contraindication
Pregnancy (first and second trimester)	Clonidine Methyldopa Hydralazine	CCB (DHP)	ABB ACEI ARB BB D RI
Premature ventricular contractions	ABB ACEI ARB BB	AB CAA CCB (DHP) RI	BB with ISA D DV
Prostatism	AB	BB	
Proteinuria	ACEI ARB RI SARA	CCB D ABB	
Pulmonary hypertension	CCB (DHP) DV	ACEI ARB	BB
Raynaud's phenomenon	CCB (DHP)	AB ACEI ARB	BB ABB
Renal insufficiency	ACEI ARB CCB RI	ABB AB BB DV Indapamide Loop D	Thiazide D
Renin Status: PRA > 0.65 = HRH and PRA < 0.65 = LRH			
High renin (HRH)	ACEI ARB RI	BB	D
Low renin (LRH)	CCB SARA	D AB CAA	ACEI ARB BB RI
Renovascular Disease (renal artery disease, bilateral)	CAA CCB AB	ABB BB	ACEI[§‖] ARB[§‖] RI[§‖]
Sexual dysfunction	ARB ACEI CCB RI	AB DV	ABB BB CAA D Reserpine
Sick sinus syndrome or atrioventricular (AV) block	ACEI ARB CCB (DHP) RI	AB D DV	ABB BB CAA CCB (non-DHP) Reserpine
Sinusitis/rhinitis	CAA	ARB ACEI AB CCB	BB Reserpine

(Continued)

Concomitant condition	Drug(s) of Choice	Alternatives	Relative or absolute contraindication
Supraventricular tachycardia	BB without ISA CAA CCB (non-DHP)	ABB AB ACEI ARB CCB (DHP) D RI	DV
Toxemia of pregnancy (eclampsia)	CAA[#] CCB (non-DHP)[#] Hydralazine Methyldopa	AB[#] ABB[#] ACEI[#] ARB[#] RI[#]	BB[#] D[#]
Use of NSAIDs	CCB	ABB AB ACEI ARB BB CAA D RI	DV
Volume overload	D SARA	ACEI ARB CCB	DV

*Watch out for volume depletion, especially hot weather.
[†]BB if compelling indications.
[‡]D as required for BP control or compelling indications.
[§]Drugs of choice for unilateral RAS.
[||]Use with caution, but can be highly effective. Need to monitor K+ and creatinine, especially initially.
[#]These products are not approved for use during pregnancy.

Demographics and Antihypertensive Drugs

Demographic profile	Drug(s) of choice	Alternatives	Relative or absolute contraindication
Young patient (<55 years)	ACEI* ARB* CCB RI*	ABB AB CAA	BB* D*
Elderly patient (>55 years)	ACEI ARB CCB CAA RI	AB ABB	BB D DV
Black patient	ACEI ARB CCB CAA Indapamide	AB ABB D CV RI	BB
White patient	ACEI ARB CCB CAA Indapamide RI	AB ABB	BB D

*Avoid during pregnancy.

Resistant Hypertension

Definition
The patient's DBP remains above 90 mm Hg despite full doses of three appropriate antihypertensive medications and has been documented on at least two separate visits in the office under proper conditions and out of the office with home BP monitoring or 24-hour ABPM.

Causes
An inadequate drug regimen and patient noncompliance account for 70% of total causes.

1. Patient noncompliance to therapy
2. Inadequate drug regimen
   (a) Drug doses too low
   (b) Drug interactions or inappropriate combinations—antihypertensive agents (two central alpha-agonists, two ACEI or BBs, and central alpha-agonist with BB) or AB with central alpha-agonist
   (c) Rapid metabolism or inactivation (hydralazine)
   (d) Other drug interactions and interfering agents.
       (i) Corticosteroids and anabolic steroids
       (ii) Aldosterone (florinef)
       (iii) Sympathomimetics and phenylpropanolamine
       (iv) NSAIDs (ACEIs, BBs, diuretics, ARBs)
       (v) Antidepressants—tricyclics and central alpha-agonist
       (vi) Decongestants—pseudoephedrine and nasal sprays
       (vii) Excess alcohol ingestion (over 30 mL/day) for 7–10 weeks
       (viii) Excess caffeine ingestion (variable)
       (ix) Excess tobacco use (variable)
       (x) Oral contraceptives
       (xi) Erythropoietin
       (xii) Cyclosporine
       (xiii) MAO inhibitors and phenothiazines
       (xiv) Cocaine and amphetamines
       (xv) Appetite suppressants
       (xvi) Omeprazole (Prilosec).
   (See other drugs listed in Secondary Hypertension section.)
3. Volume overload states
   (a) Inadequate diuretic therapy
   (b) High sodium intake (10–15 g/day)
   (c) Secondary to BP reduction with some agents (direct vasodilators) and some BBs pseudotolerance caused by reflex volume overload, tachycardia, or vasoconstriction
   (d) Nephrosclerosis and CRF.
4. Obesity and rapid weight gain
5. Secondary hypertension (10%)
   (See other drugs listed in Secondary Hypertension section.)
   (a) Renovascular hypertension (most common)
   (b) Renal insufficiency and failure

   (c) Pheochromocytoma

   (d) Primary aldosteronism and low renin hypertension with pseudo hyperaldosteronism which responds to SARA. Patients have low PRA and normal serum aldosterone levels.

   (e) Cushing's syndrome

   (f) Coarctation of aorta

   (g) Sleep apnea

   (h) Thyroid disease

   (i) Hypercalcemia

   (j) Licorice intoxication (in chewing tobacco).

6. Pseudoresistance

   (a) Using regular adult cuff on obese arm

   (b) White coat hypertension

   (c) Pseudohypertension in elderly.

7. Miscellaneous

   (a) Chronic anxiety, panic attacks

   (b) Chronic pain

   (c) Diffuse vasoconstriction (arteritis)

   (d) Insulin resistance

   (e) Inappropriate diuretic in patients with renal insufficiency and creatinine clearance below 30 cc/min (i.e., thiazide).

ISH in the Elderly

- All randomized placebo-controlled trials of antihypertensive therapy have demonstrated dramatic reductions in CV and cerebrovascular morbidity and mortality in the treatment of ISH in the elderly with a wide variety of drugs. The DHP-CCB and diuretics (+BBs) and ACEIs are efficacious as initial and in combination along with ARBs. The BB however does not reduce total mortality, CV mortality, CHD, or MI more than placebo. The reduction in CVA with BB is also less than that with other antihypertensive agents (Table 66 and Figures 81–83).
- ISH is defined as SBP >160 mm Hg with a DBP <95 mm Hg (except in SHEP where DBP <90 mm Hg).

Table 66 Patient Status at 12 Months in the Merck-Medco Study

Drug (number of patients)	No. of Patients	Patients remaining on initial therapy %	Patients switching to new therapy %
AT1 receptor blocker (5567)	64	7	29
Angiotensin-converting enzyme inhibitor (5842)	58	9	33
Calcium channel blocker (5094)	50	9	41
Beta-blocker (4994)	43	7	50
Diuretic (5226)	38	6	56

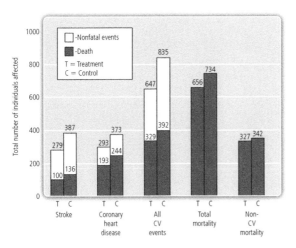

Entry BP average 174/83 mm Hg. Mean difference in treated and control: 10.4/4.1 mm Hg. Median follow-up 3.8 years. Summary results of 15 693 patients with ISH (8 trials).

Reprinted from Staessen JA, Gasowski J, Wang JG, et al. Risks of untreated and treated isolated systolic hypertension in the elderly. *Lancet* 2000; 355: 865–872, with permission.

BP = blood pressure; CV = cardiovascular.

Figure 81 ISH in the Elderly: Drug Treatment Categories Incidence of CV Events per 1000 Patient-Years.

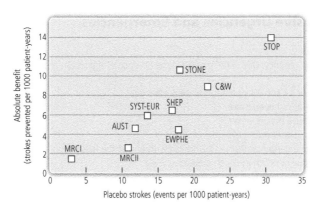

Absolute benefit of antihypertensive treatment in terms of stroke reduction is related to the stroke risk (stroke events in the placebo group) of the patient population. Each point represents data from a major placebo-controlled outcome trial.

Adapted from Meredith, P. Do pharmacologic differences among antihypertensive agents point to clinical benefits. *Am J Cardiol* 1999; 84: 22S–27S.

AUST = Australian; EWPHE = European Working Party on High Blood Pressure in the Elderly; MRC I and II = Medical Research Council I and II; SHEP = Systolic Hypertension in the Elderly program; STONE = Shanghai Trial of Nifedipine in the Elderly; STOP = The Swedish Trial in Old Patients; SYST-EUR = Systolic Hypertension in Europe.

Figure 82 ISH in the Elderly. Stroke Reduction: Absolute Benefit.

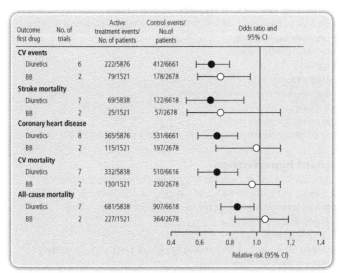

Stroke reduction: absolute benefit of antihypertension. Absolute benefit of antihypertensive treatment in terms of stroke reduction is related to the stroke risk (stroke events in the placebo group) of the patient population. Each point represents data from a major placebo-controlled outcome trial.

Adapted from Meredith, P. Do pharmacologic differences among antihypertensive agents point to clinical benefits? *Am J Cardiol* 1999; 84: 22S–27S.

BB = beta-blocker; CV = cerebrovascular.

Figure 83 Meta-Analysis of Prospective Clinical Trials in Elderly Patients with Hypertension According to First-Line Treatment Strategy.

Hypertensive Urgencies and Emergencies

Definitions
1. Hypertensive urgency: DBP ≥120 mm Hg in the absence of significant end-organ damage
   (a) Grade I or II Keith–Wagener fundoscopic changes
   (b) Postoperative hypertension
   (c) Preoperative hypertension
   (d) Pain- or stress-induced hypertension.
2. Hypertensive emergency: DBP >120 mm Hg with one of the following:
   (a) Intracranial hemorrhage or thrombotic CVA
   (b) Subarachnoid bleed
   (c) Hypertensive encephalopathy
   (d) Acute aortic dissection
   (e) Acute pulmonary edema, acute CHF, and acute LV failure
   (f) Eclampsia (toxemia of pregnancy)
   (g) Pheochromocytoma hypertensive crisis
   (h) Grade III or IV Keith–Wagener fundoscopic changes
   (i) Acute renal insufficiency or failure
   (j) Myocardial insufficiency syndromes (unstable angina pectoris, acute MI)
   (k) Hematuria.

Precipitating factors in hypertensive crisis
1. Accelerated sudden rise in BP in a patient with preexisting essential hypertension
2. Renovascular hypertension
3. Glomerulonephritis—acute
4. Eclampsia
5. Pheochromocytoma
6. Antihypertensive withdrawal syndromes
7. Head injuries
8. Renin-secreting tumors
9. Ingestion of catecholamine precursors in patients taking MAO inhibitors

Malignant hypertension
1. Fundoscopic changes of necrotizing arteriolitis (hemorrhages, exudates), disc edema, and papilledema (visual changes, nausea, vomiting, headache, confusion, somnolence, stupor, neurologic deficits, seizures, coma)
2. Hypertensive encephalopathy
3. DBP >120 mm Hg with TOD
4. Decreasing renal function, proteinuria, hematuria, casts, oliguria, azotemia
5. Microangiopathic hemolytic anemia
6. LV failure and CHF and pulmonary edema.

Factors that constitute malignant hypertension
1. Absolute level of BP
2. Rate of development of BP
3. Type and level of vasoactive substances
4. Presence of end-organ damage.

Pathophysiology (Figure 84)

Treatment: general principles
Balance the benefit of immediate reduction in BP to prevent irreversible organ damage against the risk of marked decrease in perfusion and blood flow to vital organs, particularly to the brain, myocardium, and kidney, or regional blood flow changes within each organ (Figure 84).

1. Reduce the DBP to no less than 100 mm Hg, the SBP to no less than 160 mm Hg, or the MAP to no less than 120 mm Hg the first 24–48 hours except in hypertensive emergencies as indicated. Attempt an average reduction of 25% below baseline BP or to the minimum BP indicated earlier.
2. Acute lowering of BP may decrease blood flow to the brain, myocardium, and kidneys.
3. Attempt to establish normotension within a few days.
4. Avoid hypotension or normotension during first 24 hours except in hypertensive emergencies as indicated.
5. Parenteral or oral antihypertensives are appropriate depending on the clinical setting.
6. Begin concomitant long-term therapy soon after the initial emergency treatment.
7. Assess volume status of patient. Do not overuse diuretics, and avoid sodium restriction in the early phases of malignant hypertension. Volume expansion is often indicated.
8. Reflex volume retention may occur after a few days on some nondiuretic antihypertensive drugs, such as BBs and direct vasodilators—a concept of pseudotolerance.

Treatment: rapidity of onset
1. Aortic dissection
2. Pulmonary edema (caution in acute MI)
3. Malignant hypertension in certain clinical settings with encephalopathy, papilledema—controlled reduction
4. Subarachnoid bleed or intracerebral bleed—controversial.

Nontreatment of BP may be appropriate.

Treatment: choice of drug
1. Rapidity of BP drop desired and level of BP
2. Duration of action of antihypertensive agent
3. Hemodynamic effect of drug (i.e., use in the presence of pulmonary edema, CHF, angina, MI, CVA, aortic dissection, renal insufficiency)
4. Effect on RBF, GFR, and function
5. Potential and known adverse effects.

Acute nonparenteral therapy
Table 67 summarizes acute nonparenteral therapy.

Acute parenteral therapy
Table 68 summarizes acute parenteral therapy.

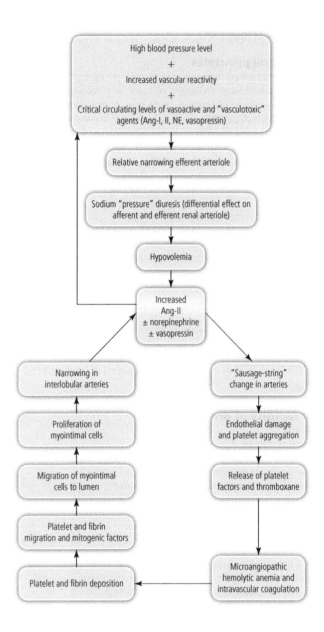

Figure 84 Pathophysiology.

Table 67 Acute Nonparenteral Therapy

Drugs	Route	Onset	Effect	Duration	Dosage
Clonidine	Oral	30 minutes	1–2 hours	8–12 hours	0.1–0.2 mg initial then 0.05–0.1 mg q hour to maximum 0.8 mg
Nitroglycerin	Sublingual	1 minute	15 minutes	1 hour	0.4 mg

Use of sublingual short-acting nifedipine is never medically appropriate.

Treatment of specific hypertensive disorders

1. Hypertension with congestive heart failure
Nitroglycerin IV
Sodium nitroprusside and loop diuretics
Fenoldopam
DHP-CCB, amlodipine
Clonidine
ACEI
ARB.

2. Hypertension with coronary insufficiency
Non-DHP-CCB
Nitroglycerin
BBs
Clonidine.

3. Aortic dissection with aneurysm
Trimethaphan + propranolol
Nitroprusside + propranolol
Labetalol or esmolol.

4. Catecholamine excess and pheochromocytoma
Phentolamine.

5. Hypertension alone
Fenoldopam
Sodium nitroprusside
Labetalol
Nicardipine
Nitroglycerin
Clonidine (urgency).

SPECIAL CONSIDERATIONS

Table 68 Acute Parenteral Therapy

Drugs	Route	Onset	Maximum effect	Duration	Dosage
Sodium nitroprusside (Nipride, Nitropress)*	IV	Seconds	1–2 minutes	3–5 minutes	16 μg/kg/min to 1–6 μg/kg/min
Fenoldopam mesylate (Corlopam)*	IV	<5 minutes	5–10 minutes	30 minutes	0.1–0.3 mg/kg/min
Trimethaphan (Arfonad)	IV	1–5 minutes	2–5 minutes	10 minutes	0.5–5 mg/min (limited availability)
Diazoxide (Hyperstat)	IV	1–5 minutes	2–3 minutes	4–24 hours	50 mg IV q 5–10 minutes
				Bolus infusion	7.5–30 mg/min 1 propranolol load
				Infusion method	
Hydralazine (Apresoline)	IV	10–20 minutes	20–40 minutes	3–8 hours	10–20 mg
Methyldopa (Aldomet)	IV	2–3 hours	3–5 hours	6–12 hours	250–500 mg q 6 hours
Phentolamine (Regitine)	IV	(for catecholamine excess)			Load 5–10 mg IV q 5 minutes, infuse 0.2–0.5 mg/min
Labetalol (Trandate, Normodyne)*	IV	5 minutes	5–10 minutes	3–6 hours	2 mg/min IV infusion or 20 mg q 10 minutes to a maximum 80 mg q 10 minutes Maximum cumulative dose 300 mg may not be effective in severely hypertensive patients already receiving other antihypertensive agents (propranolol, prazosin)
Nicardipine (Cardene)	IV	10 minutes	30 minutes	3–6 hours	5 mg/h increased 1–2.5 mg/h every 15 minutes up to 15 mg/h
Nitroglycerin	IV	1–2 minutes	–	2–3 minutes	5–100 μg/min
Dilevalol	IV	1–5 minutes	–	3–6 hours	10 mg followed by 25–100 mg every 15 minutes
Enalapril AT*	IV	10 minutes	1–4 hours	2–6 hours	1.25 μg then 2.5–10 mg every 30–60 minutes
Esmolol hydrochloride	IV	1–2 minutes	5 minutes	10–20 minutes	250–500 μg/kg/min for 1 minute then 50–100 μg/kg/min for 4 minutes; may repeat sequence

*Preferred drugs.

Hypertension in Pregnancy

Classification
1. Pregnancy-induced hypertension (PIH) or gestational hypertension
2. Chronic hypertension: preexisting, before the 20th week of gestation
3. Preeclampsia: hypertension with proteinuria and edema; occurs after the 20th week of gestation (usually after 36th week)
4. Eclampsia: preeclampsia + convulsions, coma.

Definition
1. BP usually falls during the first and second trimester.
2. PIH occurs if BP rises more than 30/15 mm Hg or MAP >25 mm Hg or to a level above 140/90 in the last trimester, MAP >95.
3. Most PIH occurs after the 35th week.
4. Preeclampsia develops after the 20th week.
5. About 10% of pregnancies are complicated by hypertension.

Pathogenesis: preeclampsia
1. Increased sensitivity to pressure effects of Ang-II
2. Reduced intravascular volume
3. Decreased PRA
4. Decreased prostacyclin/thromboxane ratio
5. Increased atrial natriuretic peptide
6. Increased endothelin
7. Decreased endothelium-derived relaxing factor (nitrous oxide)
8. Activation of coagulation
9. Increased fibrin degradation products
10. Thrombocytopenia
11. Increased factor XII
12. Decreased factors X and XI
13. Increased fibrinogen
14. High fibronectin
15. Low antithrombin III
16. Low alpha1, antiplasmin
17. Increased PAI activity
18. Vasospasm
19. Reduced cardiac output
20. Increased peripheral vascular resistance
21. Decreased sodium exchange
22. Decreased RBF
23. Decreased glomerular filtration
24. Hyperuricemia
25. Hypomagnesemia.

There is generalized reduced organ perfusion that occurs with widespread hemorrhage and necrosis in brain, liver, heart, and kidney with vascular endothelial damage and marked vasoconstriction of small arterioles. Preeclampsia may be a result of abnormal trophoblastic implantation and immunologic disorder.

Disease spectrum: preeclampsia

The clinical spectrum of coagulation disorders varies from thrombocytopenia to HELLP syndrome (hemolysis, elevated liver enzymes, low platelet count).

Predisposing factors

1. PIH
   - (a) Young primigravida
   - (b) DM
   - (c) Primary hypertension
   - (d) Renal disease.
2. Preeclampsia and eclampsia
   - (a) Extremes of reproductive age
   - (b) Chronic hypertension
   - (c) Nulliparas
   - (d) Renal disease
   - (e) Multifetal pregnancy
   - (f) Thalassemia and Rh incompatibility
   - (g) Fetal hydrops
   - (h) DM
   - (i) Family history of preeclampsia.

Management

1. PIH
   - (a) Do not restrict sodium
   - (b) Bed rest and mild sedation, hospitalization
   - (c) Avoid thiazide diuretics, BBs (except labetalol), ACEIs, ARBs, and RI.
   - (d) Use hydralazine, methyldopa, clonidine, CCBs, and labetalol.
2. Preeclampsia and eclampsia
   - (a) Calcium supplement, 1–2 g/day
   - (b) Aspirin, 60–100 mg/day
   - (c) Dipyridamole
   - (d) Dipyridamole + heparin
   - (e) Bed rest and sedation
   - (f) Liberal sodium intake
   - (g) $MgSO_4$ in eclampsia for convulsions and lower BP
   - (h) Volume expansion: controversial
   - (i) Medications to control BP: CCBs, clonidine, methyldopa, hydralazine, labetalol
   - (j) Avoid diuretics, BBs (except labetalol), ACEIs, ARBs, and RI.

Part 7
The Antihypertensive Drugs

Handbook of Hypertension. By M.C. Houston. Published 2009 by Blackwell Publishing,
ISBN: 9781-4051-8250-8

General Review of Antihypertensive Drug Classes

Antihypertensive drug compliance [193–195]

Diuretics and BBs have the lowest compliance rate and refill rate among the various antihypertensive drug classes with chronic use.

The ARBs, ACEIs, and CCB have the highest compliance rate and refill rate with chronic use. These differences are significant compared with BBs and diuretics (p < 0.001) (Figures 85 and 86 and Table 69).

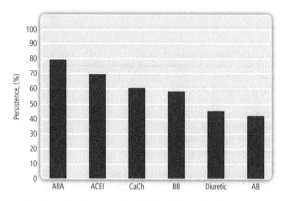

Persistence with antihypertensive therapy by drug class in the Saskatechewan Health Database. AB = alpha-blocker; ACEI = angiotensin converting enzyme inhibitor; AlIA = angiotensin antagonist; BB = beta-blocker; CaCh = calcium channel antagonist.

Figure 85 Persistence with Anti-hypertensive Therapy by Drug Class.

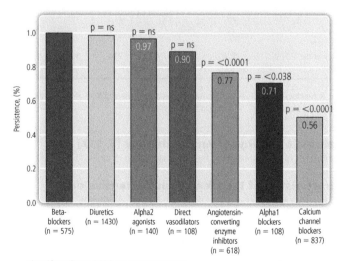

Adapted from: Elliot WJ. (1994) *Am J Hypertens,* 7:26A.
p-Values vs. beta-blockers. N = 2829 patients; 1196 patients dropped out over 7years.

Figure 86 Relative Likelihood of Discontinuing Antihypertensive Therapy Over 7 years According to Drug Class.

Table 69 Patient Status at 12 Months in the Merck-Medco Study

Drug (number of patients)	Number of patients	Patients remaining on initial therapy (%)	Patients switching to new therapy (%)
AT1 receptor blocker (5567)	64	7	29
Angiotensin-converting enzyme inhibitor (5842)	58	9	33
Calcium channel blocker (5094)	50	9	41
Beta-blocker (4994)	43	7	50
Diuretic (5226)	33	6	56

Table 70 Total Cost of Antihypertensive Therapy

1. Acquisition cost
2. Coprescription of secondary drugs
3. Office visits
4. Ancillary laboratory costs (electrolytes, glucose, lipids, ECG)
5. Costs to patient's lifestyle: QOL and adverse effects
6. Cost of increasing end-organ damage
7. Mean costs per drug cost category—1-year use [117]

	Acquisition cost ($)	Supplemental drug cost ($)	Laboratory cost ($)	Clinic visit cost ($)	Side effect cost ($)	Total cost ($)
Diuretics	133	232	117	298	263	1043
BBs	334	115	56	187	203	895
ABs	401	290	114	227	256	1288
Centrally acting alpha-agonists	285	295	125	267	193	1165
ACEIs + Ang-II receptor antagonists	444	291	95	218	195	1243
Calcium entry blockers	540	278	87	214	306	1425

ABs = alpha-blockers; ACEIs = angiotensin-converting enzyme inhibitors; Ang-II = angiotensin II; BBs = beta-blockers; ECG = electrocardiogram.

Total cost of antihypertensive therapy [5, 117]

The total cost of antihypertensive therapy is illustrated in Table 70.

Characteristics of the ideal antihypertensive drug

1. Efficacious as monotherapy in more than 50% of all patients
2. BP control during all activities for 24 hours. Avoid excessive nocturnal dipping
3. Once–a–day dosing with high trough to peak ratio
4. Hemodynamically logical and effective: reduces SVR, improves arterial compliance, preserves CO, and maintains perfusion to all vital organs
5. Lack of tolerance or pseudotolerance: no reflex volume retention or stimulation of neurohumoral mechanisms

6. Favorable biochemical effects, metabolic effects, and risk factor profile
7. Reverses structural, vascular smooth muscle, and cardiac hypertrophy; improves systolic and diastolic compliance and LV contractility and function; reduces ventricular ectopy if present
8. Reduces all end-organ damage: cardiac, cerebrovascular, renal, retinal, and large artery
9. Maintains normal hemodynamic response to aerobic and anaerobic exercise
10. Low incidence of side effects; good QOL
11. Good compliance with drug regimen
12. Good profile for concomitant diseases or problems
13. Reasonable cost (cost/benefit ratio)
14. No withdrawal symptoms and prolongation of BP control with missed dose due to long biological half-life and efficacy of drug

Combination antihypertensive therapy: selected drugs [125]

1. CCB plus
   (a) Alpha-blocker
   (b) ACEI, ARB, or RI
   (c) CCB of different class: non-DHP with DHP
   (d) Central alpha-agonist
   (e) Diuretic
   (f) BB (see comment with 6a.)
   (g) Alpha-/beta-blocker
2. AB plus
   (a) Calcium channel blocker;
   (b) ACEI, ARB, or RI;
   (c) Diuretic;
   (d) Do not generally use with central alpha-agonist (reduced response rate);
   (e) Beta-blocker.
3. Central alpha-agonist plus
   (a) Calcium channel blocker;
   (b) ACEI, ARB, or RI;
   (c) Diuretic;
   (d) Do not generally use with AB (reduced response rate);
   (e) Beta-blocker.
4. ACEI plus
   (a) Calcium channel blocker;
   (b) Alpha-blocker;
   (c) Angiotensin receptor blocker;
   (d) Central alpha-agonist;
   (e) Diuretic;
   (f) Renin inhibitor;
   (g) Beta-blocker.
5. Diuretic plus
   (a) Any other antihypertensive class.
6. BB plus
   (a) CCB-DHP best: use non–DHP-CCB with caution in the presence of systolic dysfunction or conducting problems, particularly with verapamil or diltiazem;

    (b) ACEI, ARB, or RI;
    (c) Diuretic;
    (d) Alpha-blocker;
    (e) Do not use with central alpha-agonist because of possible central antagonism and potential for severe hypertensive withdrawal syndrome.
7. ARB plus
    (a) ACEI;
    (b) Calcium channel blocker;
    (c) Central alpha-agonist;
    (d) Alpha-blocker;
    (e) Diuretic;
    (f) BB;
    (g) ABB;
    (h) RI.

Combinations of these classes of antihypertensive drugs in low doses can achieve:
1. additive or synergistic reduction in BP;
2. reduce adverse effects;
3. improvement of the structural, functional, and metabolic components of the hypertension syndrome;
4. most patients need three to four drugs to reach goal BP of $\leqslant 130/85$ mm Hg or better.

Antihypertensive therapy: efficacy of monotherapy

Drug class	White (%)	African-American (%)	Elderly (%) (both races)
Diuretic	50	60	50
Beta-blocker	50	30–40	20–30
Calcium channel blocker	75	75–80	75–80
ACEI	60	60	60
Alpha-blocker	60	60	60
Central alpha-agonist	60	60	60
Ang-II blocker	60	60	60
Alpha/beta-blocker	50	50	50
Renin inhibitor	60	60	60

Selected drug interactions with antihypertensive therapy [116]

Selected drug interactions with antihypertensive therapy are illustrated in Table 71.

Table 71 Selected Drug Interactions with Antihypertensive Therapy

Class of agent	Increase efficacy	Decrease efficacy	Effect on other drugs
Diuretics	• Diuretics that act at different sites in the nephron (e.g., furosemide + thiazides)	• Resin-binding agents • NSAIDs • Steroids	• Diuretics raise serum lithium levels • Potassium-sparing agents may exacerbate hyperkalemia due to ACEIs
BBs	• Cimetidine (hepatically metabolized BBs) • Quinidine (hepatically metabolized BBs) • Food (hepatically metabolized BBs)	• NSAIDs • Withdrawal of clonidine • Agents that induce rifampin and phenobarbital	• Propranolol hydrochloride induces hepatic enzymes to increase clearance of drugs with similar metabolic pathways • BBs may mask and prolong insulin-induced hypoglycemia • Heart block may occur with non-DHP calcium antagonists • Sympathomimetics cause unopposed alpha-adrenoreceptor-mediated vasoconstriction • BBs increase angina-inducing potential of cocaine
ACEIs ARBs RIs	• Chlorpromazine or clozapine	• NSAIDs • Antacids • Food decreases absorption (moexipril)	• ACEIs may raise serum lithium levels • ACEIs may exacerbate hyperkalemic effect of potassium-sparing diuretics
Calcium antagonists	• Grapefruit juice (some DHPs) • Cimetidine or ranitidine (hepatically metabolized calcium antagonists)	• Agents that induce hepatic enzymes, including rifampin and phenobarbital	• Cyclosporine levels increase with diltiazem hydrochloride, verapamil hydrochloride, mibefradil dihydrochloride, or nicardipine hydrochloride (but not felodipine, isradipine, or nifedipine) • Non-DHPs increase levels of other drugs metabolized by the same hepatic enzyme system, including digoxin, quinidine, sulfonylureas, and theophylline • Verapamil hydrochloride may lower serum lithium levels

(Continued)

Table 71 (Continued)

Class of agent	Increase efficacy	Decrease efficacy	Effect on other drugs
ABs	N/A		• Prazosin may decrease clearance of verapamil hydrochloride
Central alpha2-agonists and peripheral neuronal blockers		• Tricyclic antidepressants (and probably phenothiazines)	• Methyldopa may increase serum lithium levels
		• Monoamine oxidase inhibitors	• Severity of clonidine hydrochloride withdrawal may be increased by BBs
		• Sympathomimetics or phenothiazines antagonize guanethidine monosulfate or guanadrel sulfate	• Many agents used in anesthesia are potentiated by clonidine hydrochloride
		• Iron salts may reduce methyldopa absorption	

ABs = alpha-blocker; ACEIs = angiotensin-converting enzyme inhibitors; ARBs = angiotensin receptor blockers; BBs = beta-blockers; NSAID = nonsteroidal anti-inflammatory drug; RIs = renin inhibitors.

Reproduced with permission from Joint National Committee on Prevention, Detection, Evaluation, and Treatment of High Blood Pressure. The Sixth Report of the Joint National Committee on Prevention, Detection, and Treatment of High Blood Pressure. *Arch Intern Med* 1997; 157: 2413–2446.

Maximum recommended doses* of antihypertensive drugs with best treatment characteristics

	Dose/day (mg)
Calcium channel blockers	
Amlodipine (Norvasc)	10
Diltiazem (Cardizem SR and CD, Dilacor XR, Tiazac)	540
Felodipine (Plendil)	10
Isradipine (DynaCirc)	10
Nicardipine (Cardene and Cardene SR)	120
Nifedipine (Adalat Oros and CC, Procardia XL)	90
Nisoldipine (Sular)	60
Verapamil (Calan SR, Isoptin SR, Verelan)	540
ACEIs	
Benazepril (Lotensin)	40
Captopril (Capoten)	50
Enalapril (Vasotec)	40
Fosinopril (Monopril)	80
Lisinopril (Prinivil, Zestril)	40
Moexipril (Univasc)	30
Quinapril (Accupril)	80
Ramipril (Altace)	20
Trandolapril (Mavik)	8
Perindopril (Aceon)	16
Central alpha-agonists	
Clonidine (Catapres and Catapres-TTS)	0.4/TTS-3
Guanabenz (Wytensin)	16
Guanfacine (Tenex)	2
Alpha-blockers	
Doxazosin (Cardura)	10
Prazosin (Minipress)	10
Terazosin (Hytrin)	10
Diuretics	
Indapamide (Lozol)	2.5
Chlorthalidone	25
HCTZ	25
Ang-II blockers	
Losartan (Cozaar)	100
Valsartan (Diovan)	320
Irbesartan (Avapro)	300
Telmisartan (Micardis)	80
Candesartan cilexetil (Atacand)	32
Eprosartan (Teveten)	1200
Olmesartan (Benicar)	40

* Approximately 80–90% of total antihypertensive effect achieved in most patients.

ANTIHYPERTENSIVE DRUGS

Specific Review of All Antihypertensive Drug Classes

Diuretics [103–105]

The mechanism of action of diuretics is inhibition of NaCl resorption in the renal tubules (Table 72). There is an initial reduction in CO secondary to reduction in plasma volume and extracellular fluid volume, but SVR is reduced with long-term therapy (after 4–8 weeks), and volume reduction reverses to near normal over the same time frame.

Diuretics are used as monotherapy to treat mild to moderate hypertension or as an adjunct to other antihypertensive agents. The major differences among the diuretics are related to duration and site of action as well as potency of diuretic action. The adverse effects are similar, particularly among the thiazide diuretics. Lower doses of diuretics (i.e., HCTZ 12.5–25 mg/day or its equivalent) are now recommended by Joint National Committee (JNC-7) and other international committees for treatment of essential hypertension. In addition, the BHS does not recommend diuretics for first-line therapy in patients under the age of 55 and only for selected use in other patients. The maximum antihypertensive dose should not exceed 25 mg of HCTZ or its equivalent. Approximately 80% of the antihypertensive effect of HCTZ is achieved with a 12.5 mg/day dose; 95% is achieved with a 25 mg/day dose [105]. Thiazide-type diuretics (except indapamide) generally lose their effectiveness in patients with serum creatinine levels in excess of 1.7 mg/dL or a creatinine clearance of <30 cc/min. Indapamide remains effective in patients with moderate to severe chronic kidney disease. Therefore, there is a relatively flat dose–response curve for the antihypertensive efficacy of thiazide diuretics, whereas the diuretic effect may continue up to doses of 100 mg/day of HCTZ.

Indapamide offers many advantages over other diuretics. It is more potent than other diuretics in reducing BP and has mild CCB and AB effects, which may make it the diuretic of choice in treating hypertension [106, 107]. Indapamide has a better metabolic profile (lipid neutral, minimal to no glucose intolerance, and less reduction in potassium and magnesium) and is less nephrotoxic compared with thiazide and thiazide-like diuretics. It reduces LVH and platelet aggregation. There is no effect on insulin resistance. Indapamide is also effective in the presence of renal insufficiency. Indapamide was used in the PROGESS trial with significant reductions in all cardiovascular and cerebrovascular events.

1. **Classification**: Diuretic inhibition of NaCl resorption in renal tubules
2. **Mechanism**:
   (a) Initial reduction in CO secondary to reduction in plasma volume and extracellular fluid volume
   (b) Long-term reduction in SVR
   (c) Direct vasodilator action
3. **Pharmacology**: See individual diuretics listings
4. **Hemodynamics**:
   (a) MAP reduced
   (b) CO slightly reduced (1–5%)
   (c) SVR reduced
   (d) HR increased
   (e) RBF, RPF, and GFR slightly reduced

(f) Renin, aldosterone, and Ang-II increased

(g) Postural hypotension (mild) decreased IVV

(h) Glomerular pressure increased

5. **Clinical use:**

   (a) Adjunctive with other antihypertensives

   (b) Monotherapy, initial therapy in mild to moderate hypertension in absence of compelling indications for other agents (controversial)

   (c) Relatively inexpensive acquisition cost

   (d) Reduces supine and upright BP

   (e) Fairly well tolerated

   (f) No tachyphylaxis

6. **Major differences in diuretics:**

   (a) Duration and site of action

   (b) Potency of diuretic action (loop diuretics > thiazides)

   (c) Efficacy with renal insufficiency (loop > metolazone > indapamide > thiazides)

   (d) Efficacy on BP control: indapamide > thiazides > loop

   (e) Hemodynamic regulatory mechanisms

   (f) Hormonal regulatory mechanisms

7. **Most common adverse effects:**

   (a) Hypokalemia

   (b) Hypomagnesemia

   (c) Hyperuricemia

   (d) Hyperglycemia (less with loop diuretics), insulin resistance, and new onset type 2 DM (except indapamide)

   (e) Hyponatremia

   (f) Hypochloremia

   (g) Hyperlipidemia (mostly thiazides) including hypertriglyceridemia, hypercholesterolemia, increased LDL cholesterol, and decreased HDL cholesterol

   (h) Azotemia and renal insufficiency, decreased GFR. Renal vascular fibrosis, proteinuria, and MAU

   (i) Hypercalcemia (usually only thiazide-like diuretics)

   (j) Impotence—20–25% of male patients

   (k) Dermatologic reactions, rash, and purpura

   (l) Blood dyscrasias

   (m) Cardiac arrhythmias

   (n) Volume depletion and postural hypotension

   (o) Metabolic alkalosis

   (p) Hyperreninemia

   (q) Hyperaldosteronism (secondary)

   (r) Pancreatitis

   (s) Allergic disorders

   (t) Vasculitis

   (u) Homocysteinemia

   (v) Renal cell carcinoma (increased by 55%) and colon carcinoma

   (w) Increased PAI-I and PAI-I/tPA ratio

   (x) Increased fibrinogen and thrombotic risk

Table 72 Diuretics Highlights*

	Preparation	Mechanism of action	Pharmacodynamics	Hemodynamics	Adverse effects	Contr-aindications	Daily dosage	Drug interactions
Thiazides (benzothiadiazine derivatives) Chlorothiazide (Diuril)—Merck	250 mg 500 mg	See HCTZ	Duration: 6–12 hours	See HCTZ	See HCTZ	See HCTZ	250–500 mg	See HCTZ
Cyclothiazide (Anhydron)—Lilly	2 mg	See HCTZ	Duration: 12 hours	See HCTZ	See HCTZ	See HCTZ	1–2 mg on alternate days	See HCTZ
HCTZ (Oretic)—Abbott (Esidrix)—Novartis (Hydro-DIURIL)—Merck Mircozide (Watson)	25–50 mg 25–50 mg 25–100 mg 12.5 mg	Inhibits resorption of NaCl and thereby increases the quantity of Na$^+$ traversing the distal tubule and volume of water excreted. initial antihypertensive effect is due to volume contraction and lower CO. Long-term antihypertensive effect is due to lower SVR.	Duration: 6–12 hours	MAP reduced CO slightly reduced initially plasma volume reduced SVR decreased HR increased NE increased aldosterone increased PRA increased Ang-II increased PGC increased	Hyponatremia Hypokalemia Hyperuricemia Hypercalcemia Hyperglycemia Hypomagnesemia Hypochloremia Metabolic alkalosis Volume depletion Postural hypotension Hyperlipidemia Increased total cholesterol triglycerides Decreased HDL Increased LDL Not renoprotective	Anuria Hypersensitivity to sulfonamide derivatives	6.25–50 mg	Cholestyramine: decreased thiazide effect Corticosteroids: increased potassium loss Diazoxide: increased hyperglycemic effect Digitalis glycosides increased digitalis toxicity (hypokalemia and hypomagnesemia) Indomethacin: decreased antihypertensive and natriuretic effects NSAIDs: decreased diuretic and antihypertensive effects

304

Drug (Manufacturer)	Strengths/Forms	Action/Site	Pharmacokinetics	Renal effects	Adverse effects	Contraindications	Dose	Drug interactions
Methyclothiazide (Enduron)—Abbott	2.5mg, 5mg	See HCTZ	Duration: 24 hours, Peak: 2 hours	See HCTZ	See HCTZ	Renal decompensation, Hypersensitivity	2.5–5mg	See HCTZ
Polythiazide (Renese)—Pfizer	1mg, 2mg, 4mg	See HCTZ	Duration: 24–48 hours	See HCTZ	See HCTZ	See HCTZ	1–4mg	See HCTZ
Chlorthalidone (Hygroton)—Aventis (Thalitone)—BI	25mg, 50mg, 100mg, 25mg	increases excretion of Na$^+$ and H$_2$O Site of action is at the cortical diluting segment of the distal tubule	Duration: 24–72 hours, Onset: 2 hours	See Thiazides	Hypomagnesemia Increases cholesterol triglycerides, and LDL Decreases HDL	See HCTZ	12.5–50mg	See Thiazides
Loop diuretics		Decreases chloride and secondary sodium resorption in ascending limb of the loop of Henle						
Bumetanide (Bumex)—Roche	Oral: 0.5mg, 1mg, 2mg; IV: 0.25mg/mL		Onset: ½ hour, Peak: 1–1½ hours, Half-life: 4–6 hours, Metabolism: liver, Excretion: renal	GFR, RPF, RBF preserved Reduction in free water clearance	Hypokalemia, Hypochloremic alkalosis, Hyperuricemia, Ototoxicity, Muscle pain and tenderness, Dizziness, Hypotension, Weakness	See HCTZ	Average dose: 1–2mg, Range: 0.5–10mg, Maximum: 10mg	Probenecid: reduces bumetanide effectiveness, Indomethacin: blunts sodium excretion associated with bumetanide, Lithium: reduces renal clearance of bumetanide, high risk of lithium toxicity
Ethacrynic acid (Edecrin)—Merck	25mg, 50mg; IV powder: 50mg diluted to 100mL	See Furosemide	Duration: 1–4 hours, Onset: 1 hour	See Furosemide	Gastrointestinal symptoms common with larger doses Hyperuricemia	Anuria	50–100mg should not exceed 400mg	Oral anticoagulants: increased anticoagulant effect Aminoglycoside antibiotics, digitalis: see Furosemide

(Continued)

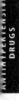

Table 72 (Continued)

Preparation	Mechanism of action	Pharmacodynamics	Hemodynamics	Adverse effects	Contraindications	Daily dosage	Drug interactions
Torsemide (Demadex)—Roche	5 mg, 10 mg, 20 mg, 100 mg, IV: 2 mL (20 mg) vial, IV: 5 mL (10 mg/mL) vial	See Furosemide	Onset: ½ hour—simultaneous food intake delays absorption, Peak: 1 hour, Half-life: 3.5 hours, Metabolism: liver, Excretion: renal, Less protein bound	GFR, RPF, RBF acid base balance preserved, Increased urinary excretion of sodium chloride + H_2O	Dizziness, Headache, Nausea, Weakness, Vomiting, Hyperglycemia, Excessive urination, Hyperuricemia, Hypokalemia, Excessive thirst	Anuria, Hypersensitivity	Initial: 5 mg qd, Range: 5–10 mg qd, Maximum: 10 mg qd	Salicylates: salicylate toxicity, NSAIDs: possible renal dysfunction, Indomethacin: blunts sodium excretion associated with torsemide, Probenecid: reduces torsemide effectiveness, Lithium: reduces renal clearance of torsemide, high risk of torsemide toxicity
Furosemide (Lasix)—Adventis	20 mg, 40 mg, 80 mg	Primarily inhibits the resorption of Cl^-, Na^+, and H_2O in the ascending loop of Henle and exerts a weak diuretic effect in the proximal and distal tubules	Duration: 1–4 hours, Onset: 1 hour, Peak: 1–2 hours, Metabolism: liver, Excretion: renal	Decreased PWP, Decreases CO, Decreases SVR, Fluid and electrolyte imbalance, Hypomagnesemia, Hypokalemia, Mild diarrhea, Nerve deafness, Decreases HDL	Anuria, Azotemia	20–150 mg	Digitalis glycosides: increased digitalis toxicity (hypokalemia and hypomagnesemia), Indomethacin: decreased antihypertensive and natriuretic effect, Prabenecid: decreased diuretic effect, NSAIDs: decreased diuretic and antihypertensive effects, Aminoglycoside antibiotics: increased ototoxicity and nephrotoxicity

	Dose	Mechanism of Action	Pharmacokinetics	Hemodynamics	Adverse Effects	Contraindications/Cautions	Dosage	Drug Interactions
Diuretic of the pyridine-sulfonylurea class (Demadex)—Boehringer Mannheim	5 mg 10 mg 20 mg 100 mg	Acts within the lumen of the thick ascending portion of the loop of Henle where it inhibits the Na$^+$/K$^+$/Cl$^-$ carrier system	Duration: oral 6–8 hours IV 6–8 hours Onset: oral 1 hour IV 10 minutes Peak: oral 1–2 hours IV 1 hour Excretions: hepatic 80% renal 20% Bioavailability: 80%	GFR, RPF preserved CO decreased SVR decreased	Fluid and electrolyte imbalance Dizziness Headache Excessive urination Rhinitis Nausea	Known sensitivity to Demadex or to sulfonylurea Use with caution: Hepatic disease with cirrhosis and ascites Ototoxicity Volume and electrolyte depletion	Hypertension: initial dose 5 mg qd Increase to 10 mg qd if inadequate BP response after 4–6 weeks Maximum recommended: 10 mg qd	Indomethacin: natriuretic effects partially inhibited Lithium: may decrease renal clearance Salicylates: salicylate toxicity Cholestyramine: decreases the absorption of oral Demadex
Potassium-sparing diuretics Amiloride (Midamor)—Merck	5 mg	Inhibits K$^+$/Na$^+$ exchange in the distal tubule—a weak diuretic antihypertensive	Duration: 24 hours Onset: 2 hours Peak: 6–10 hours Excretion: kidney		See Triamterene	Hyperkalemia Should not be used with other potassium-conserving drugs in patients with impaired renal function	5–10 mg Should not exceed 20 mg	NSAIDs: renal failure, hyperkalemia ACEIs: hyperkalemia

(Continued)

Table 72 (Continued)

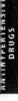

Preparation		Mechanism of action	Pharmacodynamics	Hemodynamics	Adverse effects	Contr-aindications	Daily dosage	Drug interactions
Spironolactone (Aldactone), Pharmacia	25 mg 50 mg 100 mg	Antagonist of aldosterone through competitive binding of receptors at the aldosterone-dependent Na⁺/K⁺ exchange site in the distal convoluted renal tubule; causes an increase in Na⁺ and water excreted	Duration: 12–48 hours		Gynecomastia Menstrual irregularity or amenorrhea Postmenopausal bleeding Hyperkalemia Hyponatremia Gastrointestinal symptoms impotence fever rash	Anuria Acute renal insufficiency Significant impairment of renal function Hyperkalemia	100–400 mg to treat hyperaldosteronism 50–100 mg to treat essential hypertension	Salicylates: decreased diuretic effect Anticoagulations decreased anticoagulant effect Captopril: hyperkalemia Ether, nitrous oxide: hypotension
Triamterene (Dyrenium)— Wellspring	50 mg 100 mg	Not a diuretic but has a diuretic effect on the distal renal tubules, inhibiting the resorption of Na⁺ in exchange for K⁺	Duration: 7–9 hours Onset: 2–4 hours		Blood dyscrasias Photosensitivity Skin rash Hyperkalemia Hyperglycemia Metabolic acidosis Triamterene Kidney stones	Anuria Renal insufficiency Severe hepatic disease	100 mg bid after meals Should not exceed 300 mg	Indomethacin and NSAIDs: renal failure Captopril and ACEIs: hyperkalemia (additive) Ether, nitrous oxide: hypotension (additive)
Epleronone (Pfizer) (INSPRA)	25 mg 50 mg 100 mg 200 mg 400 mg	High selectivity for aldosterone receptor			Minimal Rare Hyperkalemia (2.7%)		25–400 mg/day, effective in reducing BP, LVH, CHF, and proteinuria	Other K⁺ sparing agents

Combination diuretics HCTZ 50 mg + amiloride 5 mg (Moduretic)—Merck	Combination tablet only	Amiloride is a K$^+$-conserving diuretic with weak, natriuretic antihypertensive activity. HCTZ blocks the resorption of Na$^+$ and K$^+$, thereby increasing the quantity of Na$^+$ traversing the distal tubule and the volume of water excreted	Duration: 24 hours Onset: 1–2 hours	See Thiazides	Electrolyte imbalance elevates BUN Hyperkalemia Mild skin rash	Renal impairment, patients receiving K$^+$-conserving agents, Hyperkalemia	1–2 tablets	See HCTZ and amiloride
HCTZ 25 mg + spironolactone 25 mg (Aldactazide)—Pharmacia/Pfizer	Combination tablet only	Combination of diuretic agents with different but complementary mechanisms and sites of action, providing additive diuretic and antihypertensive effects and preserving K$^+$	Duration: 24 hours Onset: 1–2 hours	See Thiazides	Gynecomastia Gastrointestinal symptoms Hyperkalemia Rash	Anuria Acute renal insufficiency Acute, severe hepatic failure Hyperkalemia	Optimal dosage established by individual titration of the components	See HCTZ and Spironolactone

(*Continued*)

Table 72 *(Continued)*

ANTIHYPERTENSIVE
DRUGS

Preparation	Mechanism of action	Pharmacodynamics	Hemodynamics	Adverse effects	Contr- aindications	Daily dosage	Drug interactions
HCTZ 25 mg + Triamterene 50 mg (Dyazide)— GlaxoSmithKline	Combination capsule only	HCTZ blocks resorption of Na⁺ and Cl⁻ and thereby increases the quantity of Na⁺ traversing the distal tubule and volume of water excreted. Triamterene has a weak diuretic effect on the distal renal tubules, inhibiting the resorption of Na⁺ in exchange for K⁺	Duration: 7–9 hours	Reduces SVR Mild reduction in CO Mild reduction in plasma volume (see Thiazides)	Electrolyte imbalance Muscle cramps Rash Weakness Photosensitivity Gastrointestinal disturbances	Renal dysfunction azotemia hyperkalemia Anuria	1–2 capsules Not to exceed 4 capsules†	See HCTZ and Triamterene
HCTZ 50 mg + Triamterene 75 mg (Maxzide)—Bertek	Tablet (scored) 25 mg HCTZ + 37.5 mg Triamterene	HCTZ blocks NaCl resorption and later reduces SVR. Triamterene has a weak diuretic effect on distal renal tubule, preserves K⁺	Duration: 6–12 hours Onset: 2 hours Peak: 4 hours Excretion: kidney Improved bioavailability over Dyazide (Thiazides)	Reduces SVR Mild reduction in CO Mild reduction in plasma volume (see Gastrointestinal disturbances)	Electrolyte imbalance Muscle cramps Rash Weakness Photosensitivity	Renal dysfunction Azotemia Hyperkalemia Anuria	½ to 1 tablet‡	See HCTZ and Triamterene

Drug	Dose	Action	Pharmacokinetics	Hemodynamic effects	Adverse effects	Renal insufficiency	
Quinazoline diuretic derivative Metolazone (Zaroxolyn)— Celltech (Diulo) Mykrox	2.5mg 5mg 10mg 0.5mg	Acts primarily to inhibit Na$^+$ resorption at the cortical diluting site and in the proximal convoluted tubule	Duration: 12–24 hours Onset: 1 hour Peak: 24 hours Excretion: renal	See Thiazides	Azotemia Hyperglycemia Hyperuricemia Hypercalcemia Hyponatremia Hypokalemia Hypomagnesemia	Renal insufficiency 2.5–5mg Higher doses may be indicated with other disorders	see Thiazides
Indoline diuretic derivative Indapamide (Lozol) Aventis	1.25mg 2.5mg 5mg	Similar to thiazides—acts on the cortical diluting segment; may be effective in mild renal insufficiency	Duration: 24 hours Onset: 1 hour Peak: 2 hours Metabolism: liver Excretion: renal 70% bile 23%	MAP reduced CO reduced SVR reduced Minimal change in RBF, RPF, and GFR	Hypokalemia Hypomagnesemia Hyperuricemia Hyponatremia Hypochloremia	See Thiazides Average: 1.25–2.5mg Maximum: 2.5mg	See Thiazides

ACEIs = angiotensin-converting enzyme inhibitors; Ang-II = angiotensin II; BP = blood pressure; CHF = congestive heart failure; CO = cardiac output; GFR = glomerular filtration rate; HCTZ = hydrochlorothiazide; HDL = high-density lipoproteins; HR = hazard ratio; IV = intravenous; LDL = low-density lipoproteins; LVH = left ventricular hypertrophy; MAP = mean arterial pressure; NE = norepinephrine; NSAID = nonsteroidal anti-inflammatory drug; PGC = glomerular capillary pressure; PRA = plasma renin activity; PWP = pulmonary wedge pressure; RBF = renal blood flow; RPF = renal plasma flow; SVR = systemic vascular resistance.

*Consult the *Physicians' Desk Reference* for full prescribing information.

†Bioequivalence is low, with only 30% absorption.

‡Bioequivalence is improved compared with Dyazide; 60% absorption.

8. Contraindications:
 (a) Anuria
 (b) Known allergy (some sulfa-allergic patients)
9. Dose and tablet strength:
 (a) Start with a low dose (1.25 mg of indapamide and 12.5 mg of chlorthalidone
 or HCTZ or a thiazide equivalent) to control BP and titrate dose up to a
 maximum of 2.5 mg of indapamide or 25 mg of chlorthalidone or HCTZ
 per day. These doses are more effective in volume-dependent, low-renin
 hypertension. About 95% of patients respond to the low-dose regimen.
 (b) For treatment of hypertension, but not for the diuretic effect, there is a flat
 dose response over 25 mg/day of HCTZ or its equivalent.
 (c) HCTZ and other thiazides are not effective if the creatinine clearance is
 <30 mL/min.
 (d) Indapamide offers many advantages over other diuretics such as an
 improved metabolic profile, better BP control, less type 2 DM, better
 reduction in LVH, and many other effects.

Central alpha-agonists [103, 104]

The central alpha-agonists all stimulate the central postsynaptic alpha2 receptor
in the brain stem, which reduces SNS activity to the periphery (Tables 73 and 74).
These CNS effects result in a reduction in SVR, plasma, and urine NE levels, PRA,
CO, RBF, and GFR. The CO is preserved at rest and with exercise.

Common side effects are sedation and dry mouth, which are minimized with
low-dose long-term therapy. Concern about withdrawal syndrome has been
overemphasized with all these drugs, particularly clonidine. When low doses are
used, the frequency of withdrawal syndrome is minimal and probably less than
that with BBs. However, duration of treatment, dose and individual variability,
and concomitant medical diseases will determine the severity and frequency of a
withdrawal syndrome. Therefore, it is prudent to always taper any of the central
alpha-agonists over at least 2–4 weeks to avoid any potential adverse effects.

Antihypertensive efficacy is excellent and similar with all the central alpha-
agonists. Selection of therapy depends more on some of the unique side effects,
duration of action, and cost. Clonidine, guanabenz, and guanfacine all have a
neutral or favorable effect on serum lipids and glucose compared with methyldopa,
which has an unfavorable effect. Methyldopa reduces HDL cholesterol and
increases triglycerides. There is little reason to use methyldopa now because the
side effects are greater and efficacy is inferior to those of the other central alpha-
agonists [108–110]. The one exception to this is the approved and appropriate use
of methyldopa during pregnancy.
1. Clonidine (Catapres): oral and transdermal patch
2. Guanabenz (Wytensin)
3. Guanfacine (Tenex)
4. Methyldopa (Aldomet)
Alpha receptors are primarily of two types:
1. Presynaptic (prejunctional): located at the membranes of the neurons that
 contain the neurotransmitter NE. Stimulation inhibits the release of NE from the
 postganglionic sympathetic nerve ending. NE in the synaptic cleft inhibits its
 own release
2. Postsynaptic: located on the target organ. Activation results in an agonist effect
 (vasoconstriction in the periphery) but reduced sympathetic activity centrally

Table 73 Central Alpha-Agonists Highlights*

	Preparation	Mechanism of action	Pharmacodynamics	Hemodynamics	Adverse effects	Contra-indications	Daily dosage	Drug interactions
Clonidine (Catapres)— Boehringer Ingelheim	0.1 mg (oral) 0.2 mg (oral) 0.3 mg (oral) TTS 1–3	Selective stimulation of postsynaptic alpha$_2$ adrenergic receptors in depressor site of vasomotor center of medulla, nucleus tractus solitarii, and hypothalamus. Reduces efferent sympathetic tone and increases vagal tone to heart, peripheral vasculature, and kidney. Reduces SVR, causing vasodilation and lowering blood pressure. Spares peripheral reflexes. Reduces PRA	Onset: ½–1 hour Peak: 3–5 hours Plasma half-life: 12–16 hours Metabolism: liver (minimal) Excretion: renal TTS—duration of antihypertensive effect: 1 week	MAP reduced; CO unchanged; HR reduced (10%); SVR reduced; RBF, RPF, GFR: no change or increase; RVR reduced; plasma NE and urinary NE and EPI reduced; Ang-II reduced; PRA reduced; aldosterone reduced; exercise response preserved; PWP reduced; fluid retention: minimal to none; diuresis in some patients	Sedation and drowsiness, dry mouth, dizziness, withdrawal syndrome and rebound hypertension (uncommon with doses <1.2 mg qd), weakness, headache, bradycardia, constipation, impotence (uncommon— 4%), depression, nightmares	Sick sinus syndrome, second- or third-degree AV block, depression	Initial: 0.1 mg hs and increase by 0.1 mg qd, 3–4 days, giving larger bid doses at bedtime. Some qd, usually bid Average: 0.4–0.6 mg Maximum: 1.2 mg Range: 0.2–1.2 mg TTS: once per week TTS—1, 2, or 3	Tricyclic antidepressants and beta-adrenergic blockers: loss of antihypertensive effect in some patients

(Continued)

Table 73 (Continued)

Preparation		Mechanism of action	Pharmacodynamics	Hemodynamics	Adverse effects	Contra-indications	Daily dosage	Drug interactions
Guanabenz (Wytensin)— Wyeth-Ayerst	4 mg 8 mg	Stimulation of postsynaptic alpha2 receptors in medulla reduces sympathetic activity, SVR and PRA	Onset: 1 hour Peak: 4 hours Plasma and half-life: 6 hours Metabolism: 75% (site undetermined) Excretion: renal: 80%	MAP reduced; CO unchanged; HR reduced (minimal); SVR reduced; RBF, RPF, GFR: no change; RVR reduced; plasma and urinary NE and EPI reduced; aldosterone reduced; PRA reduced; Ang-II reduced; exercise response preserved; plasma volume unchanged; diuresis in some patients	Dry mouth, sedation and drowsiness, fatigue, impotence, withdrawal syndrome, rebound and overshoot hypertension, dizziness, weakness, headache, constipation	Pregnancy	Average dose: 16 mg Range: 8–48 mg Maximum: 48 mg	Potentiates central nervous system depressant drugs
Guanfacine (Tenex)— Wyeth	1 mg 2 mg	Reduces sympathetic tone, SVR, and HR	Onset: 1 hour Peak: 4 hours Plasma half-life: 12 hours Excretion: renal	MAP reduced; CO unchanged; HR reduced (10%); SVR reduced; RBF, RPF, GFR: no change or increase; RVR reduced; plasma and urinary NE and EPI reduced; Ang-II reduced; PRA reduced; aldosterone reduced; exercise response preserved; PWP reduced; fluid retention: minimal to none; diuresis in some	See Clonidine	Allergy to guanfacine	1 mg hs Maximum: 3 mg hs	See Clonidine

| Methyldopa (Aldomet)— Merck | Alpha-methylnorepinephrine stimulates a postsynaptic alpha2 adrenergic receptor in the medulla and decreases sympathetic outflow, which reduces SVR and PRA. Also has some peripheral action | Onset: 2–3 hours Peak: 5 hours Plasma half-life: 12 hours Metabolism: hepatic Excretion: renal | MAP reduced; CO unchanged or some decrease; HR slightly decreased; SVR decreased; RBF, RPR, GRF: no change; RVR reduced; Ang-II reduced; PRA reduced; aldosterone reduced; exercise response preserved; plasma volume increased | Lassitude, drowsiness and sedation, dry mouth, mild orthostasis, positive Coombs' test and anemia, positive rheumatoid factors and lupus erythematosus preparation, impotence, hepatitis, withdrawal syndrome, rebound and overshoot hypertension, altered mental acuity, depression | Active hepatic disease | Average: 250–3000 mg bid schedule Maximum: 3000 mg[†] | Beta-adrenergic blockers: loss of antihypertensive action in some patients Oral contraceptives: decreased antihypertensive effect |
| 125 mg 250 mg 500 mg Also available in elixir, 250 mg/mL | | | | | | | |

Ang-II = angiotensin II; AV = atrioventricular; CO = cardiac output; EPI = epinephrine; GFR = glomerular filtration rate; HR = hazard ratio; MAP = mean arterial pressure; NE = norepinephrine; PRA = plasma renin activity; PWP = pulmonary wedge pressure; RBF = renal blood flow; RPF = renal plasma flow; RVR = renal vascular resistance; SVR = systemic vascular resistance.

*Consult the *Physicians' Desk Reference* for full prescribing information.

†Variable oral absorption, 50–80%.

Table 74 Comparison of Commonly Used Oral Central Alpha-Agonists

Drug	Initial dose (mg)	Range of usual total daily dose (mg)	Orthostasis	Effect on RBF and GFR	Fluid retention	CO	HR	Effect on plasma renin	Insufficiency states needing dose change	Available tablet/capsule sizes (mg)
Clonidine	0.1 bid	0.2–1.2	Rare	→/↑	Minimal or none	↑	↓	↓	Renal insufficiency	0.1, 0.2, 0.3, and TTS 1, 2, 3
Guanabenz	4 bid	8–48	Rare	↑	Minimal or none	↑	→/↓	↓	Renal insufficiency	4, 8
Guanfacine	1 hs	1–3	Rare	→/↑	Minimal or none	↑	→/↓	↓	Renal insufficiency	1, 2
Methyldopa	250 bid	250–3000	Yes (mild)	↑	Yes	→/↓	→/↓	↓	Renal and hepatic insufficiency	125, 250, 500

CO = cardiac output; GFR = glomerular filtration rate; HR = hazard ratio; RBF = renal blood flow.
↑ increased; ↓ decreased; → no change.

Central alpha-agonists: similarities

1. Stimulation of central postsynaptic alpha2 receptors in the nucleus tractus solitarii of the medulla oblongata results in
   a. reduced SNS activity;
   b. reduced NE levels in serum and urine;
   c. reduced PRA owing to reduced NE levels;
   d. increased vagal stimulation (bradycardia)
      (1) Clonidine: direct
      (2) Guanabenz: direct
      (3) Guanfacine: direct
      (4) Methyldopa: indirect (alpha-methylnorepinephrine)
2. Peripheral alpha-agonist pressor response is overwhelmed by central alpha-agonist effect except rarely with:
   a. intravenous doses (transient pressor effects);
   b. high oral doses.
3. Peripheral sympathetic reflexes remain intact, so fewer problems occur with
   a. postural hypotension: methyldopa effect greater than that of clonidine, guanabenz, or guanfacine;
   b. exercise: preserved with all four drugs;
   c. sexual dysfunction: methyldopa effect greater than that of clonidine, guanabenz, or guanfacine.
4. Lowering of BP is not associated with reduction of systemic or regional blood flow.
5. Minimal to no sodium or water retention or weight gain occurs except with methyldopa. Natriuresis occurs in some patients with clonidine, guanabenz, and guanfacine.
6. Hemodynamic effects are similar.
7. Drugs are effective as monotherapy.
8. Adjunctive therapy with other antihypertensive drugs allows for additive or synergistic effects at lower doses of each drug. The recommended average maximum is
   a. Clonidine: 0.4 mg (oral); TTS-3 mg once/week;
   b. Guanabenz: 16–24 mg/day;
   c. Guanfacine: 2 mg/day;
   d. Methyldopa: 2000 mg/day.
9. Dose equivalency: clonidine 0.1 mg = guanabenz 4 mg = guanfacine 0.5 mg = methyldopa 500 mg.

Postganglionic neuronal inhibitors [103, 104]

The postganglionic neuronal inhibitors act by depleting catecholamine stores or inhibiting the release of catecholamines in peripheral sympathetic nerve endings (Table 75). The onset of action is slow except for guanadrel and the drugs have a long half-life. This class of antihypertensive drugs is best avoided unless it is necessary to treat severe refractory hypertension unresponsive to all other medications, which is very rare with the newer drugs available now. The adverse effects are similar, and they are poorly tolerated by most patients.

ANTIHYPERTENSIVE
DRUGS

Table 75 Postganglionic Neuron Inhibitors Highlights*

	Preparation	Mechanism of action	Pharmacodynamics	Hemodynamics	Adverse effects	Contraindications	Daily dosage	Drug interactions
Guanadrel (Hylorel)— Fisons	10 mg, 25 mg	Decreases adrenergic neuronal activity by inhibiting NE release and depleting NE stores in the peripheral nerve endings. Does not cross into central nervous system	Duration: 10–14 hours Onset: 2 hours Peak: 4–6 hours Excretion: renal Metabolism: hepatic	CO reduced, venous capacitance increased; SVR reduced, marked Na^+ and H_2O retention	Faintness, orthostatic hypotension, diarrhea, severe volume retention	Avoid use in CHF, angina, cerebrovascular disease	5–50 mg in divided doses	Tricyclic antidepressants: decreased antihypertensive effect, sympathomimetic amines: decreased antihypertensive effect, antihistamines: hypertensive response
Guanethidine (Ismelin)— Novartis	10 mg, 25 mg	Interferes with release of NE from sympathetic nerve terminals	Onset: 5–7 days Half-life: 7–14 days Excretion: renal	CO reduced; venous capacitance increased; SVR reduced; GFR, RBF, RPF reduced; severe Na^+ and H_2O retention	False-negative urine VMA and catecholamines, orthostatic and postexertional hypotension, severe Na^+ and H_2O retention, impotence, retrograde ejaculation, bradycardia, CHF, exacerbates angina, diarrhea	Pheochromocytoma Simultaneous use of EPI	10–25 mg Maximum: 100 mg	Tricyclic antidepressants: decreased antihypertensive effect, oral contraceptives: decreased guanethidine effect, minoxidil: severe orthostatic hypotension, phenothiazines: decreased antihypertensive effect, sympathomimetic amines: decreased antihypertensive effect, hypoglycemia drugs: enhanced hypoglycemic effect

| Reserpine | 0.1 mg, 0.25 mg, 1 mg | Depletes catecholamine stores in both peripheral SNS and central nervous system | Onset: 4–6 weeks Half-life: 7 days or more | Bradycardia, CO reduced, SVR reduced | False-negative VMA and urine catecholamines, bradycardia, premature ventricular contractions, nasal congestion, depression, Na^+ and H_2O retention, postural hypotension, weight gain, nightmares, extrapyramidal reactions, lowers HDL cholesterol | History of or current depression, active peptic ulcer, hypotension | 0.1–0.25 mg Maximum: 0.25 mg | May prolong or inhibit effects of sympathomimetic amines |

CHF = congestive heart failure; CO = cardiac output; EPI = epinephrine; GFR = glomerular filtration rate; HDL = high-density lipoproteins; NE = norepinephrine; RBF = renal blood flow; RPF = renal plasma flow; SNS = sympathetic nervous system; SVR = systemic vascular resistance; VMA = vanillylmandelic acid.
*Consult the *Physicians' Desk Reference*, for full prescribing information.

ANTIHYPERTENSIVE DRUGS

BBs—General [103, 104]

1. Proposed mechanisms of action in hypertension:
   a. Slowing of heart rate with reduction of CO
   b. Reduction of cardiac contractility and CO
   c. Block of renal renin release
   d. Sympathetic outflow reduced because of central beta effect
   e. Blockade of postsynaptic peripheral beta receptors
   f. Competitive antagonism of catecholamines at receptor site
   g. Increased prostaglandin levels in vascular tissue (indomethacin blocks)
   h. Increased baroreflex sensitivity
   i. Alpha-blocking properties (selected mixed alpha/beta-blocker)
   j. Antioxidant activity (Carvedilol)
   k. Activation of L-arginine/NO pathway (Nebivolol)
2. At equipotent doses, there is little or no difference in antihypertensive effect among the various BBs, and side effects are similar except for the new alpha/beta-blockers and the vasodilating BBs, which may be more effective in reducing central arterial pressure and have minimal adverse effects
3. Antihypertensive efficacy depends on patient profile: The exception for those situations listed below is with the alpha/beta-blockers and the vasodilating BBs.
   a. Age: not as effective in the elderly (reduced beta receptors).
   b. Race: not as effective in African-Americans (low renin and volume dependent).
   c. Renin status: best in high-renin and normal-renin patients; not as effective in low-renin patients.
   d. Duration of hypertension
      (1) Recent onset, younger patient—hyperdynamic with relatively increased CO and relatively increased SVR: possibly effective.
      (2) Established—hypodynamic with reduced CO and elevated SVR: less effective.
4. Antihypertensive effect correlates poorly with plasma levels.
5. All BBs without ISA increase SVR and decrease CO, which is the opposite hemodynamic effect desired to reduce BP. The vasodilating BB as well as those with alpha-blocking properties or with ISA decrease SVR and either do not change or actually increase CO.

BBs and Beta Receptors
Beta-1 stimulation:
1. Cardiac stimulation: increased myocardial contractility, stroke volume, and CO; tachycardia; increased AV conduction and automaticity
2. Renin release from kidneys
3. Lipolysis of FFAs
Beta-2 stimulation:
1. Bronchodilation
2. Vasodilation
3. Glycogenolysis (liver and skeletal muscle) and lactate production
4. Pancreatic insulin release
5. Smooth muscle relaxation (uterus)
6. Skeletal muscle stimulation: tremor

Beta-1 blockade:

1. Reduction in myocardial contractility and CO
2. Bradycardia and heart block, depressed automaticity
3. Decreased renin release
4. Reduced release of FFAs

Beta-2 blockade:

1. Bronchoconstriction
2. Vasoconstriction
3. Abnormal glucose metabolism (liver and skeletal muscle glycogenolysis reduced)
4. Hyperglycemia (inhibited pancreatic insulin release)
5. Smooth muscle contraction (uterus)
6. Skeletal muscle: reduced tremor

BBs differ mainly in 10 properties:

1. Cardioselectivity
2. ISA
3. Membrane-stabilizing activity (MSA)
4. Lipid solubility vs. water solubility
5. Pharmacokinetics
6. Potency
7. Platelet aggregation effect
8. Alpha-blocking properties
9. Antioxidant activity
10. Vasodilatory or vasoconstrictive effects

BBs: selectivity

1. Nonselective: blockade of both beta1 and beta2 receptors
   Nadolol
   Penbutolol
   Pindolol
   Propranolol
   Timolol
2. Cardioselective: blockade of beta1 receptor with relative sparing of blockade of beta2 receptor (susceptible to stimulation by EPI). Cardioselectivity diminishes with increasing doses.
   Acebutolol
   Atenolol
   Metoprolol
   Betaxolol
   Bisoprolol
   Nebivolol (discussed later)
3. Intrinsic sympathomimetic activity
   Acebutolol
   Pindolol
   Penbutolol
   Carteolol
4. Alpha and beta blockade
   Labetalol
   Carvedilol
5. Vasodilating BBs: Highly selective B-1 agent with endothelium-dependent vasodilation through activation of the L-arginine/NO pathway
   Nebivolol

ANTIHYPERTENSIVE DRUGS

321

Side effects and contraindications of BBs [103, 104]
The side effects and contraindications of BBs are illustrated in Table 76.

Drug interactions with BBs [103, 104]
The drug interactions with BBs are illustrated in Table 77.

BB highlights [103, 103]
BB highlights are illustrated in Tables 77–79.

Direct vasodilators [103]
The direct vasodilators have a potent relaxation effect on the vascular smooth muscle of arteries, reducing SVR. The hemodynamics of the vasodilators are similar, but the adverse effects differ. Due to increased PRA, CO, plasma volume, and reflex tachycardia, direct vasodilators require the concomitant use of either BBs or central alpha-agonists and diuretics. The direct vasodilators hydralazine and minoxidil therefore should not be used alone (as monotherapy) to treat chronic hypertension. Minoxidil is much more potent than hydralazine (Table 80).

Alpha1-blockers [103]
The alpha1-blockers (indirect vasodilators) prazosin, doxazosin, and terazosin block the peripheral postsynaptic alpha1-adrenergic receptor and reduce SVR, but usually do not cause reflex tachycardia. CO is preserved or increased, and plasma volume is usually unchanged. These favorable hemodynamic changes reverse the abnormalities in essential hypertension and preserve organ perfusion. Monotherapy with modest sodium restriction is effective in 50–60% of patients with mild hypertension. However, the ABs are not generally recommended as first-line antihypertensive drug therapy since the ALLHAT trial. Concomitant use of diuretics is not usually required.

The alpha1-blockers have favorable effects on serum lipids and no adverse effects other than CHD risk factors. Side effects are infrequent and minor. First-dose syncope and hypotension are rare (<1%) and have been overemphasized. They are more likely to occur in patients who are volume depleted, are on diuretics, or in the elderly.

Initiation at a low dose (1 mg hs) and slow titration to 10 mg/day improve compliance and minimize adverse effects while maximizing efficacy when used as initial monotherapy. The ABs are useful in BPH and may prevent or reduce progression of prostate carcinoma (Table 81).

Angiotensin-converting enzyme inhibitors [103, 104]
These agents inhibit the conversion of Ang-I to Ang-II, thus interrupting the RAAS. PRA is increased; Ang-II and aldosterone levels are decreased. The Ang-II levels tend to return to pretreatment levels over several weeks or months due to escape pathways. The net antihypertensive mechanism appears to be a decrease in fluid volume and vasodilation through various mechanisms. ACEIs may be used alone or in combination with other antihypertensive agents to enhance their effect. The agents affect the kinin-bradykinin and prostaglandin systems and increase Ang 1–7, a potent vasodilator.

Table 76 Side Effects and Contraindications of BBs [103, 104]

Contraindications
1. Sinus bradycardia
2. Heart block greater than first degree
3. Cardiogenic shock
4. Overt cardiac failure
5. Bronchial asthma/chronic obstructive pulmonary disease
6. Known hypertensitivity to product

Side effects
1. Myocardial depression: CHF, reduced CO (less with drugs with ISA), and dyspnea
2. Bradycardia and heart block (electrical depression) (less with drugs with ISA)
3. Central nervous system (due to penetration of blood-brain barrier): fatigue, lethargy, poor memory, weakness, drowsiness, emotional lability, mental depression, paresthesias, disorientation, hallucinations, psychosis, delirium, catatonia, insomnia, nightmares, dreams, headache, dizziness, and vertigo
4. Gastrointestinal: nausea, diarrhea, constipation, pain, flatulence, and ischemic colitis
5. Respiratory: bronchospasm, wheezing, exacerbation of asthma, and chronic obstructive pulmonary disease
6. Peripheral vascular constriction: Raynaud's phenomenon, claudication, and cold extremities (less with pindolol and acebutolol)
7. Inhibition of glycogenolysis
8. Withdrawal syndrome: severe hypertension, unstable angina, arrhythmias, MI, and death
9. Drug interactions: indomethacin blocks antihypertensive action
10. Hyperglycemia: exacerbated DM, inhibited insulin release, and insulin resistance
11. Hypertriglyceridemia HDL cholesterol decreased LDL cholesterol increased, HDL/LDL ratio decreased (except for drugs with ISA) and dense small-atherogenic LDL is increased
12. Hypertriglyceridemia: additive with thiazides
13. Muscle fatigue and exercise-induced fatigue
14. Impotence and decreased libido
15. Postural hypotension
16. Hyperuricemia: additive with thiazides
17. Hyperkalemia (blocks intracellular transport of K^+)
18. Hyperthyroidism symptoms after sudden withdrawal
19. Hypoglycemia in:
    a. DM: masked and prolonged symptoms
    b. Postanesthesia
    c. Dialysis
    d. Fasting (children)
    e. Prolonged exercise
20. Severe hypertensive response in hypoglycemic patients on beta blockade
21. Crosses placenta (fetal bradycardia, hypotension, and hypoglycemia)
22. Precipitates labor by increasing uterine contractions in eclampsia
23. Paradoxic hypertension in the presence of catecholamine excess owing to EPI, pheochromocytoma, hypoglycemia, withdrawal of central alpha-agonist during combined therapy, or volume-dependent hypertension
24. Reduction in GFR, RBF, RPF, which may persist for 6 months to 1 year or longer after discontinuing therapy
25. Reduced birth weight (atenolol)

BB = beta-blocker; CHF = congestive heart failure; CO = cardiac output; DM = diabetes mellitus; EPI = epinephrine; GFR = glomerular filtration rate; HDL = high-density lipoproteins; ISA = intrinsic sympathomimetic activity; LDL = low-density lipoproteins; MI = myocardial infarction; RBF = renal blood flow; RPF = renal plasma flow.

ANTIHYPERTENSIVE DRUGS

Table 77 BBs Highlights*

	Preparation	Mechanism of action	Pharmacodynamics	Hemodynamics	Adverse effects	Contraindications	Daily dosage	Drug interactions
Acebutolol (Sectra)—Wyeth-Ayerst	200 mg 400 mg	Cardioselective beta-adrenergic receptor block with weak ISA and MSA	Onset: ½–1 hour Peak: 2½ hours Half-life: 3–4 hours ISA: 1+ MSA: 1+ Lipid solubility: Low (1+) Metabolism: hepatic Excretion: renal	HR, CO, PRA, RPF, RBF, GFR, aldosterone reduced; SVR and RVR unchanged; MAP reduced; plasma volume increased or no change	See separate list of side effects	See separate list of contraindications	Initial: 400 mg Average: 600 mg Range: 200–1200 mg Maximum: 1200 mg	See separate list of drug interactions
Atenolol (Tenormin)—Astra-Zeneca	25 mg 50 mg 100 mg	Beta1 selective blocking agent without MSA or ISA. Preferential effect not absolute. Higher doses inhibit beta adrenoreceptors located in the bronchial and vascular musculature	Onset: 1 hour Peak: 2–4 hours Half-life: 6–9 hours ISA: none MSA: none Lipid solubility: low (1+), more water soluble Metabolism: minimal, hepatic (10%) Excretion: renal, unchanged	HR, CO, PRA, GFR, RBF, RPF, aldosterone reduced; SVR and RVR increased; MAP reduced; plasma volume increased	See separate list of side effects	See separate list of contraindications	Initial: 25–50 mg Average: 50 mg Maximum: 100 mg	See separate list of drug interactions
Betaxolol (Kerlone)—Pharmacia	10 mg 20 mg	Cardioselective	Onset: 1 hour Peak: 3 hours Half-life: 14–22 hours ISA: none, MSA: 1+ Lipid solubility: none Metabolism: hepatic Excretion: renal	HR, CO, PRA, GFR, RBF, RPF, aldosterone reduced; SVR and RVR increased; MAP reduced; plasma volume increased or no change	See separate list of side effects	See separate list of contraindications	Initial: 10 mg Average dose: 10 mg Maximum dose: 20 mg	See separate list of drug interactions
Metoprolol (Lopressor)—Novartis	50 mg 100 mg	Selective beta-adrenergic blocking agent with relative selectivity for beta adrenoreceptors located primarily in cardiac muscle.	Onset: 1 hour Peak: 1½–2 hours, Half-life: 3–4 hours, ISA: none, MSA: minimal (1+) to none	HR, CO, PRA, RPF, RBF, GFR, and aldosterone reduced; SVR and RVR increased; MAP reduced; plasma volume increased	See separate list of side effects	See separate list of contraindictions	Initial: 50 mg (qd or bid) Average: 200 mg (lose beta selectivity at 150 mg) Range: 50–450 mg Maximum: 450 mg	See separate list of drug interactions

Drug							
(Toprol XL)—Astra-Zeneca	25 mg 50 mg 100 mg 200 mg	Specificity is lost with large doses	Lipid solubility: moderate (3⁺) Metabolism: hepatic Excretion: hepatic to renal				Initial: 50–100 qd Maximum: 400 mg
Nadolol (Corgard)—Monarch	20 mg 40 mg 80 mg 120 mg 160 mg	Nonselective beta-adrenergic receptor antagonist	Onset: 1–2 hours Peak: 3–4 hours Half-life: 20–24 hours ISA: none MSA: none Lipid solubility: low (1⁺), more water soluble Metabolism: minimal, hepatic (27%) Excretion: renal, unchanged	HR, CO, PRA, aldosterone reduced; may not alter RPF and GFR; RVR unchanged; SVR increased; MAP reduced; plasma volume increased	See separate list of side effects	See separate list of contraindications	Initial: 40 mg Average: 160 mg Range: 40–340 mg Maximum: 340 mg See separate list of drug interactions
Carteolol (Cartrol)—Abbott Laboratories	2.5 mg 5 mg	Nonselective beta-adrenergic receptor antagonist with ISA	Onset: ½–1 hour Peak: 1–3 hours Half-life: 6 hours ISA: yes MSA: none lipid solubility: low Metabolism: 30–50% hepatic; Excretion: renal, unchanged (50–70%)	HR reduced less than with other BB (2–5 beats/min); CO reduced less than with other BB or not at all; MAP reduced; plasma volume increased; SVR unchanged or reduced; GFR, RBF, RPF preserved or slightly reduced	See separate list of side effects	See separate list of contraindications	Initial: 2.5 mg Range: 5–10 mg Maximum: 10 See separate list of drug interactions
Penbutolol (Levatol)—Schwarz Pharma	20 mg	Nonselective beta-adrenergic antagonist with mild ISA, mild partial agonist activity	Onset: ½–1 hour Peak: 1½–3 hours Half-life: 5 hours ISA: 0–1⁺, MSA: none. Lipid solubility: low (1⁺), Metabolism: hepatic Excretion: renal	HR, CO, PRA, aldosterone reduced; GFR, RBF, RPF unchanged; MAP reduced; plasma volume unchanged or increased	See separate list of side effects	See separate list of contraindications	Initial: 10 mg Average: 20–40 mg Maximum: 50 mg See separate list of drug interactions

(continued)

Table 77 (Continued)

Preparation		Mechanism of action	Pharmacodynamics	Hemodynamics	Adverse effects	Contraindications	Daily dosage	Drug interactions
Pindolol (Visken)—Novartis	5 mg 10 mg	Nonselective beta-adrenergic antagonist with ISA	Onset: ½–1 hour Peak: 1–2 hours Half-life: 3–4 hours ISA: yes (3⁺) MSA: minimal (1⁺) to none Lipid solubility: moderate (3⁺) Metabolism: hepatic (60%) Excretion: renal (40%)	HR reduced less than with other BBs (4–8 beats/min); CO reduced less than with other BBs or not at all; SVR unchanged or reduced; MAP reduced; GFR, RBF, RPF preserved or slightly reduced; RVR unchanged or reduced; plasma volume increased	Neutral effects on lipids. See separate list of side effects	See separate list of contraindications	Initial: 10 mg bid Average: 20 mg, Range: 10–50 mg Maximum: 60 mg	See separate list of drug interactions
Propranolol (Inderal)—Wyeth-Ayerst	10 mg 20 mg 40 mg 60 mg 80 mg	Nonselective beta-adrenergic receptor blocker	Onset: 1–2 hours Peak: 2–4 hours Half-life: 2½–6 hours ISA: none MSA: 3⁺	HR, CO, PRA, RPF, RBF, GFR, aldosterone reduced; SVR and RVR increased; MAP reduced	See separate list of side effects	See separate list of contraindications	Initial: 40 mg bid Average: 80 mg bid Range: 10–640 mg Maximum: 640 mg	See separate list of drug interactions
(Inderal LA)—Wyeth-Ayerst	60 mg 80 mg 120 mg 160 mg		Lipid solubility: high (4⁺) Metabolism: hepatic Excretion: hepatic to renal	Plasma volume increased				
Timolol (Blocadren)—Merck	5 mg 10 mg 20 mg	Nonselective beta-adrenergic receptor blocking agent	Onset: ½–1 hour Peak: 1–2 hours Half-life: 3–4 hours ISA: none to minimal (1⁺) MSA: none Lipid solubility: low (2⁺) Metabolism: hepatic (80%) Excretion: renal (20%)	HR, CO, PRA, RPF, RBF, GFR, aldosterone reduced; SVR, RVR increased; MAP reduced; plasma volume increased	See separate list of adverse effects	See separate list of contraindications	Initial: 10 mg bid Average: 20 mg Range: 10–60 mg Maximum: 60 mg	See separate list of drug interactions

Drug	Dose	Description	Pharmacokinetics	Hemodynamic effects	Adverse effects	Contraindications	Dosing	Drug interactions
Alpha/beta-blocker, Labetalol (Trandate)—Promethus (Normodyne)— Schering Plough	100 mg 200 mg 300 mg also intravenous 5 mg/mL	Competitive antagonist at both alpha and beta receptors. Oral: Alpha/beta ratio is 1:3, IV: Alpha/beta ratio is 1:7. Beta2 agonist; Beta1 and beta2 antagonist; alpha1-blocker; nonselective	Onset: 1 hour, Peak: 2–4 hours, Half-life: 6–8 hours, ISA: none to 1+, MSA: 1+, Lipid solubility: low (1*). Metabolism: hepatic (40%), Excretion: renal (60%)	HR, CO, PRA reduced; RPF, RBF, GFR unchanged to reduced; SVR and RVR unchanged to slightly reduced; MAP reduced; plasma volume increased or unchanged	See separate list of adverse effects	See separate list of contraindications	Initial: 100 mg bid, Average: 200–400 mg bid, Range: 400–800 mg, Maximum: 2400 mg	See separate list of drug interactions
Carvedilol (Coreg)— GlaxoSmithKline	3.125 mg 6.25 mg 12.5 mg 25 mg	Nonselective beta-adrenergic blocker with alpha1-blocking activity	Onset: ½ hour Absorption: 80%, first pass in liver 23% Peak: 1–2 hours Half-life: 7–10 hours ISA: none MSA: ? Lipid solubility: high Metabolism: hepatic (98%), P-450 enzymes Excretion: renal (2%)	Similar to labetalol, also mild CCB, antioxidant and antiproliferative actions	Dizziness (6.2%) Fatigue (4.3%)	NYHA Class IV asthma 2° or 3° AVB, bradycardia, cardiogenic shock, hepatic disease, hypersensitivity to drug	Initial: 6.25 mg bid Average: 12.5 mg bid Maximum: 25 mg bid Take with food	Catecholamine-depleting agents, Clonidine, Digoxin, Rifampin, Diltiazem, Verapamil, Insulin, Oral hypoglycemics, Climetidine
Bisoprolol (Zebeta)— Lederle	5 mg 10 mg	Beta, cardioselective adrenoreceptor blocking agent. Specificity lost with higher doses	Onset: 1 hour Peak: 2–4 hours ISA: none MSA: minimal to none Lipid solubility: low Metabolism: 50% hepatic, 50% renal Excretion: 50% renal, 50% nonrenal	HR, CO, PRA, RBF reduced; MAP reduced; SVR, RVP increased	See separate list of side effects	See separate list of contraindications	Initial: 5 mg Average: 10 mg Maximum: 20 mg	See separate list of drug interactions

BB = beta-blocker; CCB = calcium channel blocker; CO = cardiac output; GFR = glomerular filtration rate; HR = hazard ratio; ISA = intrinsic sympathomimetic activity; IV = intravenous; MAP = mean arterial pressure; MSA = membrane-stabilizing activity; NYHA = New York Heart Association; PRA = plasma renin activity; RBF = renal blood flow; RPF = renal plasma flow; RVR = renal vascular resistance; SVR = systemic vascular resistance.
*Consult the *Physician' Desk Reference* for full prescribing information.

ANTIHYPERTENSIVE DRUGS

Table 78 Coreg Pharmacologic Properties

	Preparation	Mechanism of action	Pharmacodynamics
COREG CR Carvedilol phosphate Extended-release capsules GLAXOSMITHKLINE	10 mg 20 mg 40 mg 80 mg	Carvedilol Phosphate is a nonselective B-adrenergic blocking agent with alpha1-blocking activity. No ISA activity	Onset: ½ hour when administered with food. Absorption: 85% of the bioavailability of Coreg. First pass in liver: 25–35% bioavailability due to first pass metabolism Peak: 5 hours, Half-life: S (−)-Carvedilol: 11.5 hours, R (+)-Carvedilol: 10.4 hours
Hemodynamics	**Adverse effects**	**Contraindications**	

Nonselective Beta Blockade:
Decreases: cardiac output,
  exercise-induced tachycardia,
  reflex orthostatic tachycardia;
 	
Alpha1—vasodilation reduces PVR
	Similar profile to immediate release Coreg.	Bronchial asthma or bronchospastic conditions,
		Second-or third-degree AV block,
		Sick sinus syndrome,
		Severe bradycardia (unless pacemaker is in place),
		Cardiogenic shock,
		Decompensated heart failure requiring IV inotropic therapy
		Not recommended in patients with hepatic impairment
		Hypersensitivity to any component	

Daily dosage

HF—10 mg qd for 2 weeks, increase to 20 mg, 40 mg, 80 mg over 2 week intervals.
Post-MI and Hypertension—start 20 mg qd maintain for 7–14 days then increase to 40 mg qd, 80 mg qd over 7- to 14-day intervals.
Take with food.

Drug interactions

Catecholamine-depleting agents,
Clonidine
Cyclosporine
Digoxin
Rifambin
Dilitiazem

AV = atrioventricular; HF = hazard ratio; ISA = intrinsic sympathomimetic activity; IV = intravenous; MI = myocardial infarction; PVR = peripheral vascular resistance.

Table 79 BYSTOLIC™ (Nebivolol) Package Insert

BYSTOLIC™
(nebivolol) Tablets
2.5 mg, 5 mg and 10 mg
Rx Only

Description

The chemical name for the active ingredient in BYSTOLIC (nebivolol) tablets is (1RS,1′RS)-1,1′-[(2RS,2′SR)-bis(6-fluoro-3,4-dihydro-2H-1-benzopyran-2-yl)]-2,2′-iminodiethanol hydrochloride. Nebivolol is a racemate composed of d-nebivolol and l-nebivolol with the stereochemical designations of [SRRR]-nebivolol and [RSSS]-nebivolol, respectively. Nebivolol's molecular formula is $(C_{22}H_{25}F_2NO_4 \cdot HCl)$ with the following structural formula:

SRRR-or d-nebivolol hydrochloride

RSSS-or l-nebivolol hydrochloride

MW: 441.90 g/mol

Nebivolol hydrochloride is a white powder that is soluble in methanol, dimethyl-sulfoxide, and N,N-dimethylformamide, sparingly soluble in ethanol, propylene glycol, and polyethylene glycol, and very slightly soluble in hexane, dichloromethane, and methylbenzene. BYSTOLIC as tablets for oral administration contains nebivolol hydrochloride equivalent to 2.5, 5, and 10 mg of nebivolol base. In addition, BYSTOLIC contains the following inactive ingredients: colloidal silicon dioxide, croscarmellose sodium, D&C Red #27 Lake, FD&C Blue #2 Lake, FD&C Yellow #6 Lake, hypromellose, lactose monohydrate, magnesium stearate, microcrystalline cellulose, pregelatinized starch, polysorbate 80, and sodium lauryl sulfate.

Clinical Pharmacology

General

Nebivolol is a β-adrenergic receptor blocking agent. In extensive metabolizers (most of the population) and at doses ≤10 mg, nebivolol is preferentially β_1 selective. In poor metabolizers and at higher doses, nebivolol inhibits both β_1- and β_2-adrenergic receptors. Nebivolol lacks intrinsic sympathomimetic and membrane-stabilizing activity at therapeutically relevant concentrations. At clinically relevant doses, BYSTOLIC does not demonstrate α_1-adrenergic receptor blockade activity. Various metabolites, including glucuronides, contribute to β-blocking activity.

Pharmacodynamics

The mechanism of action of the antihypertensive response of BYSTOLIC has not been definitively established. Possible factors that may be involved include (1) decreased heart rate, (2) decreased myocardial contractility, (3) diminution of tonic sympathetic outflow to the periphery from cerebral vasomotor centers, (4) suppression of renin activity, and (5) vasodilation and decreased peripheral vascular resistance.

(Continued)

ANTIHYPERTENSIVE DRUGS

Table 79 (*Continued*)

Pharmacokinetics

Nebivolol is metabolized by a number of routes, including glucuronidation and hydroxylation by CYP2D6. The active isomer (d-nebivolol) has an effective half-life of about 12 hours in CYP2D6 extensive metabolizers (most people) and 19 hours in poor metabolizers and exposure to d-nebivolol is substantially increased in poor metabolizers. This has less importance than usual, however, because the metabolites, including the hydroxyl metabolite and glucuronides (the predominant circulating metabolites), contribute to β-blocking activity.

Plasma levels of d-nebivolol increase in proportion to dose in EMs and PMs for doses up to 20 mg. Exposure to l-nebivolol is higher than to d-nebivolol but l-nebivolol contributes little to the drug's activity as d-nebivolol's beta receptor affinity is >1000-fold higher than l-nebivolol. For the same dose, PMs attain a fivefold higher C_{max} and tenfold higher AUC of d-nebivolol than do EMs. d-Nebivolol accumulates about 1.5-fold with repeated once-daily dosing in EMs.

Absorption and Distribution

Absorption of BYSTOLIC is similar to an oral solution. The absolute bioavailability has not been determined.

Mean peak plasma nebivolol concentrations occur approximately 1.5–4 hours postdosing in EMs and PMs.

Food does not alter the pharmacokinetics of nebivolol. Under fed conditions, nebivolol glucuronides are slightly reduced. BYSTOLIC may be administered without regard to meals. The in vitro human plasma protein binding of nebivolol is approximately 98%, mostly to albumin, and is independent of nebivolol concentrations.

Metabolism and Excretion

Nebivolol is predominantly metabolized via direct glucuronidation of parent and to a lesser extent via N-dealkylation and oxidation via cytochrome P450 2D6. Its stereospecific metabolites contribute to the pharmacologic activity (see **Drug Interactions**).

After a single oral administration of ^{14}C-nebivolol, 38% of the dose was recovered in urine and 44% in feces for EMs and 67% in urine and 13% in feces for PMs. Essentially all nebivolol was excreted as multiple oxidative metabolites or their corresponding glucuronide conjugates.

Drug Interactions

Drugs that inhibit CYP2D6 can be expected to increase plasma levels of nebivolol. When BYSTOLIC is co-administered with an inhibitor or an inducer of this enzyme, patients should be closely monitored and the nebivolol dose adjusted according to blood pressure response. In vitro studies have demonstrated that at therapeutically relevant concentrations, d- and l-nebivolol do not inhibit any cytochrome P450 pathways.

Digoxin: Concomitant administration of BYSTOLIC (10 mg once daily) and digoxin (0.25 mg once daily) for 10 days in 14 healthy adult individuals resulted in no significant changes in the pharmacokinetics of digoxin or nebivolol (see **PRECAUTIONS, Drug Interactions**).

Warfarin: Administration of BYSTOLIC (10 mg once daily for 10 days) led to no significant changes in the pharmacokinetics of nebivolol or R- or S-warfarin following a single 10 mg dose of warfarin. Similarly, nebivolol has no significant effects on the anticoagulant activity of warfarin, as assessed by Prothrombin time and INR profiles from 0 to 144 hours after a single 10 mg warfarin dose in 12 healthy adult volunteers.

Diuretics: No pharmacokinetic interactions were observed in healthy adults between nebivolol (10 mg daily for 10 days) and furosemide (40 mg single dose), hydrochlorothiazide (25 mg once daily for 10 days), or spironolactone (25 mg once daily for 10 days).

Ramipril: Concomitant administration of BYSTOLIC (10 mg once daily) and ramipril (5 mg once daily) for 10 days in 15 healthy adult volunteers produced no pharmacokinetic interactions.

Losartan: Concomitant administration of BYSTOLIC (10 mg single dose) and losartan (50 mg single dose) in 20 healthy adult volunteers did not result in pharmacokinetic interactions.

Fluoxetine: Fluoxetine, a CYP2D6 inhibitor, administered at 20 mg/day for 21 days before a single 10 mg dose of nebivolol to 10 healthy adults, led to an eightfold increase

Table 79 (*Continued*)

in the AUC and threefold increase in C_{max} for d-nebivolol (see **PRECAUTIONS, Drug Interactions**).

Histamine-2 Receptor Antagonists: The pharmacokinetics of nebivolol (5 mg single dose) was not affected by the co-administration of ranitidine (150 mg twice daily). Cimetidine (400 mg twice daily) causes a 23% increase in the plasma levels of d-nebivolol.

Charcoal: The pharmacokinetics of nebivolol (10 mg single dose) was not affected by repeated co-administration (4, 8, 12, 16, 22, 23, 36, and 48 hours after nebivolol administration) of activated charcoal (Actidose-Aqua®).

Sildenafil: The co-administration of nebivolol and sildenafil decreased AUC and C_{max} of sildenafil by 21% and 23%, respectively. The effect on the C_{max} and AUC for d-nebivolol was also small (<20%). The effect on vital signs (e.g., pulse and blood pressure) was approximately the sum of the effects of sildenafil and nebivolol.

Other Concomitant Medications: Utilizing population pharmacokinetic analyses derived from hypertensive patients, the following drugs were observed not to have an effect on the pharmacokinetics of nebivolol: acetaminophen, acetylsalicylic acid, atorvastatin, esomeprazole, ibuprofen, levothyroxine sodium, metformin, sildenafil, simvastatin, or tocopherol.

Protein Binding: No meaningful changes in the extent of in vitro binding of nebivolol to human plasma proteins were noted in the presence of high concentrations of diazepam, digoxin, diphenylhydantoin, enalapril, hydrochlorothiazide, imipramine, indomethacin, propranolol, sulfamethazine, tolbutamide, or warfarin. Additionally, nebivolol did not significantly alter the protein binding of the following drugs: diazepam, digoxin, diphenylhydantoin, hydrochlorothiazide, imipramine, or warfarin at their therapeutic concentrations.

Special Populations

Renal Disease: The apparent clearance of nebivolol was unchanged following a single 5 mg dose of BYSTOLIC in patients with mild renal impairment (ClCr, 50–80 mL/min; $n = 7$), and it was reduced negligibly in patients with moderate (ClCr, 30–50 mL/min; $n = 9$), but by 53% in patients with severe renal impairment (ClCr, <30 mL/min; $n = 5$). The dose of BYSTOLIC should be adjusted in patients with severe renal impairment. BYSTOLIC should be used with caution in patients receiving dialysis, since no formal studies have been conducted in this population (see **DOSAGE AND ADMINISTRATION**).

Hepatic Disease: d-Nebivolol peak plasma concentration increased threefold, exposure (AUC) increased tenfold, and the apparent clearance decreased by 86% in patients with moderate hepatic impairment (Child-Pugh Class B). The starting dose should be reduced in patients with moderate hepatic impairment. No formal studies have been performed in patients with severe hepatic impairment, and nebivolol should be contraindicated for these patients (see **DOSAGE AND ADMINISTRATION**).

Clinical Studies

The antihypertensive effectiveness of BYSTOLIC as monotherapy has been demonstrated in three randomized, double-blind, multicenter, placebo-controlled trials at doses ranging from 1.25 to 40 mg for 12 weeks (Studies 1, 2, and 3). A fourth placebo-controlled trial demonstrated additional antihypertensive effects of BYSTOLIC at doses ranging from 5 to 20 mg when administered concomitantly with up to two other antihypertensive agents (ACEIs, angiotensin II receptor antagonists, and thiazide diuretics) in patients with inadequate blood pressure control. The three monotherapy trials included a total of 2016 patients (1811 BYSTOLIC, 205 placebo) with mild to moderate hypertension who had baseline diastolic blood pressures (DBP) of 95–109 mm Hg. Patients received either BYSTOLIC or placebo once-daily for 12 weeks. Two of these monotherapy trials (studies 1 and 2) studied 1716 patients in the general hypertensive population with a mean age of 54 years, 55% males, 26% non-Caucasians, 7% diabetics, and 6% genotyped as PMs. The third monotherapy trial (study 3) studied 300 black patients with a mean age of 51 years, 45% males, 14% diabetics, and 3% as PMs.

Placebo-subtracted blood pressure reductions by dose for each study are presented in Table 1. Most studies showed increasing response to doses above 5 mg.

(*Continued*)

Table 79 (*Continued*)

Table 1 Placebo-Subtracted Least-Square Mean Reductions in Trough Sitting Systolic/Diastolic Blood Pressure (SiSBP/SiDBP mm Hg) by Dose in Studies with Once-Daily BYSTOLIC

	Nebivolol dose (mg)					
	1.25	2.5	5.0	10	20	30–40
Study 1	−6.6*/−5.1*	−8.5*/−5.6*	−8.1*/−5.5*	−9.2*/−6.3*	−8.7*/−6.9*	−11.7*/−8.3*
Study 2			−3.8/−3.2*	−3.1/−3.9*	−6.3*/−4.5*	.
Study 3†		−1.5/−2.9	−2.6/−4.9*	−6.0*/−6.1*	−7.2*/−6.1*	−6.8*/−5.5*
Study 4‡			−5.7*/−3.3*	−3.7*/−3.5*	−6.2*/−4.6*	

*p < 0.05 based on pair-wise comparison vs. placebo.
†Study enrolled only African Americans.
‡Study on top of one or two other antihypertensive medications.

Study 4 enrolled 669 patients with a mean age of 54 years, 55% males, 54% Caucasians, 29% Blacks, 15% Hispanics, 1% Asians, 14% diabetics, and 5% PMs. BYSTOLIC, 5–20 mg, administered once daily concomitantly with stable doses of up to two other antihypertensive agents (ACEIs, angiotensin II receptor antagonists, and thiazide diuretics) resulted in significant additional antihypertensive effects over placebo compared to baseline blood pressure. Effectiveness was similar in subgroups analyzed by age and sex. Effectiveness was established in blacks, but as monotherapy the magnitude of effect was somewhat less than in Caucasians. The blood pressure–lowering effect of BYSTOLIC was seen within 2 weeks of treatment and was maintained over the 24-hour dosing interval.

Indications And Usage
BYSTOLIC is indicated for the treatment of hypertension. BYSTOLIC may be used alone or in combination with other antihypertensive agents.

Contraindications
BYSTOLIC is contraindicated in patients with severe bradycardia, heart block greater than first degree, cardiogenic shock, decompensated cardiac failure, sick sinus syndrome (unless a permanent pacemaker is in place), or severe hepatic impairment (Child-Pugh >B), and in patients who are hypersensitive to any component of this product.

Warnings
Abrupt Cessation of Therapy
Patients with coronary artery disease treated with BYSTOLIC should be advised against abrupt discontinuation of therapy. Severe exacerbation of angina and the occurrence of myocardial infarction and ventricular arrhythmias have been reported in patients with coronary artery disease following the abrupt discontinuation of therapy with β-blockers. Myocardial infarction and ventricular arrhythmias may occur with or without preceding exacerbation of the angina pectoris. Even patients without overt coronary artery disease should be cautioned against interruption or abrupt discontinuation of therapy. As with other β-blockers, when discontinuation of BYSTOLIC is planned, patients should be carefully observed and advised to minimize physical activity. BYSTOLIC should be tapered over 1–2 weeks when possible. If the angina worsens or acute coronary insufficiency develops, it is recommended that BYSTOLIC be promptly reinstituted, at least temporarily.

Cardiac Failure
Sympathetic stimulation is a vital component supporting circulatory function in the setting of congestive heart failure, and β-blockade may result in further depression of myocardial contractility and precipitate more severe failure. In patients who have compensated congestive heart failure, BYSTOLIC should be administered cautiously. If heart failure worsens, discontinuation of BYSTOLIC should be considered.

Angina and Acute Myocardial Infarction
BYSTOLIC was not studied in patients with angina pectoris or who had a recent MI.

Table 79 (*Continued*)

Bronchospastic Diseases
In general, patients with bronchospastic diseases should not receive β-blockers.

Anesthesia and Major Surgery
If BYSTOLIC is to be continued perioperatively, patients should be closely monitored when anesthetic agents, which depress myocardial function, such as ether, cyclopropane, and trichloroethylene, are used. If β-blocking therapy is withdrawn before major surgery, the impaired ability of the heart to respond to reflex adrenergic stimuli may augment the risks of general anesthesia and surgical procedures.

The β-blocking effects of BYSTOLIC can be reversed by β-agonists, e.g., dobutamine or isoproterenol. However, such patients may be subject to protracted severe hypotension. Additionally, difficulty in restarting and maintaining the heartbeat has been reported with β-blockers.

Diabetes and Hypoglycemia
Beta-blockers may mask some of the manifestations of hypoglycemia, particularly tachycardia. Nonselective β-blockers may potentiate insulin-induced hypoglycemia and delay recovery of serum glucose levels. It is not known whether nebivolol has these effects. Patients subject to spontaneous hypoglycemia, or diabetic patients receiving insulin or oral hypoglycemic agents, should be advised about these possibilities, and nebivolol should be used with caution.

Thyrotoxicosis
Beta-blockers may mask clinical signs of hyperthyroidism, such as tachycardia. Abrupt withdrawal of β-blockers may be followed by an exacerbation of the symptoms of hyperthyroidism or may precipitate a thyroid storm.

Peripheral Vascular Disease
Beta-blockers can precipitate or aggravate symptoms of arterial insufficiency in patients with peripheral vascular disease. Caution should be exercised in these patients.

Nondihydropyridine Calcium Channel Blockers
Because of significant negative inotropic and chronotropic effects in patients treated with β-blockers and calcium channel blockers of the verapamil and diltiazem type, caution should be used in patients treated concomitantly with these agents and ECG and blood pressure should be monitored.

Precautions
Use with CYPZD6 inhibitors
Nebivolol exposure increases with inhibition of CYP2D6 (see **Drug Interactions**). The dose of BYSTOLIC may need to be reduced.

Impaired Renal Function
BYSTOLIC should be used with caution in patients with severe renal impairment because of decreased renal clearance. BYSTOLIC has not been studied in patients receiving dialysis.

Impaired Hepatic Function
BYSTOLIC should be used with caution in patients with moderate hepatic impairment because of decreased metabolism. Since BYSTOLIC has not been studied in patients with severe hepatic impairment, BYSTOLIC is contraindicated in this population (see **CLINICAL PHARMACOLOGY, Special Populations** and **DOSAGE AND ADMINISTRATION**).

Risk of Anaphylactic Reactions
While taking β-blockers, patients with a history of severe anaphylactic reactions to a variety of allergens maybe more reactive to repeated challenges—either accidental, diagnostic, or therapeutic. Such patients may be unresponsive to the usual doses of epinephrine used to treat allergic reactions. In patients with known or suspected pheochromocytoma, an alpha-blocker should be initiated before the use of any β-blocker.

Information for Patients
Patients should be advised to take BYSTOLIC regularly and continuously, as directed. BYSTOLIC can be taken with or without food. If a dose is missed, the patient should take the next

(Continued)

Table 79 (*Continued*)

scheduled dose only (without doubling it). Patients should not interrupt or discontinue BYSTOLIC without consulting the physician.

Patients should know how they read to this medicine before they operate automobiles, use machinery, or engage in other tasks requiring alertness.

Patients should be advised to consult a physician if any difficulty in breathing occurs, or if they develop signs or symptoms of worsening congestive heart failure such as weight gain or increasing shortness of breath or excessive bradycardia.

Patients subject to spontaneous hypoglycemia, or diabetic patients receiving insulin or oral hypoglycemic agents, should be cautioned that β-blockers may mask some of the manifestations of hypoglycemia, particularly tachycardia. Nebivolol should be used with caution in these patients.

Drug Interactions

BYSTOLIC should be used with care when myocardial depressants or inhibitors of AV conduction, such as certain calcium antagonists (particularly of the phenylalkylamine [verapamil] and benzothiazepine [diltiazem] classes) or antiarrhythmic agents, such as disopyramide, are used concurrently. Both digitalis glycosides and β-blockers slow atrioventricular conduction and decrease heart rate. Concomitant use can increase the risk of bradycardia.

BYSTOLIC should not be combined with other β-blockers. Patients receiving catecholamine-depleting drugs, such as reserpine or guanethidine, should be closely monitored, because the added β-blocking action of BYSTOLIC may produce excessive reduction of sympathetic activity. In patients who are receiving BYSTOLIC and clonidine, BYSTOLIC should be discontinued for several days before the gradual tapering of clonidine.

CYP2D6 Inhibitors: Use caution when BYSTOLIC is co-administered with CYP2D6 inhibitors (quinidine, propafenone, fluoxetine, paroxetine, etc.) (see **CLINICAL PHARMACOLOGY, Drug Interactions**).

Carcinogenesis, Mutagenesis, and Impairment of Fertility

In a 2-year study of nebivolol in mice, a statistically significant increase in the incidence of testicular Leydig cell hyperplasia and adenomas was observed at 40 mg/kg/day (five times the maximally recommended human dose of 40 mg on a mg/m^2 basis). Similar findings were not reported in mice administered doses equal to approximately 0.3 or 1.2 times the maximum recommended human dose. No evidence of a tumorigenic effect was observed in a 24-month study in Wistar rats receiving doses of nebivolol of 2.5, 10, and 40 mg/kg/day (equivalent to 0.6, 2.4, and 10 times the maximally recommended human dose). Co-administration of dihydrotestosterone reduced blood LH levels and prevented the Leydig cell hyperplasia, consistent with an indirect LH-mediated effect of nebivolol in mice and not thought to be clinically relevant in man.

A randomized, double-blind, placebo- and active-controlled, parallel-group study in healthy male volunteers was conducted to determine the effects of nebivolol on adrenal function, luteinizing hormone, and testosterone levels. This study demonstrated that 6 weeks of daily dosing with 10 mg of nebivolol had no significant effect on ACTH-stimulated mean serum cortisol $AUC_{0-120min}$, serum LH, or serum total testosterone.

Effects on spermatogenesis were seen in male rats and mice at ⩾40 mg/kg/day (10 and 5 times the MRHD, respectively). For rats, the effects on spermatogenesis were not reversed and may have worsened during a 4-week recovery period. The effects of nebivolol on sperm in mice, however, were partially reversible.

Mutagenesis: Nebivolol was not genotoxic when tested in a battery of assays (Ames, in vitro mouse lymphoma TK$^\pm$, in vitro human peripheral lymphocyte chromosome aberration, in vivo *Drosophila melanogaster* sex-linked recessive lethal, and in vivo mouse bone marrow micronucleus tests).

Pregnancy: Teratogenic Effects. Pregnancy Category C

Decreased pup body weights occurred at 1.25 and 2.5 mg/kg in rats, when exposed during the perinatal period (late gestation, parturition, and lactation). At 5 mg/kg and higher doses

Table 79 (*Continued*)

(1.2 times the MRHD), prolonged gestation, dystocia, and reduced maternal care were produced with corresponding increases in late fetal deaths and stillbirths and decreased birth weight, live litter size, and pup survival. Insufficient numbers of pups survived at 5 mg/kg to evaluate the offspring for reproductive performance.

In studies in which pregnant rats were given nebivolol during organogenesis, reduced fetal body weights were observed at maternally toxic doses of 20 and 40 mg/kg/day (5 and 10 times the MRHD), and small reversible delays in sternal and thoracic ossification associated with the reduced fetal body weights and a small increase in resorption occurred at 40 mg/kg/day (10 times the MRHD). No adverse effects on embryo-fetal viability, sex, weight, or morphology were observed in studies in which nebivolol was given to pregnant rabbits at doses as high as 20 mg/kg/day (10 times the MRHD).

Labor and Delivery

Nebivolol caused prolonged gestation and dystocia at doses ≥5 mg/kg in rats (1.2 times the MRHD). These effects were associated with increased fetal deaths and stillborn pups, and decreased birth weight, live litter size, and pup survival rate, events that occurred only when nebivolol was given during the perinatal period (late gestation, parturition, and lactation).

No studies of nebivolol were conducted in pregnant women. BYSTOLIC should be used during pregnancy only if the potential benefit justifies the potential risk to the fetus.

Nursing Mothers

Studies in rats have shown that nebivolol or its metabolites cross the placental barrier and are excreted in breast milk. It is not known whether this drug is excreted in human milk.

Because of the potential for β-blockers to produce serious adverse reactions in nursing infants, especially bradycardia, BYSTOLIC is not recommended during nursing.

Geriatric Use

Of the 2800 patients in the US-sponsored placebo-controlled clinical hypertension studies, 478 patients were 65 years of age or older. No overall differences in efficacy or in the incidence of adverse events were observed between older and younger patients.

Pediatric Use

Safety and effectiveness in pediatric patients have not been established. Pediatric studies in ages newborn to 18 years have not been conducted because of incomplete characterization of developmental toxicity and possible adverse effects on long-term fertility (see **Carcinogenesis, Mutagenesis and Impairment of Infertility**).

Adverse Reactions

The data described below reflect worldwide clinical trial exposure to BYSTOLIC in 6545 patients, including 5038 patients treated for hypertension and the remaining 1507 subjects treated for other cardiovascular diseases. Doses ranged from 0.5 to 40 mg. Patients received BYSTOLIC for up to 24 months, with over 1900 patients treated for at least 6 months and approximately 1300 patients for more than 1 year. In placebo-controlled clinical trials comparing BYSTOLIC with placebo, discontinuation of therapy due to adverse events was reported in 2.8% of patients treated with nebivolol and 2.2% of patients given placebo. The most common adverse events that led to discontinuation of BYSTOLIC were headache (0.4%), nausea (0.2%), and bradycardia (0.2%).

Adverse Reactions in Controlled Trials

Table 2 lists treatment-emergent signs and symptoms that were reported in three 12-week, placebo-controlled monotherapy trials involving 1597 hypertensive patients treated with either 5 mg, 10 mg, or 20–40 mg of BYSTOLIC, and 205 patients given placebo and for which the rate of occurrence was at least 1% of patients treated with nebivolol and greater than the rate for those treated with placebo in at least one dose group.

(Continued)

Table 79 (*Continued*)

Table 2 Treatment-Emergent Adverse Events with an Incidence (over 6 weeks) ≥1% in BYSTOLIC-treated Patients and at a Higher Frequency than Placebo-Treated Patients

	Placebo (*n* = 205) (%)	Nebivolol 5 mg (*n* = 459)(%)	Nebivolol 10 mg (*n* = 461) (%)	Nebivolol 20–40 mg (*n* = 677) (%)
Headache	6	9	6	7
Fatigue	1	2	2	5
Dizziness	2	2	3	4
Diarrhea	2	2	2	3
Nausea	0	1	3	2
Insomnia	0	1	1	1
Chest pain	0	0	1	1
Bradycardia	0	0	0	1
Dyspnea	0	0	1	1
Rash	0	0	1	1
Peripheral edema	0	1	1	1

Other Adverse Events Observed During Worldwide Clinical Trials

Listed below are other reported adverse events with an incidence of at least 1% in the more than 5300 patients treated with BYSTOLIC in controlled or open-label trials, whether or not attributed to treatment, except for those already appearing in Table 2, terms too general to be informative, minor symptoms, or events unlikely to be attributable to drug because they are common in the population. These adverse events were in most cases observed at a similar frequency in placebo-treated patients in the controlled studies.

Body as a whole: asthenia
Gastrointestinal System Disorders: abdominal pain
Metabolic and Nutritional Disorders: hypercholesterolemia and hyperuricemia
Nervous System Disorders: paraesthesia
Laboratory
In controlled monotherapy trials, BYSTOLIC was associated with an increase in BUN, uric acid, and triglycerides and a decrease in HDL cholesterol and platelet count.

Events Identified from Spontaneous Reports of BYSTOLIC Received Worldwide

The following adverse events have been identified from spontaneous reports of BYSTOLIC received worldwide and have not been listed elsewhere. These adverse events have been chosen for inclusion due to a combination of seriousness, frequency of reporting, or potential causal connection to BYSTOLIC. Events common in the population have generally been omitted. Because these events were reported voluntarily from a population of uncertain size, it is not possible to estimate their frequency or establish a causal relationship to BYSTOLIC exposure: abnormal hepatic function (including increased AST, ALT, and bilirubin), acute pulmonary edema, acute renal failure, atrioventricular block (both second and third degree), bronchospasm, erectile dysfunction, hypersensitivity (including urticaria, allergic vasculitis, and rare reports of angioedema), myocardial infarction, pruritus, psoriasis, Raynaud's phenomenon, peripheral ischemia/claudication, somnolence, syncope, thrombocytopenia, various rashes and skin disorders, vertigo, and vomiting.

Overdosage

In clinical trials and worldwide postmarketing experience, there were reports of BYSTOLIC overdose. The most common signs and symptoms associated with BYSTOLIC overdosage are bradycardia and hypotension. Other important adverse events reported with BYSTOLIC overdose include cardiac failure, dizziness, hypoglycemia, fatigue, and vomiting. Other adverse events associated with β-blocker overdose include bronchospasm and heart block.
The largest known ingestion of BYSTOLIC worldwide involved a patient who ingested up to 500 mg of BYSTOLIC along with several 100 mg tablets of acetylsalicylic acid in a suicide

Table 79 (*Continued*)

attempt. The patient experienced hyperhidrosis, pallor, depressed level of consciousness, hypokinesia, hypotension, sinus bradycardia, hypoglycemia, hypokalemia, respiratory failure, and vomiting. The patient recovered.

Due to extensive drug binding to plasma proteins, hemodialysis is not expected to enhance nebivolol clearance.

If overdose occurs, BYSTOLIC should be stopped and general supportive and specific symptomatic treatment should be provided. Based on expected pharmacologic actions and recommendations for other β-blockers, the following general measures should be considered when clinically warranted:

Bradycardia: Administer IV atropine. If the response is inadequate, isoproterenol or another agent with positive chronotropic properties may be given cautiously. Under some circumstances, transthoracic or transvenous pacemaker placement may be necessary.

Hypotension: Administer IV fluids and vasopressors. Intravenous glucagon may be useful.

Heart Block (second or third degree): Patients should be carefully monitored and treated with isoproterenol infusion. Under some circumstances, transthoracic or transvenous pacemaker placement may be necessary.

Congestive Heart Failure: Initiate therapy with digitalis glycoside and diuretics. In certain cases, consideration should be given to the use of inotropic and vasodilating agents.

Bronchospasm: Administer bronchodilator therapy such as a short-acting inhaled β_2-agonist and/or aminophylline.

Hypoglycemia: Administer IV glucose. Repeated doses of IV glucose or possibly glucagon may be required.

In the event of intoxication where there are symptoms of shock, treatment must be continued for a sufficiently long period consistent with the 12–19-hour effective half-life of BYSTOLIC. Supportive measures should continue until clinical stability is achieved.

Call the National Poison Control Center (800-222-1222) for the most current information on β-blocker overdose treatment.

Dosage and Administration

The dose of BYSTOLIC should be individualized to the needs of the patient. For most patients, the recommended starting dose is 5 mg once daily, with or without food, as monotherapy or in combination with other agents. For patients requiring further reduction in blood pressure, the dose can be increased at 2-week intervals up to 40 mg. A more frequent dosing regimen is unlikely to be beneficial.

Renal Impairment

In patients with severe renal impairment (ClCr <30 mL/min), the recommended initial dose is 2.5 mg once daily; upward titration should be performed cautiously if needed. BYSTOLIC has not been studied in patients receiving dialysis (see **CLINICAL PHARMACOLOGY, Special Populations**).

Hepatic Impairment

In patients with moderate hepatic impairment, the recommended initial dose is 2.5 mg once daily; upward titration should be performed cautiously if needed. SYSTOLIC has not been studied in patients with severe hepatic impairment and therefore it is not recommended in that population (see **PRECAUTIONS** and **CLINICAL PHARMACOLOGY, Special Populations**).

Geriatric Patients

It is not necessary to adjust the dose in the elderly (see above and PRECAUTIONS, Geriatric Use)

CYP2D6 Polymorphism (see **CLINICAL PHARMACOLOGY, Pharmacokinetics**)

No dose adjustments are necessary for patients who are CYP2D6 poor metabolizers. The clinical effect and safety profiles observed in poor metabolizers were similar to those of extensive metabolizers.

(Continued)

ANTIHYPERTENSIVE DRUGS

Table 79 *(Continued)*

How Supplied

BYSTOLIC is available as tablets for oral administration containing nebivolol hydrochloride equivalent to 2.5, 5, and 10 mg of nebivolol.

BYSTOLIC tablets are triangular-shaped, biconvex, unscored, differentiated by color, and are engraved with "**FL**" on one side and the number of mg (2½, 5, or 10) on the other side. BYSTOLIC tablets are supplied in the following strengths and package configurations:

BYSTOLIC

Tablet Strength	Package Configuration	NDC #	Tablet Color
2.5 mg	Bottle of 30	0456-1402-30	Light Blue
	Bottle of 100	0456-1402-01	
5 mg	Bottle of 30	0456-1405-30	
	Bottle of 100	0456-1405-01	Beige
	10 × 10 Unit Dose	0456-1405-63	
10 mg	Bottle of 30	0456-1410-30	
	Bottle of 100	0456-1410-01	Pinkish-Purple
	10 × 10 Unit Dose	0456-1410-63	

Store at 20–25°C (68–77°F). (See USP for Controlled Room Temperature.)

Dispense in a tight-resistant container as defined in the USP using a child-resistant closure.

Forest Pharmaceuticals, Inc.
Subsidiary of Forest Laboratories, Inc.
St. Louis, MO 63045, USA
Licensed from Mylan Laboratories, Inc.
Under license from Janssen
Pharmaceutica N.V., Beerse, Belgium

Actidose-Aqua® is a registered trademark of Paddock Laboratories, Inc.

Rev. 12/07
©2007 Forest Laboratories, Inc.

ACE = angiotensin-converting enzyme; ACTH = adrenocorticotropic hormone; ALT = alanine aminotransferase; AST = aspartate aminotransferase; AV = atrioventricular; HDL = high-density lipoprotein; IV = intravenous; LH = luteinizing hormone; MI = myocardial infarction; MRHD = maximum recommended human dose.

ACEIs are effective in all forms of hypertension (HRH, NRH, and LRH) but are most effective in HRH. Side effects are minor and infrequent, and most patients tolerate these agents well. Cough occurs in 10–15% of patients and is more common in women. Patients who cough tend to have the best antihypertensive effect. The cough is due to increased levels of bradykinin and substance P. ACEIs are useful as initial therapy and as monotherapy. They are effective in African-Americans, elderly, Caucasians and young patients. Higher doses are often needed in the African-American patients to achieve equal BP reduction. However, higher doses are now recommended for most patients to achieve not only good BP control but also some of the beneficial nonhypertensive effects on the vascular system.

ACEIs also have a favorable effect in preserving renal function in both nondiabetic and diabetic hypertensives and in diabetic patients without hypertension with proteinuria to reduce proteinuria and IGCP.

Table 80 Direct Vasodilators Highlights*

	Preparation	Mechanism of action	Pharmacodynamics	Hemodynamics	Adverse effects	Contraindications	Daily dosage	Drug interactions
Hydralazine (Apresoline)— Novartis	10 mg 25 mg 50 mg 100 mg 20 mg/mL IV	Peripheral vasodilator that acts by direct relaxation on the vascular smooth muscles	Rapid absorption, Duration: 6 hours Onset: 20–30 minutes (IV) 1 hour (oral) Peak: 2–4 hours Excretion: renal Metabolism: liver	Peripheral vasodilation SVR, PVR reduced HR, CO increased PRA increased GFR increased RBF, RPF increased	Postural hypotension, headaches, reflex tachycardia, nausea, palpitations, fatigue, fluid retention, Lupus syndrome, nasal congestion	Aortic aneurysm, coronary artery disease, mitral valve or rheumatic heart disease	Initial:10 mg bid Range: 40–400 mg, Usual dose: 100–200 mg bid schedule	Diazoxide: severe hypotension Digoxin: decreased digoxin effect with IV hydralazine Beta-adrenergic blockers: enhanced hydralazine effect
Minoxidil (Loniten)— Pharmacia & Upjohn	2.5 mg 5 mg 10 mg	Direct relaxation of arterial smooth muscle. Reduces SVR and PVR (little effect on venous smooth muscle)	Duration: 12 hours Onset: 1 hour Peak: 4–8 hours Excretion: renal Metabolism: liver	SVR, PVR reduced Reflex tachycardia HR, CO increased PRA, NE, Ang-II, aldosterone increased RPF, RBF, GFR increased	Hypertrichosis, fluid retention and weight gain, precipitation of angina, cardiac tamponade, ECG changes, reflex tachycardia, ↓T-cell function, ↑ RVH, ↑ LVH	CHF, Pheochromocytoma	Initial: 5 mg single dose Range: 10–40 mg bid schedule	Guanethidine: severe orthostatic hypotension

Ang-II = angiotensin II; CHF = congestive heart failure; CO = cardiac output; ECG = electrocardiogram; GFR = glomerular filtration rate; HR = hazard ratio; IV = intravenous; PRA = plasma renin activity; PVR = peripheral vascular resistance; RBF = renal blood flow; RPF = renal plasma flow; SVR = systemic vascular resistance.
*Consult the *Physicians' Desk Reference* for full prescribing information.

Table 81 Alpha1-Blockers Highlights*

	Preparation	Mechanism of action	Pharmacodynamics	Hemodynamics	Adverse effects	Contraindications	Daily dosage	Drug interactions
Doxazosin (Cardura)— Pfizer	1 mg 2 mg 4 mg 8 mg,	Selective blockade of alpha1 receptor. Antagonizes pressor effect of phenylephrine and NE	Duration: 24 hours Onset: 1 hour Peak: 2–6 hours Metabolism: liver Excretion: urinary and fecal	HR unchanged or increased; CO unchanged; SVR reduced; venous capacitance increased; PRA unchanged; RBF, RPF, GFR increased or unchanged; PWP reduced or unchanged	Syncope (rare), dizziness, increased sweating, fatigue, palpitations, edema	Hypersensitivity to quinazolines	Initial: 1 mg hs, Maximum: 16 mg, Average: 4–6 mg	Vardenafil (Levitra and Tadalafil Cialis), hypotension
Prazosin (Minipress)— Pfizer	1 mg 2 mg 5 mg 10 mg	Vasodilator effect is related to blockade of peripheral postsynaptic alpha adrenoreceptors	Duration: 8–12 hours Onset: 1 hour Peak: 2–3 hours Metabolism: liver Excretion: biliary, feces	HR and CO unchanged or increased; SVR reduced; venous capacitance increased; PRA unchanged; RPF, RBF, GFR unchanged or slightly increased; PWP reduced or unchanged	Syncope with first doze (rare, <1%), postural hypotension (uncommon), palpitations, dizziness, weakness, headache	None	Initial 1 mg bid with first dose at bedtime Maintenance: 5–15 mg in divided doses (bid) Maximum: 40 mg	Beta-adrenergic blockers: increased hypotensive effect of the first dose, Indomethacin: decreased hypotensive effect, Vardenafil, Tadalafil
Terazosin (Hytrin)—Abbott	1 mg 2 mg 5 mg 10 mg	Postsynaptic alpha1 blockade	Duration: 18–24 hours Onset: 1 hour Peak: 1–2 hours Metabolism: liver Excretion: biliary, feces	See Prazosin	Syncope postural hypotension, headache, tachycardia, asthenia, edema, dry mouth, nasal congestion, dizziness	None	Initial: 1 mg Average: 1–5 mg Maximum: 40 mg; may require bid dosing	See Prazosin, Vardenfil, Tadalafil

CO = cardiac output; GFR = glomerular filtration rate; HR = hazard ratio; NE = norepinephrine; PRA = plasma renin activity; PWP = pulmonary wedge pressure; RBF = renal blood flow; RPF = renal plasma flow; SVR = systemic vascular resistance.

*Consult the *Physicians' Desk Reference* for full prescribing information.

A triphasic BP response may occur with high renin levels:
1. Initial abrupt fall (occasionally to hypotensive levels) for several hours.
2. Return of BP but below pretreatment levels.
3. Chronic gradual reduction of BP over several days, but not as low as with initial therapy. The maximum effect occurs at 2–4 weeks and is predicted by the initial response. Patients with normal or low renin levels have a more prolonged and gradual decrease in BP. Volume depletion or concurrent antihypertensive therapy exaggerates the response (Figure 87).

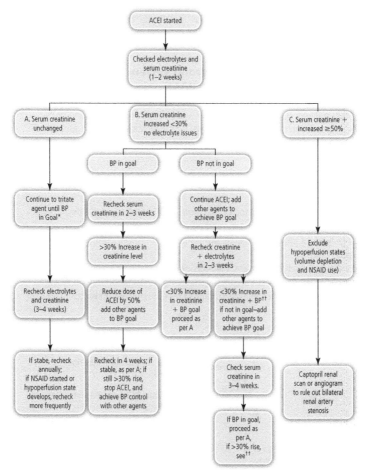

Adapted from *ARCH intern Med* (2000) Vol 160, March 13, 692.

A schematic approach to patient with renal, insufficiency started on therapy with an angiotensin-converting enzyme inhibitor (ACEI).

*Blood pressure (BP) less than 130/85 mm Hg for those with renal insufficiency or diabetes;
††If serum creatinine level increases more than 30%, reduce ACEI dose by 50% and add other BP-lowering agents and if serum creatinine rise is greater than 30% and less than 50% within the first month of therapy, causes for hypoperfusion are eliminated and nonsteroidal anti-inflammatory drugs (NSAIDs) are not given, treat as if bilateral renal arterial disease is present.

Figure 87 Approach to Initiation of ACEI Therapy.

ACE is the key enzyme in the RAAS and kinin system. ACE is found primarily in tissues such as the endothelium and blood vessels, where it stems from local synthesis secondary to gene expression. The adverse effects of ACE are related to its conversion of

Ang-I to Ang-II and its degradation of bradykinin. The ACE thus induces vasoconstriction, increases Ang-II levels, PAI-1, EDCF, and endothelin, which promote vascular smooth muscle growth and migration, matrix synthesis, platelet aggregation, and thrombosis. Degradation of bradykinin inhibits its vasodepressor, antiproliferative, and fibrinolytic effects due to decreases in endothelium-derived relaxing factor (EDRF)/NO, prostacyclin, and t-PA. The processes mediated byAng-II and bradykinin occur primarily at the tissue level and are implicated in a number of CV conditions, including hypertension, ischemia, atherosclerosis, vascular hypertrophy, and restenosis after vascular injury.

Renin–angiotensin–aldosterone system
General and major points: two RAAS

1. Classic RAAS: BP regulation and circulating ACE (10%)
2. Tissue RAAS: regulates vascular and cardiac structure and function (90%)
The general and major points of the two RAAS are shown in the Figures 88–90.

ACE is an ectoenzyme that faces lumen of vascular system (i.e., protrudes from cell membranes into extracellular space)

ACE is located on
1. vascular endothelial cells: lumen and vasa vasorum;
2. media of VSMC.

Ang-II is a potent vasoconstrictor and a growth promoter and is a thrombogenic, pro-oxidant, proinflammatory, and atherogenic hormone
Other types of angiotensins exist with variable CV effects, both qualitatively and quantitatively
Aldosterone produces similar CV effects as Ang-II
Alternate pathways exist for conversion of Ang-Ito Ang-II other than ACE
Alternate pathways become quantitatively more important under conditions of disease

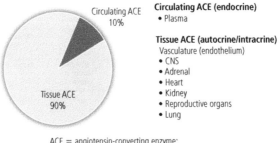

Figure 88 Circulating vs. Tissue ACE.

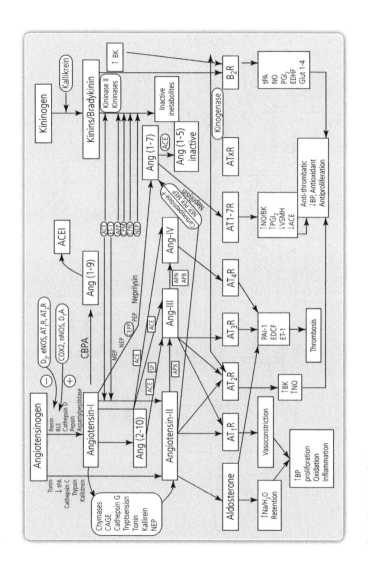

Figure 89 RAAS Pathway.

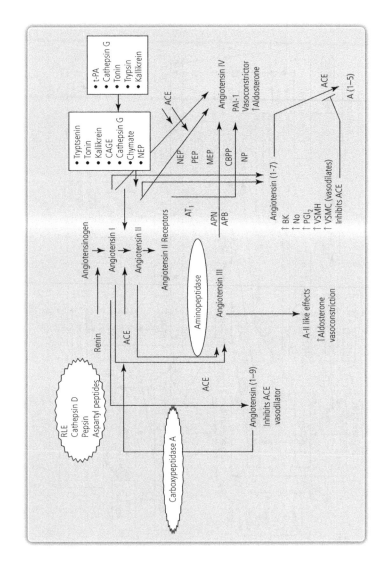

Figure 90 Formation of Angiotensins—Alternative Pathways.

ACE and ACEI: clinical basic science correlations

Extracellular engagement of ACEI to ACE is a function of
1. affinity (tissue selectivity and lipophilicity);
2. tissue blood flow.

ACEIs differ in
1. enzyme binding affinities (tissue selectivity);
2. on and off rates;
3. duration of action.

Tissue ACE and conversion of A-I to A-II is an autocrine and an intracrine function.

   ACEIs interact differently with ACE active sides, depending on their structural configurations (ACE and other endogenous degradation).

Potency of ACEIs in plasma and tissue

Plasma		Tissue
Quinaprilat (400)	High	Quinaprilat (33)
Cilazaprilat (28)		Benazeprilat (27)
Benazeprilat (17)		Perindoprilat (17)
Fosinoprilat (14)		Ramiprilat (11)
Ramiprilat (12)		Lisinopril (6)
Lisinopril (5)		Enalaprilat (2.3)
Enalaprilat (5)		Fosinoprilat (1.7)
Captopril (1)	Low	

Adapted from Fabris B, et al. *Br Pharmacol* 1990; 100: 651–655; Fabris B, et al. *I Cardiovasc Pharmacol* 1990; 15(suppl. 21–56):513; Johnston C1, et al. *Hypertension* 1989; 7(suppl. 5): 511–516.

Content points
- Radioligand inhibitor binding studies demonstrate a wide range of ACE binding affinity among the available ACEIs.
- Quinaprilat, the active metabolite of quinapril, possesses the highest ACE binding affinity in both tissue and plasma.
- Tissue ACE and the endothelium appear to play important roles in the development of atherosclerosis. It is plausible that differences in ACE binding affinity could translate into differential clinical responses.

Combination of ACEI and ARB

There is increasing evidence that the combination of ACEI and ARB may not only provide additional BP reduction but also increase vascular and renal protection and reduce proteinuria better than either agent alone (Figure 91). Clinical trials are in progress to prove this concept.

Highlights of the various ACEI

The highlights of the various ACEI are illustrated in Table 82.

Nonhypertensive effects of ACEI

The nonhypertensive effects of ACEI are illustrated in Table 83.

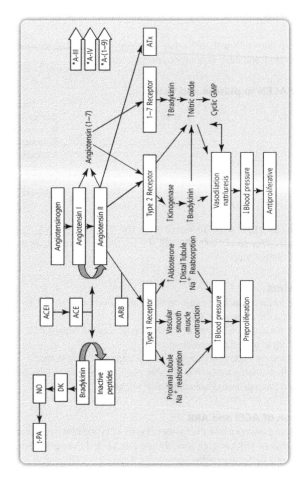

Figure 91 Rationale for Therapy: ACEI + ARB

Table 82 ACEIs Highlights*

	Preparation	Mechanism of action	Pharmacodynamics	Hemodynamics	Adverse effects	Contraindications	Daily dosage	Drug interactions
Benazepril (Lotensin)— Novartis	5 mg 10 mg 20 mg 40 mg	ACEI	Onset: 1 hour Peak: 2–4 hours Plasma half-life: 10–11 hours Metabolism: hepatic, renal Excretion: renal Absorption: unaffected by food	Exercise response preserved Ang-II and aldosterone reduced PRA and Ang-I increased GFR, RPF, RBF unchanged or increased RVR reduced HR unchanged or rarely increased SVR reduced MAP reduced	Headache, dizziness, fatigue, cough, nausea, angioedema (rare)	Similar to lisinopril	Initial: 10 mg Average 10–40 mg Maximum: 80 mg Interval: qd	Lithium, K$^+$ supplements, K$^+$ sparing diuretics: risk of hyperkalemia
Captopril (Capoten)— PAR	12.5 mg 25 mg 50 mg 100 mg	A specific inhibitor of ACE; interrupts the renin–angiotensin system and formulation of Ang-II	Onset: 1–2 hours Peak: 4 hours Plasma half-life: 8–12 hours (increases with dose) Metabolism: liver (15%) Excretion: renal (85%—unchanged 50%, metabolites 35%) Absorption: reduced by food	See Benazepril	Taste disturbances, cutaneous rash, proteinuria, leukopenia, renal insufficiency, cough, angioedema (rare)	Renal impairment, renal artery stenosis (caution), connective tissue disease (caution)	Initial: 25 mg bid or tid Average: 100–150 mg Range: 75–450 mg Maximum: 450 mg Intervals: bid or tid Lower doses now recommended	Cimetidine: severe neuropathies in patients with renal impairment, Indomethacin: decreases hypotensive effect, Spironolactone and triamterene: hyperkalemia (monitor K$^+$ concentration), Lithium: increased lithium levels, K$^+$ supplements, K$^+$ sparing diuretics (combination, i.e., Dyazide, Maxzide): risk of hyperkalemia (Continued)

Table 82 (Continued)

	Preparation	Mechanism of action	Pharmacodynamics	Hemodynamics	Adverse effects	Contraindications	Daily dosage	Drug interactions
Enalapril (Vasotec)— Biovail	5 mg 10 mg 20 mg	ACEI	Onset: 1 hour Peak: 3–4 hours Plasma half-life: 12–24 hours Metabolism: liver Excretion: renal (40%) Absorption: unaffected by food	See Benazepril	Less rash and loss of taste than with captopril, other side effects are similar	Renal impairment, renal artery stenosis (caution), connective tissue disease (caution)	Initial: 5 mg Average: 20 mg Range: 10–140 mg Maximum: 40 mg Intervals: qid or bid	
Fosinopril (Monopril)— Bristol-Myers Squibb	10 mg 20 mg 40 mg	ACEI	Onset: 1 hour Peak: 2–6 hours Plasma half-life: 12 hours Metabolism: hepatic, renal Excretion: renal, feces Absorption: unaffected by food	See Benazepril	Headache, dizziness, fatigue, cough, nausea, diarrhea, angioedema[†]	Similar to lisinopril	Initial: 10 mg Average: 20–40 mg Maximum: 80 mg Interval: qd	See above, Digoxin: may cause false low digoxin levels
Quinapril (Accupril)— Pfizer	5 mg 10 mg 20 mg 40 mg	ACEI	Onset: 1 hour Peak: 1–2 hours Plasma half-life: 25 hours Metabolism: hepatic Excretion: renal (96%) Absorption: 60% decreased by food	See Benazepril	Headache, fatigue, nausea, dizziness, cough, angioedema[†]	Hypersensitivity to drug	Initial: 10 mg Average: 20–40 mg Maximum: 80 mg Interval: bid	See Captopril

	Doses	Class	Mechanism	Pharmacokinetics	Side effects	Contraindications	Dosage	Interactions
Lisinopril (Prinivil)— Merck (Zestril)— Astra-Zeneca	2.5 mg 5 mg 10 mg 20 mg 30 mg 40 mg	ACEI	See Benazepril	Onset: 1 hour Peak: 6 hours Plasma half-life: 12–24 hours Metabolism: none Excretion: renal (100%) Absorption: unaffected by food	Dizziness, headache, fatigue, diarrhea, cough, Interval: qd, Angioedema[†], Hypotension[†], Neutropenia[†],	Hypersensitivity to drug, renal impairment, renal artery stenosis (caution), connective tissue disease (caution)	Initial: 5–10 mg monotherapy Average: 20–40 mg Maximum: 80 mg Interval: qd	Diuretics: hypotension, Indomethacin renal insufficiency, K⁺ sparing agents and K⁺ supplements: increased risk of hyperkalemia
Ramipril (Altace)— Monarch	1.25 mg 2.5 mg 5 mg 10 mg	ACEI	See Benazepril	Onset: 1 hour Peak: 3–6 hours Plasma half-life: 13–17 hours Metabolism: liver Excretion: renal (60%), hepatic (feces) (40%) Absorption: reduced by food	Headache, dizziness, fatigue, cough, nausea, angioedema[†]	Hypersensitivity to drug	Initial: 2.5 mg Average: 2.5–20 mg Maximum: 20 mg Interval: qd	Benazepril
Moexipril (Univasc)— Schwarz Pharma	7.5 mg 15 mg	ACEI	See Benazepril	Onset: 1 hour Peak: 1½ hours Plasma half-life: 12–14 hours Metabolism: liver Excretion: bile and urine Absorption: reduced by food	As above	As above	Initial: 7.5 mg Maximum: 30 mg Interval: qd	As above
Trandolapril (Mavik)— Abbott	1 mg 2 mg 4 mg	ACEI	See Benazepril	Onset: 1 hour Peak: 4–10 hours Plasma half-life: 6–10 hours Metabolism: hepatic Excretion: urine, feces, bile	Cough, dizziness, diarrhea, headache, fatigue	As above	Initial: 1–2 mg Average: 2–4 mg Maximum: 4 mg Interval: qd or bid	As above

(Continued)

Table 82 (Continued)

	Preparation	Mechanism of action	Pharmacodynamics	Hemodynamics	Adverse effects	Contraindications	Daily dosage	Drug interactions
Perindopril (Aceon)— Solvay	2 mg 4 mg 8 mg	ACEI	Onset: 1 hour Peak: 3–7 hours Plasma half-life: 3–10 hours Metabolism: liver Excretion: renal Absorption: unaffected by food	See Benazepril	Dizziness, headache, asthenia, rhinitis, dyspepsia, proteinuria, palpitations	History of angioedema related to previous ACEI, pregnancy renal impairment (caution), renal artery stenosis (caution)	Initial: 4 mg qd Average: 4–8 mg Maximum: 16 mg Intervals: qd or bid	Diuretic: hypotension K$^+$ sparing agents and K$^+$ supplements may increase risk of hyperkalemia, Gentamicin use with caution

ACE = angiotensin-converting enzyme; ACEI = angiotensin-converting enzyme inhibitor; Ang-II = angiotensin II; GFR = glomerular filtration rate; HR = hazard ratio; MAP = mean arterial pressure; PRA = plasma renin activity; RBF = renal blood flow; RPF = renal plasma flow; RVR = renal vascular resistance; SVR = systemic vascular resistance.
*Consult the Physicians' Desk Reference for full prescribing information.
†Rare

Table 83 Nonhypertensive Treatment Effects of ACEIs

- ↑ BK
- ↑ NO
- ↑ EDHF
- ↓ Vasopressin
- ↓ ET-1
- ↑ PGI-2
- ↑ Enkephalins
- ↑ EDV
- ↓ CAMS
- ↓ PAI-1 and ↑ t-PA (↑ Fibrinolysis)
- ↓ Growth factors and VSMH
- ↓ ROS/O_2
- ↑ AC_1, ↑ C_1AC, ↑ C_2AC, ↓ PWV, ↑ AGI, ↓ ASI, ↑ PP, ↓AD, ↓ ASI
- ↓ Plaque rupture
- Angiogenesis (myocardial)
- ↓ Atherosclerosis
- ↓ Platelets effects
- ↑ Ang 1–7
- ↓ Ang-II – transient
- ↓ Microalbuminuria (MAU) and proteinuria
- ↓ MLR
- ↓ Fibrinogen

ACEI = angiotensin-converting enzyme inhibitor; Ang = angiotensin; BK = bradykinin; CAMS = cellular adhesion molecules; EDHF = endothelium-dependent hyperpolarization; EDV = end-diastolic volume; ET-1 = endothelin; MLR = mixed lymphocyte responses; NO = nitric oxide; PAI-1 = plasminogen activator inhibitor-I; PGI-2 = prostacyclin-2; t-PA = tissue plasminogen activator; VSMH = vascular smooth muscle hyperplasia.

Calcium channel blockers [149]

CCBs inhibit the influx of calcium ions through slow channels in vascular smooth muscle tissue and cause relaxation of the arterioles. These agents are useful in the treatment of all degrees of hypertension (mild, moderate, or severe).

1. The higher the BP, the greater the therapeutic reduction in BP
2. Low-renin hypertensive patients (volume-dependent patients) have the best response (75–80% response rate as monotherapy), but most patients respond well
3. African-Americans and elderly patients also respond well (75–80% with monotherapy)
4. Mild edema in the absence of weight gain may be seen with long-term use. Diuretic and natriuretic effects occur. ACEI and ARB will counteract this edema. The edema is due to an increase in interstitial fluid related to dilation of the afferent arteriole of the capillary bed. Diuretics are not effective treatment for CCB-induced edema; ARBs and ACEIs are the best treatment for this type of interstitial edema as they dilate the efferent arteriole preferentially
5. The antihypertensive effect is enhanced by most other antihypertensive agents
6. The effect on lipids is neutral or favorable. No adverse effect is seen on K+, Mg2+, glucose, uric acid, homocysteine, or other metabolic parameters
7. There is a low adverse effect profile

ANTIHYPERTENSIVE DRUGS

8. CCBs preserve renal function and actually reduce microalbuminuria and proteinuria if the initial values or proteinuria are below 400 mg/day.
9. LVH is reduced.
10. CCBs are very effective as monotherapy.
11. CCBs have been shown to reduce the incidence of dementia (cognitive function improves with reduction in BP). (Forette F, Seux ML, Staessen JA, et al. Prevention of dementia in randomized double-blind placebo-controlled Systolic Hypertension in Europe (Syst-Eur) trial. Lancet 1998; 352: 1347–1351.)
12. Amlodipine (ALLHAT) and other CCBs in numerous meta-analysis studies may reduce CVA better than any other antihypertensive drug classes. Amlodipine was equal to chlorthalidone in reduction of fatal CHD and nonfatal MI as well as all-cause mortality (ALLHAT) and equal to Valsartan in reducing combined cardiac morbidity and mortality (VALUE).

CCB highlights
The CCB highlights are illustrated in Table 84.

Treatment: nonhypertensive effects of some CCBs [155A]
- Counteracts Ang-II via an increase in NO bioavailability
- Counteracts ET-1
- Increases eNOS and NO
- Antioxidant (membrane lipid) (decreases ROS and decreases superoxide anion)
- Enhances EDHF
- Interferes with cyclooxygenase-derived contracting factors
- Increases EDV
- Endothelial cell cytoprotection (reduces cytokines and reduces CAMs)
- Modifies VCMC membrane defect
- Inhibits VSMC proliferation and migration
- Inhibits ACAT in macrophages and inhibits cholesterol esterification and oxidation of LDL via lipid peroxide
- Decreases insulin resistance
- Improves AC, increases C1AC, increases C2AC, decreases PP, increases aortic distensibility (AD), decreases aortic stiffness index (ASI), decreases PVW, and decreases AGI
- Reduces atherosclerosis
- Antiplatelet effect
- Inhibits TNF
- Inhibits platelet-derived growth factor
- Decreases media/lumen ratio (MLR)
- Decreases xanthine oxidase and catalase
- Decreases beta fibroblastic growth factor (bFGF)
- Decreases leukotrienes
- Decreases thromboxane B2
- Decreases fibrinogen

Ang-II receptor blockers
ARBs like ACEIs interfere with the RAAS. ACEIs block the conversion of Ang-I to Ang-II, whereas ARBs block the binding of Ang-II to one of its receptor sites, AT1. It is thought that the actions of Ang-II are more effectively blocked by direct AT1

Table 84 CCBs Highlights*

	Preparation	Mechanism of action	Pharmacodynamics	Hemodynamics	Adverse effects	Contraindications	Daily dosage	Drug interactions
Amlodipine (Norvasc)— Pfizer	2.5 mg 5 mg 10 mg	Coronary and vascular smooth muscle vasodilation	Absorption: 100% unchanged unaltered by food, Bioavailability: 64–90% Onset: 6 hours, Peak: 6–12 hours Half-life: 30–50 hours, Protein binding: 93% Metabolism: hepatic: 90% Excretion: urine (60%); metabolites. No alteration with renal insufficiency	SVR reduced; HR palpitations; CO unchanged or increased; RBF, RPF, GFR preserved, increased; no effect on sinoatrial (SA) or AV node; coronary vasodilation; afterload reduction	Dizziness, flushing, edema	Hypersensitivity to amlodipine	Initial: 5 mg Average: 5 mg Maximum: 10 mg Interval: qd, Long T ½—intrinsic, High trough to peak ratio	None yet established
Diltiazem SR (Cardizem SR, Cardizem CD)—Biovail (Cardizem LA)	60 mg 90 mg 120 mg 180 mg 240 mg 300 mg 360 mg 420 mg	Selective relaxation of smooth muscle prevents proteinuria	Absorption: well absorbed > 90%, Bioavailability: 45–67% (first pass-hepatic) Onset: 1 hour Peak: 3 hours, Half-life: 4 hours Protein binding: 80%	Dilates coronary and peripheral arteries, depresses SA and AV nodal function, negative inotropic effect, reduces HR	Headache, AV block disorders and sinus arrest, dizziness, pedal edema, bradycardia	Sick sinus syndrome, AV block (second-degree, third-degree), severe CHF, digitalis toxicity	Average: 240–360 mg Range: 120–360 mg Maximum: 360 mg Interval: bid or tid	Beta-adrenergic blockers: cardiac failure (additive effects on contractility and blockade of compensating reflexes)

(Continued)

Table 84 (Continued)

	Preparation	Mechanism of action	Pharmacodynamics	Hemodynamics	Adverse effects	Contraindications	Daily dosage	Drug interactions
(Tiazac)—Forest/UAD	120 mg 180 mg 240 mg 300 mg 360 mg 420 mg	Relaxation of smooth muscle, reduces proteinuria	Metabolism: hepatic (60% fecal excretion) Excretion: renal (35%) Plasma levels: 40–200 ng/mL	Reduces SVR, Increases MVO$_2$, CO unchanged	Electrocardiographic abnormalities, asthenia, constipation, dyspepsia, nausea, palpitations	Acute MI and pulmonary congestion, additive effects with BBs and digoxin	Initial: 120–240 mg Average: 180–360 mg Maximum: 540 mg Interval: once daily	AV conduction disturbances and sinus bradycardia (additive)
(DilacorXR)—Watson	180 mg 240 mg 360 mg	Relaxation of smooth muscle						
Tiamate	120 mg 240 mg	Relaxation of smooth muscle, reduces proteinuria						
Isradipine (DynaCirc, DynaCirc SR†)—Novartis Reliant	2.5 mg 5 mg 10 mg	Selective relaxation of smooth muscle in systemic vasculature. Mild diuretic activity	Absorption: 90–95% Bioavailability: 15–24% Onset of action: 20 minutes Peak: 2–3 hours, Food increases time to peak by 1 hour, Half-life: biphasic; early: 1½–2 hours terminal: 8 hours, Protein binding: 95% Excretion: urine 60–65%, feces 25–30%	Vasodilation with increased coronary, cerebral, and skeletal muscle blood flow, SVR reduced, HR increased, CO increased	Headache, dizziness, edema, palpitations, fatigue, flushing	Hypersensitivity to drug	Initial: 2.5 mg bid Average: 5–10 mg in divided doses Maximum: 20 mg	

Drug	Dose	Action	Pharmacologic effects	Pharmacokinetics	Side effects	Contraindications	Dosage	Comments/Interactions
Nicardipine (Cardene)—Roche	20mg 30mg	Selective relaxation of vascular smooth muscle. More selective on smooth muscle than myocardium. Greater effect on cerebral and coronary vessels than peripheral vessels	SVR reduced, reflex increase in HR, MAP reduced, RBF, RPF, GFR preserved, CO unchanged or increased, no effect on SA or AV nodal conduction, coronary artery vasodilation	Absorption: >95% Bioavailability: 35% Onset: 30 minutes Peak: 1 hour Half-life: 8.6 hours Protein binding: 95% Metabolism: liver Excretion: urine 60%, feces 35% Plasma levels: 10–100 ng/mL	Flushing, headache, pedal edema, asthenia, palpitations, dizziness, tachycardia	Advanced aortic stenosis, hypersensitivity to drug	Initial: 20mg tid Average: 30mg tid Maximum: 40mg tid	Food: increases time to peak by 1 hour Cimetidine: increases nicardipine levels Cyclosporine: increases cyclosporine plasma levels BBs: CHF
(Cardene SR)—Roche	30mg 45mg 60mg							
Nifedipine (Adalat CC)—Bayer; (Procardia XL)—Pfizer	30mg 60mg 90mg extended-release tablets	Selective relaxation of vascular smooth muscle by reducing intracellular calcium concentration	SVR reduced; PRA decreased; MAP reduced; RBF, RPF, GFR preserved; CO increased or unchanged by reflex sympathetic activity and decreased SVR; no effect on SA or AV nodal function; smooth muscle relaxation (generalized)	Absorption: 90% Bioavailability: 75% Onset: immediate, First peak: 2.5–5 hours Second peak: 6–12 hours Half-life: 2 hours Protein binding: 92–98% Metabolism: liver—complete Excretion: renal (60–80%) Plasma levels: C_{max} is 36% greater average concentration, 70% greater in subjects age >60 years 6–120 ng/mL	Headache, dizziness, lightheadedness, tachycardia, tremor, nervousness, palpitations, leg cramps, fatigue, weakness, nausea, diarrhea, edema, flushing, orthostatic hypotension, tinnitus	Hypersensitivity to drug	Initial: 30mg Average: 30mg Range: 30–90mg Maximum: 90mg Interval: qd on empty stomach	Beta-adrenergic blockers: cardiac failure (additive effects on contractility and blockade of compensating reflexes) Digoxin: increases digoxin effect (rare), Hypoglycemics, sulfonylurea: increased hypoglycemic effect with oral nifedipine (decreased glucose metabolism), Cimetidine: increased nifedipine plasma levels

(Continued)

Table 84 (Continued)

	Preparation	Mechanism of action	Pharmacodynamics	Hemodynamics	Adverse effects	Contraindications	Daily dosage	Drug interactions
Nisoldipine (Sular)— Astra-Zeneca	10 mg 20 mg 30 mg 40 mg	Inhibits calcium influx into vascular smooth muscle and cardiac muscle	Absorption: 87% Bioavailability: 5% Onset: 2 hours Peak: 6–12 hours Half-life: 7–12 hours Protein binding: 99%, Metabolism: liver, Excretion: urine (60–80%)	Similar to nifedipine	Similar to nifedipine	Allergy	Average: 20 mg, Range: 10–60 mg qd, Maximum: 60 mg	Cimetidine: increased plasma levels Quinidine: decreased bioavailability
Verapamil (Calan SR)— Pharmacia (Isoptin SR)—Abbott (Verelan)— Wyeth-Ayerst, Verelan PM— (Schwarz) Pharma	Oral: 120 mg, 180 mg, 240 mg, SR tab, 40 mg, 80 mg, 120 mg, 180 mg, 240 mg, 180 mg, 200 mg, 300 mg	Selective relaxation of smooth muscle by reducing intracellular calcium concentration in coronary and peripheral vasculature and inhibiting slow-channel Ca^{2+} transport, Reduces proteinuria	Absorption: 95%, Bioavailability: 10–20% (extensive hepatic first pass) Onset: 1 hour Peak: 2 hours Half-life: 3–6 hours (up to 9 hours with long-term therapy) Protein binding: 90% Metabolism: hepatic (85%) fecal (15%); accumulates in liver disease Excretion: renal (70%), biexponential elimination (fast/ slow), Plasma levels: 80–300 ng/mL	SA and AV nodal function depressed reentrant pathways, ventricular response slowed, SVR arterial reduced (no venous effect), MAP reduced—less pronounced, CO reduced, negative inotropic action, mild bradycardia, myocardial oxygen supply increased by increasing coronary blood flow	Constipation: most common, headache, vertigo, dizziness, lightheadedness, weakness, nervousness, pruritus, flushing, gastric disturbances, Hepatitis, SGOT, alkaline phosphatase, orthostatic hypotension, AV block, AV dissociation	Sick sinus syndrome, second-degree or third-degree AV block, digitalis toxicity, cardiogenic shock	Average: 240 mg Range: 120–480 mg Maximum: 540 mg Interval: qd, bid	Beta-adrenergic blockers: cardiac failure (additive effects on contractility and blockade of compensating reflexes) Digoxin: increased digoxin toxicity (possibly decreased renal excretion) Hypoglycemics, sulfonylurea: increased hypoglycemic effect (increased glucose metabolism), Lithium: increased lithium levels

Drug—Manufacturer	Dosage	Comments	Pharmacokinetics	Mechanism	Side effects	Contraindications	Dosage	Drug interactions
(Covern HS)—Pharmacia	180 mg 240 mg	See above. Unique delivery system designed for 4–5 hours delay to be taken at bedtime for maximum concentration in the A.M.	Absorption: 65%, Bioavailability: 33–65% Onset: 4–5 hours Peak: 11 hours Half-life: 14–16 hours Protein binding: 94% Metabolism: hepatic Excretion: renal (70%), fecal (16%)	Myocardial oxygen demand reduced by decreasing HR and reducing afterload, no adverse effect on pulmonary function, smooth muscle relaxation—generalized (vascular, gut, bronchial)	Aystole, sinus arrest, pedal edema, pulmonary edema and CHF, paresthesias (cold, numbness), hyperprolactinemia and galactorrhea		Average: 240 mg, Range 180–480 mg, Maximum: 540 mg, Interval: qhs (swallow whole)	Rifampin: reduced bioavailability of Calan, Carbamazepine: increased carbamazepine concentrations, Neuromuscular-blocking agents: Calan may protentiate their effects
Felodipine (Plendil)—Astra-Zeneca	2.5 mg 5 mg 10 mg	Selective relaxation of vascular smooth muscle, more than on myocardium	Absorption: 95%, Bioavailability: 20% Onset: 1/2–1 hour Peak 2.5–5 hours Half-life: 11–16 hours Protein binding: 99% Metabolism: liver Excretion: urine 70%, feces 10%	SVR reduced; HR increased; RBF, RPF, GFR preserved; CO unchanged or increased; No effect on SA or AV conduction; Coronary artery vasodilation	Edema, headache, flushing, dizziness, asthenia, tachycardia, fatigue, extrasystoles, nausea, palpitations	Hypersensitivity to drug	Initial: 5 mg, Average 5–10 mg, Maximum: 20 mg. Adjust every 2 weeks if necessary. Take tablet whole	Cimetidine: increased felodipine levels, Digoxin: increased digoxin levels, Phenytoin, carbamazepine, phenobarbital: decreased felodipine levels

AV = atrioventricular; BB = beta-blocker; CCB = calcium channel blocker; CHF = congestive heart failure; CO = cardiac output; GFR = glomerular filtration rate; HR = hazard ratio; MAP = mean arterial pressure; MVO2 = myocardial oxygen consumption; PRA = plasma renin activity; RBF = renal blood flow; RPF = renal plasma flow; SA = sinoatrial; SGOT = serum glutamic oxaloacetic transaminase; SVR = systemic vascular resistance.

*Consult the *Physicians' Desk Reference* for full prescribing information.

†Not found in *Physicians' Desk Reference*.

receptor antagonism. Blockade of the AT1 receptor allows Ang-II to stimulate the AT2 receptors, which induces vasodilation and other beneficial vascular effects. In addition, there is an increase in NO and slight increase in bradykinin. There may be an increase in Ang 1–7, which also induces vasodilation and favorable vascular effects (Figures 92 and 93).

ARBs have a more favorable safety and tolerability profile than ACEIs. They do not cause the adverse effects, such as cough and angioedema, that are attributed to ACEI interactions with the bradykinin system.

Ang-II receptors and the effects of blockade

From Weber MA. Interrupting the renin-angiotensin system: The role of angiotensin-converting enzyme inhibitors and angiotensin II receptor antagonists in the treatment of hypertension. *Am J Hypertens* 1999; 12: 189S–194S.

Vascular AT1 receptors
Constantly expressed
Mediate vasoconstriction
Mediate Ang-II arterial wall growth effects

Vascular AT2 receptors
Expressed only after injury (sustained hypertension might provoke expression)
Mediate vasodilation
Mediate antiproliferative actions
Activate other factors (e.g., NO)

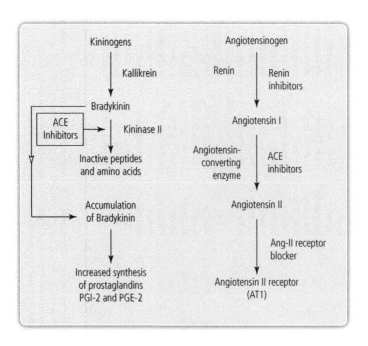

Figure 92 Renin Angiotensin and Kinin/Bradykinin Pathways.

Potential double action of selective AT1 blockers
Directly block vasoconstrictor and growth actions of Ang-II at AT1 receptors
Increase circulating Ang-II levels
Unblocked AT2 receptors (if expressed), stimulated by increased Ang-II activity, mediate vasodilation and growth inhibition
Net effects: AT1 blockade + AT2 stimulation
Unknown effect on other AT receptors

Highlights of ARBs
The highlights of ARBs are illustrated in Tables 85 and 86.

Examples of genes that can be regulated by Ang-II
Early genes/proto-oncogene: fos, myc, myb, jun, jun-B, egr-1

Growth factor genes: Transforming growth factor $\beta1$, platelet-derived growth factor-A chain, fibroblast Growth factor-2, insulin-like growth factor-1 receptor

Cell matrix factor genes: Fibronectin, collagen type I-α_1, collagen type III-α_1, laminin-β_1, and laminin-β_2

Hypertrophic marker: Atrial natriuretic peptide, brain natriuretic peptide, and skeletal muscle action-alpha-1

Fibrinolytic system genes: PAI, types 1 and 2

Miscellaneous genes: Aldosterone synthase (CYP11B2), endothelial NO synthase

From Kurtz TW, Gardner DG. Transcription-modulating drugs: A new frontier in the treatment of essential hypertension. *Hypertension* 1998; 32: 380–386, 1999; 12(12), Part 3, with permission.

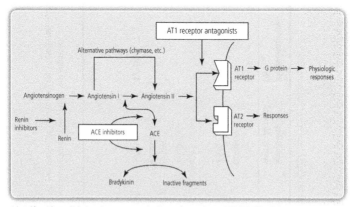

Adapted from Johnston CI: Angiotensin receptor antagonists: Focus on losartan. *Lancet* 1995; 346: 1403–1407.
Site of angiotensin II type 1 (AT1) receptor antagonists and angiotensin-converting enzyme
(ACE) inhibitors in the renin-angiotensin-aldosterone system.

Figure 93 Interrupting the Renin System.

Table 85 Pharmacologic Properties of Available ARB

Compound	Solubility in water/alcohol	Bioavailability (%)	Food effect	Active metabolite	Half-life (h)	Protein binding (%)	Dosing (mg)
Irbesartan [8]	−/low solubility	60–80	No	No	11–15	90	150–300 daily
Losartan [9]	+/+	33	Minimal	Yes	2 (6–9)	98.7 (99.8)	50–100 daily, twice daily
Valsartan [10]	low solubility/+	25	40–50% decrease	No	6	95	80–320 daily
Candesartan [11]	−/low solubility	15	No	Yes	9	>99	8–32 daily, twice daily
Telmisartan [12]	−/NR	42–58	6–20% decrease	No	24	99.5	40–80 daily
Eprosartan	−	13	Yes minimal <25%	No	20	98	400–1200 daily
Olmesartan	−	25	No	No	13	99	20–40 daily

ARB = angiotensin receptor blocker; NR = not reported.
From Zusman RM. Are there differences among angiotensin receptor blockers? *Am J Hypertens* 1999;12: 231S–235S, with permission.

Table 86 ARBs Highlights*

	Preparation	Mechanism of action	Pharmacodynamics	Hemodynamics	Adverse effects	Contraindications	Daily dosage	Drug interactions
Candesartan cilexetil (Atacand)— Astra-Zeneca	4 mg 8 mg 16 mg 32 mg	Selective AT1 angiotensin II receptor antagonist (see Irbesartan)	Onset: 0.5 hour Peak: 3–4 hours Plasma half-life: 9 hours Metabolism: hepatic and renal Excretion: urine and feces	(see Irbesartan)	Headache, dizziness, upper respiratory infections, pharyngitis, rhinitis	Pregnancy, hypersensitivity to drug	Initial: 16 mg qd Range: 8–32 mg Maximum: 32 mg qd	No significant interactions reported
Eprosartan (Teveten)— Unimed	400 mg 600 mg	Vascular and presynaptic AT1 blockade	Peak: 1–2 hours T ½ 20 hours Metabolism: none Excretion: bile Absorption: 13%	Similar to other ARBs	Rare facial edema, similar to other ARBs	Pregnancy, hypersensitivity	400–1200 mg	None
Irbesartan (Avapro)— Bristol-Myers Squibb	75 mg 150 mg 300 mg	Blocks vasoconstrictor- and aldosterone-secreting effects of Ang-II by selectively binding to the AT1 Ang-II receptor	Peak: 1.5–2 hours Plasma half-life: 11–15 hours Metabolism: biliary and renal Excretion: urine 20%, feces 80% Absorption: (not affected by food) 60–80%	Exercise response preserved; All and PRA increased; Aldosterone reduced; No effect on bradykinin; GFR, RPF, RBF unchanged; MAP reduced; HR unchanged	Diarrhea, dyspepsia/heartburn, musculoskeletal trauma, fatigue, upper respiratory infection	Hypersensitivity to drug, pregnancy	Initial: 150 mg qd Range: 150–300 mg qd Maximum: 300 mg qd	May be administered with other hypertensives. HCTZ has shown additive effect

(Continued)

Table 86 *(Continued)*

	Preparation	Mechanism of action	Pharmacodynamics	Hemodynamics	Adverse effects	Contraindications	Daily dosage	Drug interactions
Losartan (Cozaar)— Merck	25 and 50 mg 1000 mg	Blocks vasoconstrictor- and aldosterone-secreting effects of Ang-II	Onset: 1 hour Peak: 3–4 hours (active metabolite) Plasma half-life: 6–9 hours (active metabolite) Metabolism: hepatic and renal Excretion: renal and biliary Absorption: food slows absorption	Exercise response preserved; Ang-II and PRA increased; Aldosterone reduced; No effect on bradykinin; GFR, RPF, RBF unchanged; MAP reduced; HR unchanged	Dizziness, aesthenia/ fatigue, headache, cough	Pregnancy, hypersensitivity, caution with decreased liver function	Initial: 25–50 mg Range: 25–100 mg qd or bid Maximum: 100 mg qd or bid	May be administered with other hypertensives
Telmisartan (Micardis)— Boehringer Ingelheim	40 mg 80 mg	(see Irbesartan)	Peak: 0.5–1 hour Plasma half-life: 24 hours Metabolism: gut wall Excretion: feces (>97%) Absorption: slightly affected by food	(see Irbesartan)	Upper respiratory infection, back pain, sinusitis, diarrhea, pharyngitis	Pregnancy, nursing mothers, hypersensitivity to drug, caution with biliary obstruction and hepatic insufficiency	Initial: 40 mg qd Range: 20–80 mg qd Maximum: 80 mg qd	Digoxin: ↑ peak plasma concentration

Drug	Forms	Mechanism	Pharmacokinetics	Side effects	Contraindications	Dosing	Interactions
Valsartan (Diovan)— Novartis	80 mg caps 160 mg caps 320 mg	Blocks the vasoconstrictor- and aldosterone- secreting effects of Ang-II by selectively blocking binding of Ang-II to AT1 receptor tissues	Onset: 2 hours Peak: 2–4 hours Half-life: 6 hours Metabolism: liver and renal. Absorption: 30–50% Excretion: urine 13%, feces 83%	Exercise response preserved; Ang-II and PRA increased; aldosterone reduced; no effect on bradykinin; GFR, RPF, RBF unchanged; MAP reduced; HR unchanged	Headache, dizziness, viral infections, fatigue, abdominal pain	Hypersensitive to drug, pregnancy, caution with liver function tests	Initial: 80 mg qd Average: 80–160 mg qd 320 mg qd, Maximal BP reduction seen in 4 weeks	No significant interactions reported
Olmesartan (Benicar)— Sanyko	50 mg 20 mg 40 mg	High affinity and specific binding at AT1R, insurmountable inhibition of Ang-II	Onset: 2 hours, Peak: 2–4 hours T ½ 13 hours, Bioavailability 25% Albumin bound 99% Not metabolized by CYP450 Renal: 35–50% Hepatic: 50–65%, 24 hours duration	Similar to other ARBs	Similar to placebo dizziness in 3% withdrawal rate less than placebo	Hypersensitive to drug, pregnancy, no dose adjustment for – elderly, – hepatic disease, – renal disease, – food	Initial: 20 mg qd Average: 20 mg qd Maximum 40 mg qd	None No dose adjustments needed for – digoxin – warfarin – antacids

Ang-II = angiotensin II; ARB = angiotensin receptor blocker; AT1 = angiotensin type-I; AT1R = angiotensin type-I receptor; GFR = glomerular filtration rate; HCTZ = hydrochlorothiazide; HR = hazard ratio; MAP = mean arterial pressure; PRA = plasma renin activity; RBF = renal blood flow; RPF = renal plasma flow.
*Consult the *Physicians' Desk Reference* for full prescribing information.

Renin inhibitors (*Hypertension* 2003; 42: 1137–1143)

The direct RI (Aliskiren) (Tekturna) decreases PRA and inhibits the conversion of angiotensinogen to Ang-I. This results in a decrease in PRA, Ang-I and Ang-II. There are significant reductions in both SBP and DBP, and additive effects are seen with virtually all other classes of antihypertensive agents including diuretics, CCB, ARBs, ACEIs, and BB. Aliskiren results in a conformational change in renin, which reduces PRA. This is a different result in PRA compared with ACEI and ARB, which increase PRA. Recent studies have documented the presence of renin receptors in the vasculature and the kidney, which mediate hypertension, oxidative stress, vascular inflammation, and vascular damage. The reduction in PRA may reduce stimulation of these renin receptors.

Pharmacologic properties of aliskiren

Compound	Solubility water/alcohol	Bioavailability	Food effects	Active metabolites
Aliskiren	Minimal/+	2.6%	71–85% decrease	No

Half-life	Protein binding	Dosing (mg)
24 hours accumulation	NR	150–300 daily
40 hours elimination		

Preparation	Mechanism of action	Pharmacodynamics	Hemodynamics
150 mg; 300 mg	Direct inhibitor of renin reducing PRA, Ang-I, and Ang-II production	Peak: 1–3 hours; Metabolism: CYP3A4; Elimination: Y4 of dose eliminated unchanged in the urine	PRA, Ang-I, and Ang-II reduced

Adverse effects	Contraindications
Overall similar to placebo	NR

AEs >1% and more frequent than placebo: cough (1.1%), diarrhea (2%)
NR = not reported.

Drug interactions

Irbesartan reduces aliskiren C_{max} up to 50%
Atorvastatin increases aliskiren C_{max} 50% and AVC with multiple dosing
Ketaconazole increases aliskiren C_{max} ~80%
Cyclosporine increases aliskiren AVC fivefold and C_{max} 2.5-fold

Arterial Compliance: Structure/Function: Treatment Considerations [199–201]

Human trials with gluteal artery biopsies to assess vascular wall structure and function (Figure 94).
- Correct both structure and function and reduce BP. Increase small artery diameter, increase arterial compliance, decrease media/lumen ratio, decrease SVR, and BP remodeling or arterioles
  - ACEI
  - ARB
  - CCB
  - RI

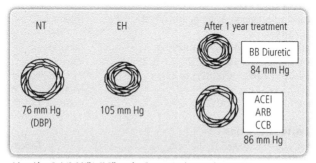

Adapted from Park JB, Schiffrin EI. Effects of antihypertensive therapy on hypertensive vascular disease. *Curr Hypertens Reports.* 2000; 2: 280–288.
ACEI = angiotensin-converting enzyme inhibitor; ARB = angiotensin receptor blocker; CCB = calcium channel blocker; BB = beta-blocker; EH = essential hypertension, NT = normotensive.

Figure 94 Antihypertensive Drug Effects on Vascular Remodeling in Humans.

- Correct BP but no functional or structure changes. (No change on ED, AC M/L ratio, and arterial diameter)
  - Diuretic
  - BB (nonselective, selective, and those with ISA)

Nitroglycerin
- Increases the AC (C-1)
  - Decreases PWV
  - No change in SVR, distensibility, EM
  - Lowers SBP and PP (10%), no change in DBP

Selected Combination Antihypertensive Drugs

Beta-adrenergic blockers and diuretics
Atenolol, 50 or 100 mg/chlorthalidone, 25 mg   Tenoretic
Bisoprolol fumarate, 2.5, 5, or 10 mg/HCTZ, 6.25 mg   Ziac
Metoprolol tartrate, 50 or 100 mg/HCTZ 25 and 50 mg   Lopressor/
HCTZ
Nadolol, 40 or 80 mg/bendroflumethiazide, 5 mg   Corzide
Propranolol hydrochloride, 40 or 80 mg/hydrochlorothiazide, 25 mg   Inderide
Propranolol hydrochloride (extended release), 80, 120, or 160 mg/HCTZ,   Inderal LA
50 mg
Timolol maleate, 10 mg/HCTZ, 25 mg   Timolide

ACEI and diuretics
Benazepril hydrochloride, 5, 10, or 20 mg/HCTZ, 6.25,   Lotensin/HCT
12.5, or 25 mg
Captopril, 25 or 50 mg/HCTZ, 15 or 25 mg   Capozide
Enalapril maleate, 5 or 10 mg/HCTZ, 12.5 or 25 mg   Vaseretic
Lisinopril, 10 or 20 mg/HCTZ, 12.5 or 25 mg   Prinzide, Zestoretic
Moexipril 7.5 or 15 mg + HCTZ   Miretic 12.5 or 25 mg
Quinapril 10 or 20 mg + HCTZ   Accuretic 12.5 or 25 mg

ARBs and diuretics
Valsartan, 80 or 160 mg/HCTZ, 12.5 mg   Diovan HCT
Losartan potassium, 50 mg/HCTZ, 12.5 mg and 100 mg/HCTZ 25 mg   Hyzaar
Candesartan 16 or 32 mg + HCTZ 25 mg   Atacand-HCT
Irbesartan 150 or 300 mg + HCTZ 12.5 mg   Availide
Telmisartan 40 mg + HCTZ 12.5 mg   Micardis/HCT
Eprosartan 600 mg + HCTZ 12.5 mg   Teveten HCT

Calcium antagonists and ACEIs
Amlodipine besylate, 2.5 or 5 mg/benazepril + hydrochloride, 10 or   Lotrel
20 mg
Diltiazem hydrochloride, 180 mg/enalapril maleate, 5 mg   Teczem
Verapamil hydrochloride (extended release), 180 or 240 mg/trandolapril,   Tarka
1, 2, or 4 mg
Felodipine, 5 mg/enalapril maleate, 5 mg   Lexxel

Calcium channel antagonists and ARBs
Amlodipine, 5 or 10 mg with valsartan, 160 or 320 mg   Exforge
Amlodipine, 5 or 10 mg with olmesartan, 20 or 40 mg   Azor

RIs with diuretics
Aliskirin, 150 or 300 mg, with HCTZ, 12.5 or 25 mg   Tekturna HCT

CCB with statin
Amlodipine, 5 or 10 mg with atorvastatin, 10, 20, 40, 80 mg   Caduet

See ASCOT trial for discussion of CVD risk reductions with the combination of amlodipine and other antihypertensive drugs with atorvastatin. See amlodipine section for pharmacodynamics.

Other combinations

Triamterene, 37.5, 50, or 75 mg/HCTZ, 25 or 50 mg	Dyazide, Maxide
Spironolactone, 25 or 50 mg/HCTZ, 25 or 50 mg	Aldactazide
Amiloride hydrochloride, 5 mg/HCTZ, 50 mg	Moduretic
Guanethidine monosulfate, 10 mg/HCTZ, 25 mg	Esimil
Hydralazine hydrochloride, 25, 50, or 100 mg/HCTZ, 25 or 50 mg	Apresazide
Methyldopa, 250 or 500 mg/HCTZ, 15, 25, 30, or 50 mg	Aldoril
Reserpine, 0.125 mg/HCTZ, 25 or 50 mg	Hydropres
Reserpine, 0.10 mg/hydralazine hydrochloride, 25 mg/HCTZ, 15 mg	Ser-Ap-Es
Clonidine hydrochloride, 0.1, 0.2, or 0.3 mg/chlorthalidone, 15 mg	Combipres
Methyldopa, 250 mg/chlorothiazide, 150 or 250 mg	Aldochlor
Reserpine, 0.125 or 0.25 mg/chlorthalidone, 25 or 50 mg	Demi-Regroton
Reserpine, 0.125 or 0.25 mg/chlorothiazide, 250 or 500 mg	Diupres
Prazosin hydrochloride, 1, 2, or 5 mg/polythiazide, 0.5 mg	Minizide

Hypertension Drug Selection: Summary

- CCBs, ARBs, ACEIs, RIs, SARAs, the newer vasodilating BBs, and the newer BBs with alpha-blocking properties have the best overall profile based on the eight parameters in the subsets of approach to hypertension
- Combination therapy with CCBs, ACEIs, ARBs, RIs, indapamide, SARAs, vasodilating BBs, and combined alpha/beta-blockers may provide synergistic antihypertensive effects, reduce side effects, and improve surrogate endpoints as well as TOD
- Clinical trials in hypertension with CCBs (especially amlodipine) reduce CHD, MI, and CVA equal to diuretics and better than the older BBs, ACEI, and possibly ARBs. See VALUE and ALLHAT trials comparing these classes
- ACEIs are equal to diuretics and BBs in reducing cardiovascular and cerebrovascular morbidity and mortality in recent clinical trials, with the exception of lisinopril in ALLHAT (see controversies) related to CHF and CVA in non-black patients. However, CHD and MI morbidity and mortality are equally reduced
- Clinical trials in hypertension with ARBs proved superior to BB in CVA reduction at equal BP levels in the LIFE trial. Valsartan was similar to amlodipine in reducing primary endpoints of combined cardiac morbidity and mortality (VALUE). Clinical trials in CHF show benefit with ACEIs and ARBs, and clinical trials in MI show benefit with ACEIs
- Diuretics may be used as initial or add-on therapy but should never exceed 25 mg/day of HCTZ or its equivalent. Their impact on CHD and MI is suboptimal in all clinical trials except ALLHAT. Diuretics reduces CVA and CHF. HCTZ and chlorthalidone may be nephrotoxic, induce renal cell carcinoma, and increase vascular inflammation (HS-CRP) long-term, which may limit their usefulness

  Indapamide, however, appears to stabilize or improve renal function, is more potent in reducing BP and LVH, and in general has a more potent antihypertensive effect and a better metabolic, vascular, and clinical profile. It is the preferred diuretic. HCTZ and chlorthalidone increase insulin resistance and increase the incidence of new onset type 2 DM
- The older BBs (nonselective, selective, and those with ISA) when given as monotherapy do not reduce CHD or MI in the elderly population, and their efficacy in younger populations is also questionable. BBs reduce CVA but are less effective than all other classes of drugs. The BBs do not reduce total mortality in the primary treatment of hypertension. The BBs are effective in reducing morbidity after an acute MI. They increase insulin resistance and new onset type 2 DM. The BBs do not reduce central arterial pressure as well as other antihypertensive agents
- Central alpha-agonists and ABs are effective as monotherapy or as add-on therapy with favorable metabolic profiles but may be limited due to side effects unless kept at very low doses

  The SARAs show great promise in cases of resistant hypertension, especially in those with low-renin hypertension and those with increased aldosterone production. These agents reduce BP and improve vascular function similar to the other RAAS drugs

  The RIs are excellent antihypertensive agents equal to all other antihypertensive classes and they have a very low incidence of adverse effects.

Clinical trials are ongoing to evaluate their effect on CV and renal events. They have excellent metabolic, structural, and vascular effects

- In patients with DM and hypertension, recent clinical trials indicate that CCBs, ACEIs, and ARBs are superior to diuretics and the older BBs in reducing cardiovascular, cerebrovascular, and renal morbidity and mortality. New studies with RI vasodilating BBs and alpha/beta-blockers indicate good overall BP, glucose, metabolic, renal, and other CV effects
- In ISH, a CCB/ACEI prevents CVA and other CV events better than D/BB combination (STOP-2 trial)

The summary of the hypertension drug selection is illustrated in Table 87.

In high-risk hypertensive patients (ASCOT), the combination of a statin (atorvastatin) with amlodipine or amlodipine with perindopril resulted in better CV event reduction than addition of other antihypertensive drugs. These reductions occurred with LDL cholesterol as low as 100 mg/dL. It is recommended that a statin

Table 87 Effects on Structural and Functional Changes in Compliance Appear to Vary Among Antihypertensive Drug Classes*

Drug class	No. of agents tested	No. of studies	No. of patients	Increase in arterial compliance yielded
ACEIs	8	15	~273	With agents studied (perindopril was most used agent)[†]
Calcium channel blockers	8	11	~150	With agents studied
β-blockers	7	10	~326	With none, except "vasodilating" BBs
Diuretics	4	5	~75	Little effect beyond that associated with ↓ BP (an attempt was made methodologically to separate pressure-dependent from direct effects)

ACEI = angiotensin-converting enzyme inhibitor.

*Studies are primarily cross-sectional and short term. Thus, these studies can only be used for information regarding directional effects and by and large cannot distinguish functional from structural changes. The number of published studies using nitrovasodilators, ABs, and clonidine are too few for inclusion.

[†]Certain studies of ACEIs included evaluation of biopsy-demonstrated improvement in vascular remodeling.

Modified from Glasser SP et al. *J Clin Pharmacol* 1998; 38: 202–212.

be used routinely in these high-risk hypertensive patients. In addition, the CCB/ACEI combination was superior to the BB/diuretic combination in reducing all CV events. The addition of the statin improved outcomes more in the CCB/ACEI group.

New Antihypertensive Drug Classes

1. Vasopressin antagonists
2. Neuropeptidase inhibitors
3. Serotonin receptor antagonists (ketanserin)
4. Prostaglandin analogs (PGI2-iloprost)
5. Lipoxygenase inhibitors (phenidone)
6. Cicletanine
7. Potassium channel activators (BRL-34915)
8. Sodium channel blockers (6-iodoamiloride)
9. Endothelin antagonists (bosentan)

Subset Selection of Antihypertensive Therapy

1. Pathophysiology and vascular biology
2. Hemodynamics
3. End-organ damage and risk factor reduction
4. Concomitant medical diseases or problems
5. Demographic selection
6. Adverse effects and QOL with therapy
7. Compliance
8. Total health care cost

Conclusions

1. The treatment of mild hypertension (DBP ,110mm Hg) with certain antihypertensive agents (some diuretics or older BB) may induce metabolic functional or structural changes in the vascular system or vascular biology and adversely affect other risk factors that partially or completely negate the beneficial effects of lowering BP. Optimal reduction in CHD, MI, CVA, CHF, and CVD is dependent not only on blood pressure control but also on specific non–blood pressure mechanisms. CCB, ACEI, and ARB show superiority over most diuretics and older BB in many surrogate as well as clinical CV outcomes. RI, vasodilating BB, and AB/BB show great promise pending more clinical trials.

2. Diuretic agents (except spironolactone, epleronone, amiloride, and indapamide), older BB without ISA, reserpine, and methyldopa have adverse effects on the hypertensive-atherosclerotic syndrome and other risk factors for end-organ damage. These agents also have significant clinical side effects with a corresponding poor QOL and reduced compliance rate.

3. The only antihypertensive agents available to date that do not adversely affect serum lipids, glucose, and insulin sensitivity are CCBs, alpha-1-blockers, central alpha-agonists (except methyldopa), ACEI, indapamide, ARBs, vasodilating BB, and AB/BB. All these agents are effective as initial monotherapy in about 50–60% or more of patients with mild hypertension. All are well tolerated (in .90% of patients) if dosed appropriately (start low, go slow) and have a low side-effect profile. Combination therapy is 90–95% effective.

4. Diuretic agents (HCTZ or chlorthalidone) may induce hypokalemia, hypomagnesemia, or other electrolyte and acid-base abnormalities, insulin resistance, hyperglycemia, new onset type 2 DM or other metabolic abnormalities. There may also be an increase in the incidence of sudden death in predisposed patients secondary to cardiac arrhythmias. These predisposing factors include exercise, the presence of LVH, abnormal ECGs, silent or clinical ischemia, acute stress, or digitalis treatment. These diuretics should not be administered in high doses.

5. The use of lower doses of diuretics (HCTZ 12.5–25 mg/day or chlorthalidone) is effective for the treatment of hypertension and may have fewer adverse effects. A dose of 25 mg/day achieves 95% of the antihypertensive effect and 12.5 mg achieves 80% of the antihypertensive effect [108]. However, indapamide is the preferred diuretic, and SARAs show excellent results as well.

6. The selection of nonpharmacologic therapy or antihypertensive drugs that have a neutral or favorable effect on serum lipids, glucose, electrolytes, and other risk factors and improve endothelial function and arterial compliance (improve vascular biology) may reduce the risk of CHD and other end-organ damage in patients with hypertension. Optimal treatment aims to reduce all risk factors, thereby reducing all end-organ damage.

7. Selection of drug therapy should be individualized and based on the subsets of hypertension approach and reversing the components of the hypertension–atherosclerotic syndrome.

8. An optimal goal BP may be as low as 110/70mm Hg. Newer noninvasive vascular function and compliance tests will allow for better evaluation and treatment of hypertension.

References

1. Levy RI. Lipid regulation. A new era in the prevention of coronary heart disease. *Am Heart J* 1985;110: 1099–1100.
2. Collins JG. Physician visits. Volume and interval since last visit, United States, 1980. U.S. Department of Health and Human Services (PHS) publication 83–1572, Series 10, No. 144, 1983.
3. Kannel WB. Some lessons in cardiovascular epidemiology from Framingham. *Am J Cardiol* 1976; 37: 269–282.
4. Appel LJ, Moore TJ, Obarzanek E, et al. A clinical trial of the effects of dietary patterns on blood pressure. *N Engl J Med* 1997; 336: 1117–1124.
5. Houston MC. New insights and approaches to reduce end organ damage in the treatment of hypertension: Subsets of hypertension approach. *Am Heart J* 1992; 123: 1337–1367.
6. The Fifth Report of the Joint National Committee on Detection, Evaluation, and Treatment of High Blood Pressure (JNC V). *Arch Intern Med* 1993; 153: 154–183.
7. Kirkendall WM, Feinleib M, Freis ED, Mark AL. Recommendations for human blood pressure determination by sphygmomanometers: Subcommittee of the AHA Postgraduate Education Committee. *Circulation* 1980; 62: 1146A–1155A.
8. Final Report of the Subcommittee on Nonpharmacological Therapy of the 1984 Joint National Committee on Detection, Evaluation, and Treatment of High Blood Pressure: Nonpharmacological approaches to the control of high blood pressure. *Hypertension* 1986; 8: 444–467.
9. Houston MC. New insights and new approaches for the treatment of essential hypertension: Selections of therapy based on coronary heart disease risk factor analysis, hemodynamic profiles, quality of life, and subsets of hypertension. *Am Heart J* 1989; 117: 911–951.
10. Hollifield JW, Slaton P. Demographic approach to initiation of antihypertensive therapy: Treatment strategies in hypertension. Miami: Symposium Specialists, Inc. 1981: 51–58.
11. Woods JW, Pittman AW, Pulliam CC, et al. Renin profiling in hypertension and its use in treatment with propranolol and chlorthalidone. *N Engl J Med* 1976; 294: 1137–1143.
12. Buhler FR, Bolli P, Kiowski W, et al. Renin profiling to select antihypertensive baseline drugs: Renin inhibitors for high-renin and calcium entry blockers for low-renin patients. *Am J Med* 1984; 77: 36–42.
13. Letcher RL, Chien S, Laragh JH. Changes in blood viscosity accompanying the response to prazosin in patients with essential hypertension. *J Cardiovasc Pharmacol* 1979; 1(suppl. 6): S8–S20.
14. Lund-Johansen P. Hemodynamic changes at rest and during exercise in long-term prazosin therapy for essential hypertension. In: *Prazosin Clinical Symposium Proceedings. Special Proceedings by Postgraduate Medicine.* New York: Custom Communications, McGraw-Hill Co, 1975: 45–52.
15. Okun R. Effectiveness of prazosin as initial antihypertensive therapy. *Am J Cardiol* 1983; 51: 644–650.
16. Itskovitz HD. Hemodynamic effects of antihypertensive drugs. *Am Fam Physician* 1983; 27: 137–142.

17. van Zwieten PA, Thoolen MJ, Timmermans PB. The hypertensive activity and side effects of methyldopa, clonidine and guanfacine. *Hypertension* 1984; 6: 1128–1133.
18. Lund-Johansen P. Hemodynamic changes in long-term diuretic therapy of essential hypertension: A comparative study of chlorthalidone, polythiazide and hydrochlorothiazide. *Acta Med Scand* 1970; 187: 509–518.
19. Ventura HO, Frohlich ED, Messerli FH, et al. Immediate regional blood flow distribution following angiotensin converting enzyme inhibition in patients with essential hypertension. *Am J Med* 1984; 76: 58–61.
20. Frohlich ED. Hemodynamic effects of calcium entry-blocking agents in normal and hypertensive rats and man. *Am J Cardiol* 1985; 56: 21H–27H.
21. Halperin AK, Cubeddu LX. The role of calcium channel blockers in the treatment of hypertension. *Am Heart J* 1986; 111: 363–382.
22. Ekelund LG, Ekelund C, Rossner S. Antihypertensive effects at rest and during exercise of a calcium blocker, nifedipine, alone and in combination with metoprolol. *Acta Med Scand* 1982; 212: 71–75.
23. Lund-Johansen P. Hemodynamic effects of verapamil in essential hypertension at rest and during exercise. *Acta Med Scand* 1984; 681(suppl.): 109–115.
24. Hansson L. Hemodynamics of metoprolol and pindolol in systemic hypertension with particular reference to reversal of structural vascular changes. *Am J Cardiol* 1986; 57: 29C–32C.
25. Lund-Johansen P. Central hemodynamic effects of beta-blockers in hypertension: A comparison between atenolol, metoprolol, timolol, penbutolol, alprenolol, pindolol and bunitrolol. *Eur Heart J* 1983; 4(suppl. D): 1–12.
26. Trap-Jensen J, Clausen JP, Noer I, et al. The effects of beta-adrenoceptor blockers on cardiac output, liver blood flow and skeletal muscle blood flow in hypertensive patients. *Acta Physiol Scand* 1976; 440(suppl.): 30.
27. Pedersen EB. Abnormal renal hemodynamics during exercise in young patients with mild essential hypertension without treatment and during long-term propranolol therapy. *Scand J Clin Lab Invest* 1978; 30: 567–571.
28. Hansson L, Pascual A, Julius S. Comparison of guanadrel and guanethidine. *Clin Pharmacol Ther* 1973; 14: 204–208.
29. Woosley RL, Nies AS. Guanethidine. *N Engl J Med* 1976; 295: 1053–1057.
30. Lund-Johansen P. Exercise and antihypertensive therapy. *Am J Cardiol* 1987; 59: 98A–107A.
31. Kannel WB, Wolf PA, Verter J, McNamara PM. Epidemiologic assessment of the role of blood pressure in stroke: The Framingham Study. *JAMA* 1970; 214: 301–310.
32. *Mortality Experience According to Blood Pressure after Treatment: Blood Pressure Study*. Chicago: Society of Actuaries and Association of Life Insurance Medical Directors of America, 1979.
33. Hypertension Detection and Follow-up Program Cooperative Group. Five-year findings of the Hypertension Detection and Follow-Up Program: I. Reduction in mortality of persons with high blood pressure including mild hypertension. *JAMA* 1979; 242: 2562–2571.
34. Veterans Administration Cooperative Study Group on Antihypertensive Agents. Effects of treatment on morbidity in hypertension: II. Results in patients with diastolic blood pressure averaging 90 through 114 mmHg. *JAMA* 1970; 213: 1143–1152.

35. Smith WM. Treatment of mild hypertension: Results of a ten-year intervention trial. *Circ Res* 1977; 40(suppl. I): 198–205.
36. Perry HM Jr. Treatment of mild hypertension: Preliminary results of a two-year feasibility trial. *Circ Res* 1977; 40(suppl. I): 1180–1187.
37. Helgeland A. Treatment of mild hypertension: A five year controlled drug trial. The Oslo Study. *Am J Med* 1980; 69: 725–732.
38. The Australian Therapeutic Trial in Mild Hypertension. Report by the Management Committee. *Lancet* 1980; 1: 1261–1267.
39. Greenberg G, Brennan PJ, Miall WE. Effects of diuretic and beta-blocker therapy in the Medical Research Council Trial. *Am J Med* 1984; 76: 45–51.
40. Multiple Risk Factor Intervention Trial Research Group. Multiple Risk Factor Intervention Trial: Risk factor changes and mortality results. *JAMA* 1982; 248: 1465–1477.
41. Amery A, Birkenhäger W, Brixko P, et al. Mortality and morbidity results from the European Working Party on High Blood Pressure in the Elderly Trial. *Lancet* 1985; 1: 1349–1354.
42. Miettinen TA, Huttunen JK, Naukkarinen V, et al. Multifactorial primary prevention of cardiovascular diseases in middle-aged men: Risk factor changes, incidence, and mortality. *JAMA* 1985; 254: 2097–2102.
43. Wilhelmsen L, Tibblin G, Werkö L. A primary preventive study in Gothenburg, Sweden. *Prev Med* 1972; 1: 153–160.
44. MRC Working Party. Medical Research Council trial of treatment of hypertension in older adults: Principal results. BMJ *1992*; 304: 405–412.
45. Sacks FM, Svetkey LP, Vollmer WM, Appel LJ, Bray GA, et al. Effects on blood pressure of reduced dietary sodium and the dietary approaches to stop hypertension (DASH) diet. *N Engl J Med* 2001; 344: 3–10.
46. Perry HM Jr, Goldman AI, Lavin MA, et al. Evaluation of drug treatment in mild hypertension: VA-NHLBI feasibility trial. *Ann N Y Acad Sci* 1978; 304: 267–288.
47. IPPPSH Collaborative Group. Cardiovascular risk and risk factors in a randomized trial of treatment based on the beta-blocker oxprenolol: The International Prospective Primary Prevention Study in Hypertension (IPPPSH). *J Hypertens* 1985; 3: 379–392.
48. Coope J, Warrender TS. Randomised trial of treatment of hypertension in elderly patients in primary care. *BMJ* 1986; 293: 1145–1151.
49. Wilhelmsen L, Berglund G, Elmfeldt D, et al. Beta-blockers versus diuretics in hypertensive men: Main results from the HAPPHY trial. *J Hypertens* 1987; 5: 561–572.
50. Wikstrand J, Warnold I, Olsson G, et al. Primary prevention with metoprolol in patients with hypertension: Mortality results from the MAPHY study. *JAMA* 1988; 259: 1976–1982.
51. SHEP Cooperative Research Group. Prevention of stroke by antihypertensive drug treatment in older persons with isolated systolic hypertension (SHEP): Final results of the Systolic Hypertension in the Elderly Program. *JAMA* 1991; 265: 3255–3264.
52. Dahlöf B, Lindholm LH, Hansson L, et al. Morbidity and mortality in the Swedish Trial in Old Patients with Hypertension (STOP-Hypertension). *Lancet* 1991; 338: 1281–1285.
53. Castelli WP. Epidemiology of coronary heart disease: The Framingham Study. *Am J Med* 1984; 76: 4–12.

54. Castelli W, Leaf A. Identification and assessment of cardiac risk: An overview. *Cardiol Clin* 1985; 3: 171–178.
55. Kannel WB. Status of risk factors and their consideration in antihypertensive therapy. *Am J Cardiol* 1987; 59: 80A–90A.
56. Kannel WB, Schatzkin A. Risk factor analysis. *Prog Cardiovasc Dis* 1983; 26: 309–332.
57. Bush TL, Barrett-Connor E, Cowan LD, et al. Cardiovascular mortality and noncontraceptive use of estrogen in women: Results from the Lipid Research Clinics Program Follow-Up Study. *Circulation* 1987; 75: 1102–1109.
58. Deutsche RS. The effect of heavy drinking on ischemic heart disease. *Primary Cardiol* 1986; 12: 40–48.
59. Fitzgerald DJ, Roy L, Catella F, Fitzgerald GA. Platelet activation in unstable coronary disease. *N Engl J Med* 1986; 315: 983–989.
60. Meade TW, Mellows S, Brozovic M, et al. Haemostatic function and ischaemic heart disease: Principal results of the Northwick Park Heart Study. *Lancet* 1986; 2: 533–537.
61. Spence JD. Hemodynamic effects of antihypertensive drugs: Possible implications for the prevention of atherosclerosis. *Hypertension* 1984; 6: 163–168.
62. Brunner HR, Laragh JH, Baer L, et al. Essential hypertension: Renin and aldosterone, heart attack and stroke. *N Engl J Med* 1972; 286: 441–449.
63. Giese J. Renin, angiotensin and hypertensive vascular damage: A review. *Am J Med* 1973; 55: 315–332.
64. Chobanian AV. The influence of hypertension and other hemodynamic factors in atherogenesis. *Prog Cardiovasc Dis* 1983; 26: 177–196.
65. Letcher RL, Chien S, Pickering TG, et al. Direct relationship between blood pressure and blood viscosity in normal and hypertensive subjects: Role of fibrinogen and concentration. *Am J Med* 1981; 70: 1195–1202.
66. Reaven GM, Huffman BB. A role for insulin in the aetiology and course of hypertension. *Lancet* 1987; 2: 435–437.
67. Ferrannini E, Buzzigoli G, Bonadonna R, et al. Insulin resistance in essential hypertension. *N Engl J Med* 1987; 317: 435–437.
68. Ames RP, Hill P. Elevation of serum lipid levels during diuretic therapy of hypertension. *Am J Med* 1976; 61:748–757.
69. Lasser NL, Grandits G, Caggiula AW, et al. Effects of antihypertensive therapy on plasma lipids and lipoproteins in the Multiple Risk Factor Intervention Trial. *Am J Med* 1984; 76: 52–66.
70. Helgeland A, Hjermann L, Leren P, Holme I. Possible metabolic side effects of beta-adrenergic blocking drugs. *BMJ* 1978; 1: 828.
71. Ames RP. The effects of antihypertensive drugs on serum lipids and lipoproteins: I. Diuretics. *Drugs* 1986; 32: 260–278.
72. Ames RP, Hill P. Increase in serum lipids during treatment of hypertension with chlorthalidone. *Lancet* 1976; 1: 721–723.
73. Glück Z, Weidmann P, Mordasini R, et al. Increased serum low-density lipoprotein cholesterol in men treated short-term with the diuretic chlorthalidone. *Metabolism* 1980; 29: 240–245.
74. Boehringer K, Weidmann P, Mordasini R, et al. Menopause-dependent plasma lipoprotein alterations in diuretic-treated women. *Ann Intern Med* 1982; 97: 206–209.

75. Mauersberger H. Effect of prazosin on blood pressure and plasma lipids in patients receiving a beta-blocker and diuretic regimen. *Am J Med* 1984; 76: 101–104.

76. Goldman AI, Steele BW, Schnaper HW, et al. Serum lipoprotein levels during chlorthalidone therapy: A Veterans Administration—National Heart, Lung, and Blood Institute cooperative study on antihypertensive therapy: Mild hypertension. *JAMA* 1980; 224: 1691–1695.

77. Koskinen P, Manninen V, Eisalo A. Quinapril and blood lipids. *Br J Clin Pharmacol* 1988; 26: 478–480.

78. Ames RP. Metabolic disturbances increasing the risk of coronary heart disease during diuretic-based antihypertensive therapy: Lipid alterations and glucose intolerance. *Am Heart J* 1983; 106: 1207–1214.

79. Ames RP. Negative effects of diuretic drugs on metabolic risk factors for coronary heart disease: Possible alternative drug therapies. *Am J Cardiol* 1983; 51: 632–638.

80. Grimm RH Jr, Leon AS, Hunninghake DB, et al. Effects of thiazide diuretics on plasma lipids and lipoproteins in mildly hypertensive patients: A double-blind controlled trial. *Ann Intern Med* 1981; 94: 7–11.

81. Flamenbaum W. Metabolic consequences of antihypertensive therapy. *Ann Intern Med* 1983; 98: 875–880.

82. Weinberger MH. Antihypertensive therapy and lipids: Evidence, mechanisms, and implications. *Arch Intern Med* 1985; 145: 1102–1105.

83. Drayer JI, Gardin JM, Weber MA, Aronow WS. Changes in ventricular septal thickness during diuretic therapy. *Clin Pharmacol Ther* 1982; 32: 283–288.

84. Lowenthal DT. Hypertension and exercise physiology: Clinical and therapeutic applications. In: Lowenthal DT, Bharadwaja K, Oaks WW, eds. *Therapeutics Through Exercise*. New York: Grune & Stratton, 1981: 133–144.

85. Loaldi A, Polese A, Montorsi P, et al. Comparison of nifedipine, propranolol and isosorbide dinitrate on angiographic progression and regression of coronary arterial narrowings in angina pectoris. *Am J Cardiol* 1989; 64: 433–439.

86. Lichtlen PR, Hugenholtz PG, Rafflenbeul W, et al. Retardation of angiographic progression of coronary artery disease by nifedipine: Results of the International Nifedipine Trial on Antiatherosclerotic Therapy (INTACT). *Lancet* 1990; 335: 1109–1113.

87. Kober G, Schneider W, Kaltenbach M. Can the progression of coronary sclerosis be influenced by calcium antagonists? *J Cardiovasc Pharmacol* 1989; 13(suppl. 4): 52–56.

88. The MIDAS Research Group. Multicenter Isradipine Diuretic Atherosclerosis Study (MIDAS). *Am J Med* 1989; 86(suppl. 4A): 37–39.

89. Waters D, Lespérance J. Interventions that beneficially influence the evolution of coronary atherosclerosis: The case for calcium channel blockers. *Circulation* 1992; 86(suppl. III): III 111–116.

90. Rostand SG, Brown G, Kirk KA, et al. Renal insufficiency in treated essential hypertension. *N Engl J Med* 1989; 320: 684–688.

91. Brazy PC, Fitzwilliam JF. Progressive renal disease: Role of race and antihypertensive medications. *Kidney Int* 1990; 37: 1113–1119.

92. Eliahou HE, Cohen D, Hellberg B, et al. Effect of the calcium channel blocker nisoldipine on the progression of chronic renal failure in man. *Am J Nephrol* 1988; 8: 285–290.

93. Alcazar JM, Rodicio JL, Ruilope LM. Long-term diuretic therapy and renal function in essential arterial hypertension. *Am J Cardiol* 1990; 65: 51H–54H.

94. Warram JH, Laffel LMB, Valsania P, et al. Excess mortality associated with diuretic therapy in diabetes mellitus. *Arch Intern Med* 1991; 151: 1350–1356.

95. Croog SH, Levine S, Testa MA, et al. The effects of antihypertensive therapy on the quality of life. *N Engl J Med* 1986; 314: 1657–1664.

96. Jachuck SJ, Brierly J, Jachuck S, Willcox PM. The effect of hypotensive drugs on the quality of life. *J R Coll Gen Pract* 1982; 32: 103–105.

97. Curb JD, Borhani NO, Blaszkowski TP, et al. Long-term surveillance for adverse effects of antihypertensive drugs. *JAMA* 1985; 253: 3263–3268.

98. Avorn J, Everitt DE, Weiss S. Increased antidepressant use in patients prescribed β-blockers. *JAMA* 1986; 255: 357–360.

99. Testa MA, Hollenberg HK, Anderson RB, Williams GH. Assessment of quality of life by patient and spouse during antihypertensive therapy with atenolol and nifedipine gastrointestinal therapeutic system. *Am J Hypertens* 1991; 4: 363–373.

100. Os I, Bratland B, Dahlof B, et al. Lisinopril or nifedipine in essential hypertension? A Norwegian multicenter study on efficacy, tolerability and quality of life in 828 patients. *J Hypertens* 1991; 9: 1097–1104.

101. Croog SH, Kong BW, Levine S, et al. Hypertensive black men and women. Quality of life and effects of antihypertensive medications. *Arch Intern Med* 1990; 150: 1733–1741.

102. Fletcher AE, Bulpitt CJ, Hawkins CM, et al. Quality of life on antihypertensive therapy: A randomized double-blind controlled trial of captopril and atenolol. *J Hypertens* 1990; 8: 463–466.

103. Gerber JC, Nies AS. Pharmacology of antihypertensive drugs. In: Genest J, Kuchel O, Hamet P, et al., eds. *Hypertension*, 2nd edn. New York, NY: McGraw-Hill. 1983: 1093–1127.

104. Wollam GL, Gifford RW, Tarazi RC. Antihypertensive drugs. *Clin Pharmacol Ther Drugs* 1977; 14: 420–460.

105. Carney S, Gillies AI, Morgan T. Optimal dose of a thiazide diuretic. *Med J Aust* 1976; 2: 692–693.

106. Campbell DB, Brackman F. Cardiovascular protective properties of indapamide. *Am J Cardiol* 1990; 65: 11H–27H.

107. Clarke RJ. Indapamide: A diuretic of choice for the treatment of hypertension? *Am J Med Sci* 1991; 301(3): 215–220.

108. Oster JR, Epstein M. Use of centrally acting sympatholytic agents in the management of hypertension. *Arch Intern Med* 1991; 151: 1638–1644.

109. Beers MH, Passman LJ. Antihypertensive medications and depression. *Drugs* 1990; 40: 792–799.

110. Ames RP. The effects of antihypertensive drugs on serum lipids and lipoproteins. Part II. Non-diuretic drugs. *Drugs* 1986; 32: 335–357.

111. Kaplan NM. Resistant hypertension: What to do after trying "the usual? " *Geriatrics* 1995; 50: 24–38.

112. Houston MC. Pathophysiology, clinical aspects diagnosis and treatment of hypertensive crisis. *Prog Cardiovasc Dis* 1989; 32: 99–148.

113. Cunningham FG, Lindheimer H. Hypertension in pregnancy. *N Engl J Med* 1992; 326: 927–932.

114. Sabatini S. Pathophysiology of and therapeutic strategies for hypertension in pregnancy. *Curr Opin Nephrol Hypertens* 1993; 2: 763–774.

115. Kincaid-Smith, P. Hypertension in pregnancy. *Blood Press* 1994; 3: 18–23.
116. Joint National Committee on Prevention, Detection, Evaluation, and Treatment of High Blood Pressure. The Sixth Report of the Joint National Committee on Prevention, Detection, Evaluation, and Treatment of High Blood Pressure. *Arch Intern Med* 1997; 157: 2413–2446.
117. Hilleman DE, Mohiuddin SM, Lucas D Jr, et al. Cost-minimization analysis of initial antihypertensive therapy in patients with mild to moderate essential diastolic hypertension (ABST). *Circulation* 1992; 88(Part 2): 263.
118. Himmelmann, A, Hansson L, et al. ACE inhibition prescribes renal function better than beta-blockade in the treatment of essential hypertension. *Blood Press* 1995; 4: 85–90.
119. Saruta T, Kanns Y, et al. Renal effects of amlodipine. *J Hum Hypertens* 1995; 9(suppl. I): 811–816.
120. Reeves RA. Does this patient have hypertension? How to measure blood pressure. *JAMA* 1995; 273: 1211–1218.
121. Drugs for Hypertension. *Med Lett* 1995; 37: 45–50.
122. Eberhardt RT, Kevak RM, Kang PM, Frishman WH. Angiotensin II receptor blockade: An innovative approach to cardiovascular pharmaco-therapy. *J Clin Pharmacol* 1993; 33: 1023–1038.
123. Gradman AH, Arcuri KE, Goldberg AI, et al. A randomized, placebo-controlled, double-blind, parallel study of various doses of losartan potassium compared with enalapril maleate in patients with essential hypertension. *Hypertension* 1995; 25: 1345–1350.
124. Bakris, GL, Griffen KA. Combined effects of an angiotensin converting enzyme inhibitor and a calcium antagonist on renal injury. *J Hypertens* 1997; 15: 1181–1185.
125. Bakris GL, Houston MC, Messerli FH. Effective use of combination therapy in hypertension. *Patient Care* 1997; Fall(suppl.): 10–21.
126. Gong L, Zhang W. Shanghai Trial of Nifedipine in the Elderly (STONE). *J Hypertens* 1996; 14: 1237–1245.
127. Staessen J, Facard R, et al. Systolic Hypertension in Europe Trial (SYST–EUR). *Lancet* 1997; 350: 757–764.
128. Liu L, Wang JG, Gong L, et al. Comparison of active treatment and placebo in older Chinese patients with isolated systolic hypertension: Systolic Hypertension in China (Syst-China) Collaborative Group. *J Hypertens* 1998; 16: 1823–1829.
129. Hansson L. Zanchetti A, Carruthers SG, et al. Effects of intensive blood pressure lowering and low-dose aspirin in patients with hypertension: Principal results of the Hypertension Optimal Treatment (HOT) randomized trial. *Lancet* 1998; 351: 1755–1762.
130. Messerli FH, Grossman E, Goldbourt U. Are beta-blockers efficacious as first-line therapy for hypertension in the elderly? A systematic review. *JAMA* 1998; 279: 1903–1907.
131. Bakris GL. Progression of diabetic nephropathy: A focus on arterial pressure level and methods of reduction. *Diabetes Res Clin Pract* 1998; 39(suppl.): S35–S42.
132. Epstein M. The benefits of ACE inhibitors and calcium antagonists in slowing progressive renal failure. Focus on fixed-dose combination antihypertensive therapy. *Ren Fail* 1996; 18: 813–832.

133. Hansson L, Lindholm LH, Niskanen L, et al. Effect of angiotensin-converting enzyme inhibition compared with conventional therapy on cardiovascular morbidity and mortality in hypertension: The Captopril Prevention Project (CAPPP). *Lancet* 1999; 611–616.
134. Tuomilehto J, Rastenyte D, Birkenhäger W, et al. Effects of calcium-channel blockade in older patients with diabetes and systolic hypertension. *N Engl J Med* 1999; 340: 677–684.
135. National Intervention Cooperative Study in Elderly Hypertensives Study Group. Randomized double-blind comparison of a calcium antagonist and a diuretic in elderly hypertensives. *Hypertension* 1999; 34: 1129–1133.
136. Hansson L, Lindholm LH, Ekbom T, et al., for the STOP-Hypertension-2 Study Group. Randomized trial of old and new antihypertensive drugs in elderly patients: Cardiovascular mortality and morbidity the Swedish Trial in Old Patients with Hypertension-2 study. *Lancet* 1999; 354: 1751–1756.
137. US Renal Data System. USRDS 1997 Annual Data Report. Bethesda, MD, National Institute of Health, National Institute of Diabetes and Digestive and Kidney Diseases, 1997.
138. Klag MJ, Whelton PK, et al. Blood pressure and incidence of end stage renal disease in men. A prospective study. *Circulation* 1994; 18: 941.
139. National High Blood Pressure Education Program Working Group. 1995 update of the working group reports on chronic renal failure and renovascular hypertension. *Arch Int Med* 1996; 156: 1938–1947.
140. Bauer JH, Reams GP, Lai SM. Renal protective effects of strict blood pressure control with enalapril therapy. *Arch Intern Med* 1987; 147: 1387–1400.
141. Wee PM, De Mitchell AG, Epstein M. Effects of calcium antagonists on renal hemodynamics and progression of nondiabetic chronic renal disease. *Arch Intern Med* 1994; 154: 1185–1202.
142. Hannedouche T, Landais P, et al. Randomised controlled trial of enalapril and beta-blockers in non-diabetic chronic renal failure. *BMJ* 1994; 309: 833–837.
143. GISEN Study Group. Randomized placebo controlled trial of the effect of ramipiril on decline in glomerular filtration rate and risk of terminal renal failure in proteinuric nondiabetic nephropathy. *Lancet* 1997; 349: 1857–1863.
144. Maschio G, Alberti D, Hanin G, et al. Effect of the angiotensin-converting enzyme inhibitor benazapril on the progression of renal insufficiency. *N Engl J Med* 1996; 334: 939–945.
145. Tarif N, Bakris GL. Angiotensin II receptor blockade and progression of renal disease in non-diabetic patients. *Kidney Int* 1997; 52(suppl. 63): S67-S70.
146. Bakris GL (ed). The renin-angiotensin system in diabetic nephropathy: From bench to bedside. *Miner Electrolyte Metab* 1998; 24(6): 361–438.
147. Neutel JM, Smith DHG, Weber MA. Is high blood pressure a late manifestation of the hypertension syndrome? *Am J Hypertens* 1999; 12: 215S–223S.
148. Messerli FH, Grossman E. B-blockers and diuretics: To use or not to use? *Am J Hypertens* 1999; 12: 157S–163S.
149. Abernethy, DR, Schwartz JB. Calcium antagonist drugs. *N Engl J Med* 1999; 341: 1447–1457.

150. ALLHAT Collaborative Research Group. Major outcomes in high-risk hypertensive patients randomized to angiotensin-converting enzyme inhibitor or calcium channel blocker vs. diuretic. The antihypertensive and lipid-lowering treatment to prevent heart attack trial (ALLHAT). *JAMA* 220; 288: 2981–2997.

151. Houston, MC. The role of vascular biology, nutrition and nutraceuticals in prevention of hypertension. *J Am Nutraceut Assoc* 2002; April(suppl.): 1–71.

152. Vlachopoulos C, O'Rouke M. Diastolic pressure, systolic pressure or pulse pressure? *Curr Hypertens Rep* 2000; 2: 271–279.

153. Franklin SS. Aging and Hypertension: The assessment of blood pressure indices in predicting coronary heart disease. *J Hypertens* 1999; 17(suppl. 5): S29–S36.

154. Kannel WB. Elevated blood pressure as a cardiovascular risk factor. *Am J Cardiol* 2000; 85: 251–255.

155. Blacher J, Staessen JA, Girerd X, et al. Pulse pressure not mean pressure determines cardiovascular risk in older patients. *Arch Intern Med* 2000; 160: 1085–1089.

155A. Houston M. *Vascular Biology in Clinical Practice.* Philadelphia, PA: Hanley and Belfus, 2002.

156. Staessen JA, Wang JG, Thijs, L. Cardiovascular protection and blood pressure reduction: A meta-analysis. *Lancet* 2001; 358: 1305–1315.

157. Psaty, BM, Smith NL, Siscovick DS, et al. Health outcomes associated with antihypertensive therapies used as first-line agents. *JAMA* 1997; 277: 739–745.

158. Blood Pressure lowering treatment trials collaboration. Effects of ACE inhibitors, calcium antagonists and other blood pressure lowering drugs: Results of prospectively designed overview of randomized trials. *Lancet* 2000; 355: 1955–1964.

159. Pahor M, Psaty BM, Alderman MH, et al. Health outcomes associated with calcium antagonists compared with other first line antihypertensive therapies: A meta-analysis of randomized controlled trials. *Lancet* 2000: 356: 1949–1954.

160. Neal B, MacMahon S. The World Health Organization – International Society of Hypertension. Blood Pressure Lowering Treatment Trials Collaboration: Prospective collaborative overview of major randomized trial of blood pressure–lowering treatments. *Curr Hypertens Rep* 1999; 1: 346–356.

161. Carter AB. Hypotensive therapy in stroke survivors. *Lancet* 1970; I: 485–489.

162. Barraclough M, Joy MD, Macgregor GA, et al. Control of moderately raised blood pressure. *BMJ* 1973; 3: 434–443.

163. Hypertension-Stroke Cooperative Study Group. Effect of antihypertensive treatment on stroke recurrence. *JAMA* 1974: 229: 409–418.

164. Kuramoto K, Matsushita S, Kuwajima I, et al. Prospective study on the treatment of mild hypertension in the aged. *JPN Heart J* 1981; 22: 75–85.

165. Perry HM, Smith WM, McDonald RH, et al. Morbidity and mortality in the systolic hypertension in the elderly program (SHEP) pilot study. *Stroke* 1989; 20: 4–13.

166. Medical Research Council Working Party. Medical research council trial of treatment of hypertension in older adults. *BMJ* 1992: 304: 405–423.

167. Veterans Administration Cooperative Study Group on Antihypertensive Agents. Effects of treatment on morbidity in hypertension. *JAMA* 1967; 202: 1028–1034.
168. Brown MJ, Palmer CR, Castaisne A. Morbidity and mortality in patients randomised to double-blind treatment with a long-acting calcium-channel blocker or diuretic in the international nifedipine GITS study: Intervention as a goal in hypertension treatment (INSIGHT). *Lancet* 2000; 356: 366–372.
169. Hansson L, Hedner T, Lund Johnson P, et al. Randomised trial of effects of calcium antagonists compared with diuretics and beta-blockers on cardiovascular morbidity and mortality in hypertension: The Nordic Diliazem (NORDIL) Study. *Lancet.* 2000; 356: 359–365.
170. Black HR, Elliot WJ, Grandits G, et al. Principal results of the controlled onset verapamil investigation of cardiovascular endpoints (convince trial). *JAMA* 2003; 289: 2073–2082.
171. Pitt B, Byington RP, Furberg CD, et al. Effect of amlodipine on the progression of atherosclerosis and the occurrence of clinical events. *Circulation* 2000; 102: 1503–1510.
172. Zanchetti A, Rosei EA, Plau CD. The verapamil in hypertension and atherosclerosis study (VHAS): Results of long-term randomized treatment with either verapamil or chlorthalidone on carotid intima-media thickness. *J Hypertens* 1998; 16: 1667–1676.
173. Ohihara T. Practitioner's Trial on the Efficacy of Antihypertensive Treatment in the Elderly on Hypertension (The PATE Hypertension Study) in Japan. *Am J Hypertens* 2000; 13: 461–467.
174. The GLANT Study Group. A 12-month comparison of ACE inhibitor and CA antagonist therapy in mild to moderate essential hypertension: The GLANT Study. *Hypertens Res* 1995; 18: 235–244.
175. Omae T, Matsuoka H, Arakawa K, Imura O, Ishii M, Ogihara T, Kaneko Y, Kuramochi M, Kokubu T, Takeda R, Hiwada K, Fukiyama K, Fujishima M, Yamada K, Yoshinaga K, Shimuzu U, Nobutomo K. GLANT Study. *Nipppon Iji-shinpo* 1993; 3630: 26–34 [in Japanese].
176. Hanson L, Lindhol LH, Ekbom T, et al., for the STOP-Hypertension-2 Study Group. Randomized trial of old and new hypertensive drugs in elderly patients: Cardiovascular mortality and morbidity. The Swedish trial in old patients with hypertension-2 study. *Lancet* 1999; 354: 1751–1756.
177. Lewis, EJ. The role of angiotensin receptor blockers in preventing the progression of renal disease in patients with type 2 diabetes. *Am J Hypertens* 2002; 15: 1235–1285.
178. Wright JT, Bakris G, Green T, et al. Effect of blood pressure lowering and antihypertensive drug class on progression of hypertensive kidney disease. Results from the AASK trial. *JAMA* 2002; 288: 2421–2431.
179. Estacio RO, Jeffer BW, Giffird N, Schrier RW. Effect of blood pressure control on diabetic microvascular complications in patients with hypertension and type 2 diabetes. *Diabetes Care* 2000 April; 23(suppl. 2): B54–B64.
180. Tatti P. Pahor M, Byington RP, et al. Outcome results of the fosinopril vs. amlodipine cardiovascular events randomized trial (FACET) in patients with hypertension and NIDAM. *Diabetics Care* 1998; 21(4): 597–603.
181. Zanchetti A, Bond MG, Henniq M, et al. Risk factors associated with alterations in carotid intima-media thickness in hypertension: Baseline data from the European lacidipine study on atherosclerosis. *J Hypertens* 1998; 16: 949–996.

182. Conti CR, Cooper-Deltoff RM. How will INVEST and other hypertension trials change clinical practices? *Clin Cardiol* 2001; 24(suppl. II): V24–V29.
183. Pepine CJ, Handberg-Thurmond E, Marks RG. Rationale and design of the International Verapamil SR/Trandolapril Study (INVEST): An internet based randomised trial in coronary artery disease patients with hypertension. *J Am Coll Cardiol* 1998; 32: 1228–1237.
184. Malacco E, Gnemmi AE, Romagnoli A, et al. Systolic hypertension in the elderly: Long-term lacidipine treatment. Objective protocol and organization. SHELL Study Group. *J Cardiovasc Pharmacol* 1994; 23(suppl. 5): 562–566.
185. Borhani NO, Mercuri M, Borhani PA, et al. Final outcome results of the multicenter Isradipine diuretic atherosclerosis study (MIDAS). A randomised controlled trial. *JAMA* 1996; 276: 785–791.
186. Devereux RB, Palmier V, Sharpe N, et al. Effects of once-daily angiotensin-converting enzyme inhibition and calcium channel blockade-based antihypertensive treatment regiments on left ventricular hypertrophy and diastolic filling in hypertension: The prospective randomized enalapril study evaluating regression of ventricular enlargement (preserve) trial. *Circulation* 2001; 104: 1248–1254.
187. PROGRESS Collaborative Group. Randomized trial of a perindopril-based blood-pressure lowering regimens among 6105 individuals with previous stroke or transient ischaemic attack. *Lancet* 2001; 358: 1033–1041.
188. Hanson L, Lindholm LH, Niskanew L. Effect of angiotensin-converting enzyme inhibition compared with conventional therapy on cardiovascular morbidity and mortality in hypertension: The captopril prevention project (CAPPP) randomized trial. *Lancet* 1999; 353: 611–616.
189. Kjelosen SE, Dahlof B, Devereux RB. Effects of Losartan on cardiovascular morbidity and mortality in patients with isolated systolic hypertension and left ventricular hypertrophy. *JAMA* 2002; 288: 1491–1498.
190. Dahlof B, Devereux RB, Kjelds: The LIFE Study Group. Cardiovascular morbidity and mortality in the losartan intervention for endpoint reduction in hypertension study (LIFE): A randomized trial against atenolol. *Lancet* 2002 March; 359(9311): 995–1003.
191. Zanchetti A, Rulope LM. Antihypertensive treatment in patients with type-2 diabetes mellitus: Guidelines from recent controlled randomized trials. *Hypertension* 2002; 20: 2099–2110.
192. Nosadini R, Tonolo G. Cardiovascular and renal protection in type 2 diabetes mellitus: The role of calcium channel blockers. *J Am Soc Nephrol* 2002; 13(suppl. 3): 5216–5223.
193. Zarnke KB, Marentetle MA, Gert WC. Saskatchewan health and database analysis of antihypertensive persistence. Paper presented at 2nd international forum on angiotensin antagonists, Monte Carlo, January 2001.
194. Bloom BS. Continuation of initial antihypertensive medication after 1 year of therapy. *Clin Ther* 1998; 20: 671–681.
195. Caro JJ, Speckman JL, Salas M, et al. Effect of initial drug choice on persistence with antihypertensive therapy: The importance of actual practice data. *Can Med Assoc J* 1999; 160: 41–46.
196. Grossman E, Messerli FH, Goldbourt U. Does diuretic therapy increase the risk of renal cell carcinoma? *Am J Cardiol* 1999; 83: 1090–1093.

197. Prospective studies collaboration. Age-specific relevance of usual blood pressure to vascular mortality: A meta-analysis of individual data for 1 million adults in 61 prospective studies. *Lancet* 2002; 360: 1903–1913.

198. Messerlu FH, Grossman E. Beta-blockers and diuretics: To use or not to use? *Am J Hypertens.* 1999; 12: 1573–1635.

199. Cohn IN. ACE-inhibition and vascular remodeling of resistance vessels. Vascular compliance and cardiovascular implications. *Heart Dis* 2000; 2: S2–S6.

200. Park JB, Schiffrin EL. Effects of antihypertensive therapy on hypertensive vascular disease. *Curr Hypertens Rep* 2000; 2: 280–288.

201. Oparil S, Weber MA. Hypertension: A Companion to Brenner and Rector's The Kidney. Philadelphia, PA: WB Saunders, 2000.

202. Collins R, Peto R, MacMahon S, et al. Blood pressure, stroke, and coronary heart disease. Part 2, short-term reductions in blood pressure: Overview of randomised drug trials in their epidemiologies context. *Lancet* 1990; 335: 827–838.

203. MacMahon S, Rodgers A. The effects of antihypertensive treatment on vascular disease: Reappraisal of the evidence in 1994. *J Vasc Med Biol* 1993; 4: 265–271.

204. Collins R, MacMahon S. Blood pressure, antihypertensive drug treatment and the risks of stroke and of coronary heart disease. *Br Med Bull* 1994; 50: 272–298.

205. Gueyffier F, Boutitie F, Boissel JP, et al. Effect of antihypertensive drug treatment on cardiovascular outcomes in women and men: A meta-analysis of individual patient data from randomised controlled trials. *Ann Intern Med* 1997; 126: 761–767.

206. Psaty B, Smith N, Siscovick D, et al. Health outcomes associated with antihypertensive therapies used as first-line agents: A systematic review and meta-analysis. *JAMA* 1997; 277: 739–745.

207. Zanchetti A, Bond MG, Hennig M, et al. Calcium antagonist lacidipine slows down progression of a symptom ate carotid atherosclerosis principal results of the European Lacidipine Study of Artherosclerosis (ELSA), a randomised, double-blind, long-term trial. *Circulation* 2002; 106(19): 2422–2427.

208. Malacco E, Mancia FG, Rappelli S, et al. Treatment of isolated systolic hypertension: The SHELL study results. *Blood Press* 2003; 12: 160–167.

209. Lindon MH, Wing MB, Reid CM, et al. A comparison of outcomes with angiotensin-converting enzyme-inhibitors and diuretics for hypertension in the elderly. *N Engl J Med* 2003; 348: 583–592.

210. Black HR, Elliot WJ, Grandits G. Principal results of the controlled onset verapamil investigation of cardiovascular endpoints (CONVINCE) trial. *JAMA* 2003; 289: 2073–2082.

211. PREMIER Collaborative Research Group. Effects of comprehensive lifestyle modification on blood pressure control. Main results of the PREMIER clinical trial. *JAMA* 2003; 289: 2083–2093.

212. Bakris GI, Weir MR, Shanifar S. Effects of blood pressure level on progression of diabetic nephropathy. Results from renal study. *Arch Int Med* 2003; 163: 1555–1565.

213. Chobanian AV, Bakru GL, Black HR, et al. The Seventh Report of the Joint National Committee on Prevention, Detection, Evaluation and Treatment of High Blood Pressure. The JNC 7 report. *JAMA* 2003; 289: 2560–2572.

214. The Canadian Hypertension Education Program of the management of hypertension. Available at http://www.chs.mdlindex2.html
215. Guidelines Committee. 2003 European Society of Hypertension, European Society of Cardiology guidelines for the management of arterial hypertension. *Hypertension* 2003; 21: 1011–1053.
216. Douglas JG, Bakris GL, Epotein M, et al. Management of high blood pressure in African Americans. *Arch Intern Med* 2003; 163: 525–541.
217. Hajjar I, Kotchen TA. Trends in prevalence, awareness, treatment and control of hypertension in the United States, 1988–2000. *JAMA* 2003; 290: 199–206.
218. Laragh JH, Sealey JE. Relevance of the plasma renin hormonal control system that regulates blood pressure and sodium balance for correctly treating hypertension for evaluating ALLHAT. *Am J Hypertens* 2003; 16: 407–413.
219. Psaty BM, Lumley T, Furberg CD. Health outcomes associated with various antihypertensive therapies used as first-line agents. A network meta-analysis. *JAMA* 2003; 289: 2534–2544.
220. Law MR, Walp NJ, Morris JK, Jordan RE. Value of low dose combination treatment with blood pressure lowering drugs: Analysis of 354 randomized trials. *BMJ* 2003; 326: 1427–1435.
221. Lasaridis AN, Sarafidis PA. Diabetic nephropathy and hypertensive treatment: What are the lessons from clinical trials? *Am J Hypertens* 2003; 16: 687–697.
222. Messerli FH, Williams B, Ritz E. Essential hypertension. *Lancet* 2007; 370: 591–603.
223. British Cardiac Society, British Hypertension Society, Diabetes UK, Heart UK, Primary Care Cardiovascular Society, the Stroke Association. JBS 2: Joint British Societies' guidelines on prevention of cardiovascular disease in clinical practice. *Heart* 2005; 91: 1–52.
224. Williams B. Beta-blockers and the treatment of hypertension. *J Hypertens* 2007; 25: 1351–1353.
225. Williams B. The obese hypertensive: The weight of evidence against beta-blockers. *Circulation* 2007; 115: 1973–1974.
226. Williams B. The year in hypertension. *J Am Coll Cardiol* 2006; 48: 1698–1711.
227. Williams B, Lacy PS, Thom SM, et al. Differential impact of blood pressure-lowering drugs on central aortic pressure and clinical outcomes: Principal results of the Conduit Artery Function Evaluation (CAFÉ) study. *Circulation* 2006; 113: 1213–1225.
228. Patel A, ADVANCE Collaborative Group, MacMahon S, et al. Effects of a fixed combination of perindopril and indapamide on macrovascular and microvascular outcomes in patients with type 2 diabetes mellitus (the ADVANCE trial): A randomised controlled trial. *Lancet* 2007; 370: 829–840.
229. Mason JM, Dickinson HO, Nicolson DJ, Campbell F, Ford GA, Williams B. The diabetogenic potential of thiazide-type diuretic and beta-blocker combinations in patients with hypertension. *J Hypertens* 2005; 23: 1777–1781.
230. Shargorodsky M, Boaz M, Davidovitz I, Asherov J, Gavish D, Zimlichman R. Treatment of hypertension with thiazides: Benefit or damage-effect of low- and high-dose thiazide diuretics on arterial elasticity and metabolic parameters in hypertensive patients with and without glucose intolerance. *J Cardiometab Syndr* 2007; 2: 16–23.

231. Kuti EL, Baker WL, Michael C. The development of new-onset type 2 diabetes associated with choosing a calcium channel blocker compared to a diuretic or beta-blocker. *Curr Med Res Opin* 2007; April 23 [Epub ahead of print].

232. Sarafidis PA, McFarlane SI, Bakris GL. Antihypertensive agents, insulin sensitivity, and new-onset diabetes. *Curr Diab Rep* 2007; 7: 191–199.

233. Ostergren J. Renin-angiotensin-system blockade in the prevention of diabetes. *Diabetes Res Clin Pract* 2007; 76: S13–S21.

234. Bakris GL, Sowers JR. When does new onset diabetes resulting from antihypertensive therapy increase cardiovascular risk? *Hypertension* 2004; 43: 941–942.

235. Sowers JR, Bakris GL. Antihypertensive therapy and the risk of type 2 diabetes mellitus. *N Engl J Med* 2000; 342: 969–970.

236. Hawkins RG, Houston MC. Is population-wide diuretic use directly associated with the incidence of end-stage renal disease in the United States? A hypothesis. *Am J Hypertens* 2005; 18: 744–749.

237. Hawkins RG. Is population-wide diuretic use directly associated with the incidence of end-stage renal disease in the United States? *Curr Hypertens Rep* 2006; 8: 219–225.

238. Houston MC, Hawkins RG. *Hypertension Handbook for Clinicians and Students*. Birmingham, Alabama: ANA Publishing, 2005.

239. Epstein BJ, Vogel K, Palmer BF. Dihydropyridine calcium channel antagonists in the management of hypertension. *Drugs* 2007; 67: 1309–1327.

240. Safar ME, Smulyan H. Blood pressure components in clinical hypertension. *J Clin Hypertens* 2006; 8: 659–666.

241. Mancia G, De Backer G, Dominiczak A, et al. 2007 Guidelines for the Management of Arterial Hypertension: The Task Force for the Management of Arterial Hypertension of the European Society of Hypertension (ESH) and of the European Society of Cardiology (ESC). *J Hypertens* 2007; 25: 1105–1187.

242. Mancia G, De Backer G, Dominiczak A, et al. 2007 Guidelines for the Management of Arterial Hypertension: The Task Force for the Management of Arterial Hypertension of the European Society of Hypertension (ESH) and of the European Society of Cardiology (ESC). *Eur Heart J* 2007; 28: 1462–1536.

243. 2007 ESH-ESC Practice Guidelines for the Management of Arterial Hypertension: ESH-ESC Task Force on the Management of Arterial Hypertension. *J Hypertens* 2007; 25: 1751–1762.

244. Rosendorff C, Black HR, Cannon CP, et al. Treatment of hypertension in the prevention and management of ischemic heart disease: A scientific statement from the American Heart Association Council for High Blood Pressure Research and the Councils on Clinical Cardiology and Epidemiology and Prevention. *Circulation* 2007; 115: 2761–2788.

245. Williams B, Poulter NR, Brown MJ, et al. British Hypertension Society guidelines for hypertension management 2004 (BHS-IV): Summary. *BMJ* 2004; 328: 634–640.

246. Williams B, Poulter NR, Brown MJ, et al. Guidelines for management of hypertension: Report of the fourth working party of the British Hypertension Society, 2004-BHS IV. *J Hum Hypertens* 2004; 18: 139–185.

247. Khan NA, Hemmelgarn B, Padwal, et al. The 2007 Canadian Hypertension Education Program recommendations for the management of hypertension: Part 2 – therapy. *Can J Cardiol* 2007; 23: 539–550.

248. Houston MC, Basile J, Bestermann WH, et al. Addressing the global cardiovascular risk of hypertension, dyslipidemia, and insulin resistance in the southeastern United States. *Am J Med Sci* 2005; 329: 276–291.
249. Bestermann W, Houston MC, Basile J, et al. Addressing the global cardiovascular risk of hypertension, dyslipidemia, diabetes mellitus, and the metabolic syndrome in the southeastern United States, part II: Treatment recommendations for management of the global cardiovascular risk of hypertension, dyslipidemia, diabetes mellitus, and the metabolic syndrome. *Am J Med Sci* 2005; 329: 292–305.
250. Wilson PWF, D'Agostino RB, Levy D, Belanger AM, Silbershatz H, Kannel WB. Prediction of coronary heart disease using risk factor categories. *Circulation* 1998; 97: 1837–1847.
251. Conroy RM, Pyorala K, Fitzgerald AP, et al. Estimation of ten-year risk of fatal cardiovascular disease in Europe: The SCORE project. *Eur Heart J* 2003; 24: 987–1003.
252. Yusuf S, Hawken S, Ounpuu S, et al. Effect of potentially modifiable risk factors associated with myocardial infarction in 52 countries (the INTERHEART study): Case-control study. *Lancet* 2004; 364: 937–952.
253. Houston MC. Nutraceuticals, vitamins, antioxidants, and minerals in the prevention and treatment of hypertension. *Prog Cardiovasc Dis* 2005; 47: 396–449.
254. Houston MC. Treatment of hypertension with nutraceuticals, vitamins, antioxidants and minerals. *Expert Rev Cardiovasc Ther* 2007; 5: 681–691.
255. Lewington S, Clarke R, Qizilbash N, Peto R, Collins R. Age-specific relevance of usual blood pressure to vascular mortality: A meta-analysis of individual data for one million adults in 61 prospective studies. *Lancet* 2002; 360: 1903–1913.
256. Vasan RS, Larson MG, Leip EP, et al. Impact of high-normal blood pressure on the risk of cardiovascular disease. *N Engl J Med* 2001; 345: 1291–1297.
257. MacMahon S, Meal B, Rodgers A. Hypertension: Time to move on. *Lancet* 2005; 365: 1108–1109.
258. Whelton SP, Chin A, Xin X, He J. Effect of aerobic exercise on blood pressure: A meta-analysis of randomized, controlled trials. *Ann Intern Med* 2002; 136: 493–503.
259. Cutler JA, Follmann D, Allender PS. Randomized trials of sodium reduction: An overview. *Am J Clin Nutr* 1997; 65: 643S–651S.
260. Xin X, He J, Frontini MG, Ogden LG, Motsamai OI, Whelton PK. Effects of alcohol reduction on blood pressure: A meta-analysis of randomized controlled trials. *Hypertension* 2001; 38: 1112–1117.
261. Whelton PK, He J, Cutler JA, et al. Effects of oral potassium on blood pressure: Meta-analysis of randomized controlled clinical trials. *JAMA* 1997; 277: 1624–1632.
262. Julius S, Nesbitt SD, Egan BM, et al. Feasibility of treating prehypertension with an angiotensin-receptor blocker. *N Engl J Med* 2006; 354: 1685–1697.
263. Anonymous. [PHARAO Study of the Hypertension League. Can development of hypertension be prevented with drugs?]. *MMW Fortschr Med* 2000; 142: 35–36.
264. Sever PS, Dahlof B, Poulter NR, et al., for the ASCOT Investigators. Prevention of coronary and stroke events with atorvastatin in hypertensive patients who

have average or lower-than-average cholesterol concentrations, in the Anglo-Scandinavian Cardiac Outcomes Trial – Lipid Lowering Arm (ASCOT-LLA): A multicentre randomised controlled trial. *Lancet* 2003; 361: 1149–1158.

265. Dahlof B, Sever PS, Poulter NR, et al., for the ASCOT Investigators. Prevention of cardiovascular events with an antihypertensive regimen of amlodipine adding perindopril as required versus atenolol adding bendroflumethiazide as required, in the Anglo-Scandinavian Cardiac Outcomes Trial – Blood Pressure Lowering Arm (ASCOT-BPLA): A multicentre randomised controlled trial. *Lancet* 2005; 366: 895–906.

266. Sever PS, Dahlof B, Poulter N, et al., on behalf of the ASCOT Steering Committee Members. Potential synergy between lipid-lowering and blood-pressure-lowering in the Anglo-Scandinavian Cardiac Outcomes Trial. *Eur Heart J* 2006; 27: 2982–2988.

267. Julius S, Kjeldsen SE, Weber M, et al. Outcomes in hypertensive patients at high cardiovascular risk treated with regimens based on valsartan or amlodipine: The VALUE randomised trial. *Lancet* 2004; 363: 2022–2031.

268. Logan A. BENEDICT in the treatment of hypertension. *Curr Hypertens Rep* 2005; 7: 121–123.

269. Solomon SD, Lin J, Solomon CG, et al. Influence of albuminuria on cardiovascular risk in patients with stable coronary artery disease. *Circulation* 2007; 116: 2687–2693.

270. Pitt B, O'Neill B, Feldman R, et al. The QUinapril Ischemic Event Trial (QUIET): Evaluation of chronic ACE inhibitor therapy in patients with ischemic heart disease and preserved left ventricular function. *Am J Cardiol* 2001; 87: 1058–1063.

271. Zanchetti A, Crepaldi G, Bond G, on behalf of PHYLLIS Investigators. The Plaque Hypertension Lipid-Lowering Italian Study (PHYLLIS). Program of Hypertension Prague 2002 – Joint 19th Scientific Meeting of the International Society of Hypertension and 12th European Meeting on Hypertension, June 23–27, 2002, Prague, Czech Republic. Plenary session LCT3.

272. Patel A, ADVANCE Collaborative Group, MacMahon S, et al. Effects of a fixed combination of perindopril and indapamide on macrovascular and microvascular outcomes in patients with type 2 diabetes mellitus (the ADVANCE trial): A randomised controlled trial. *Lancet* 2007; 370: 829–840.

273. Fox KM; EURopean trial on reduction of cardiac events with Perindopril in stable coronary Artery disease Investigators. Efficacy of perindopril in reduction of cardiovascular events among patients with stable coronary artery disease: Randomised, double-blind placebo-controlled, multicentre trial (the EUROPA study). *Lancet* 2003; 362: 782–788.

274. Teo KK, Burton JR, Buller CE, et al. Long-term effects of cholesterol lowering and angiotensin-converting enzyme inhibition on coronary atherosclerosis: The Simvastatin/Enalapril Coronary Atherosclerosis Trial (SCAT). *Circulation* 2000; 102: 1748–1754.

275. Stumpe KO, Ludwig M, Heagerty AM, et al. Vascular wall thickness in hypertension: The Perindopril Regression of Vascular Thickening European Community Trial: PROTECT. *Am J Cardiol* 1995; 76: 50E–54E.

276. Stratton J, Manley S, Holman R, Turner R. Hypertension in diabetes Study III. *Diabetologica* 1996; 39: 1554–1561.

277. MacMahon S, Sharpe N, Gamble G, et al. Randomized, placebo-controlled trial of the angiotensin-converting enzyme inhibitor, ramipril, in patients with coronary or other occlusive arterial disease. PART-2 Collaborative Research Group. Prevention of Atherosclerosis with Ramipril. *J Am Coll Cardiol* 2000; 36: 438–443.

278. Yusuf S, Sleight P, Pogue J, Bosch J, Davies R, Dagenais G. Effects of an angiotensin-converting-enzyme inhibitor, ramipril, on cardiovascular events in high-risk patients. The Heart Outcomes Prevention Evaluation Study Investigators. *N Engl J Med* 2000; 342: 145–153.

279. Schrader J, Luders S, Kulschewski A, et al. Morbidity and Mortality After Stroke, Eprosartan Compared with Nitrendipine for Secondary Prevention: Principal results of a prospective randomized controlled study (MOSES). *Stroke* 2005; 36: 1218–1226.

280. Julius S, Kjeldsen SE, Weber M, et al. Outcomes in hypertensive patients at high cardiovascular risk treated with regimens based on valsartan or amlodipine: The VALUE randomised trial. *Lancet* 2004; 363: 2022–2031.

281. Zanchetti A, Elmfeldt D. Findings and implications of the Study on COgnition and Prognosis in the Elderly (SCOPE) – a review. *Blood Press* 2006; 15: 71–79.

Index

Garlic, dietary supplement, 66
Geriatric/elderly
  BYSTOLIC™ for, 335, 337
GGTP. *See* Gamma-glutamyl transpeptidase
    (GGTP)
GLANT trial
  details of, 99
  results, 180
Global CV risk calculation, 41–49
Glomerular filtration rate (GFR). *See* Renal
    function
Growth factor genes, 359

H

HCTZ. *See* Hydrochlorothiazide (HCTZ)
HDS trial
  details of, 99
  results of, 203
Heart Outcomes Prevention Evaluation Study.
    See HOPE trial
Hemodynamic effects of antihypertensive drugs,
    85–86
Hemodynamic progression, of hypertension, 83
Hemodynamics
  logical and preferred method to reduce BP, 83
Hepatic disease
  BYSTOLIC™ to patient with, 331, 333, 337
HEP trial
  in renal function, 241
High blood pressure
  African-American patients with, 34
  in US adults, 21, 22
Histamine-2 receptor antagonists, interaction
    with BYSTOLIC™, 331
HOPE trial
  and cardiovascular events, 209–210
  details of, 100
HOT trial
  details of, 100
  results of, 147–148
Hydrochlorothiazide (HCTZ), 19
  doses of, 303
  risk of renal injury, 240–241
Hyperlipoproteinemia, CHD risk, 227
Hypertension
  antihypertensive drugs selection for, 368–370
  classification, 21–22
  consequences, 3
  diabetes mellitus (DM), 250–274
    CAPPP study, 267
    cardiovascular events, 266
    causes of death, 250
    effects of different drug classes in
      treatment of hypertension in, 262–263

JNC-7 recommendations for patients
    with, 250
  mortality, 268
  nephropathy meta-analysis, 264
  patients, 269
  primary trials of hypertension control in,
    260–261
  trials comparing different antihypertensive
    regimens, 258–259
  UK prospective, 251, 266
end-organ damage and, 19–20
essential, 3, 16
factors influencing prognosis of, 29–30
guidelines and recommendations, 24–40
hemodynamic progression of, 83
hemodynamics in, 83
JNC 7 recommendations for, 24
large clinical trials in, 266
malignant, 286
masked, 53–54
new treatment approach to, 14–15
NHANES IV key findings, 22
normotensive. *See* Normotensive
    hypertension
in pregnancy, 291–292
prevalence of, 3, 24, 25–26
  by age and race/ethnicity, 24, 25
  association with demographic factors and
    BMI, 26
renal disease. *See* Hypertensive
    nephrosclerosis
resistant, 282–283
secondary. *See* Secondary hypertension
selection of antihypertensive drugs based on
    subsets, 275–280
syndrome, 4
treatment, 26–27, 30–38, 59–86
  DASH diets, 75–77
  nonpharmacologic, 61–62
  nutritional and nutraceutical supplements,
    63–71
  the premier clinical trial, 78–79
in United States, 21–24
  age-specific and age-adjusted prevalence,
    25
Hypertension–atherosclerotic syndrome, 55–56
Hypertension in Diabetes Study. *See* HDS trial
Hypertension in Elderly Patients in Primary Care
    trial. *See* HEP trial
Hypertension in the Very Elderly Trial. *See* HYVET
    trial
Hypertension Optimal Treatment Trial. *See* HOT
    trial
Hypertension-related end-organ damage, 89

Metabolism, of BYSTOLIC™, 330
MIDAS trial
    details of, 100
    results, 179
Morbidity and Mortality After Stroke: Eprosartan
        vs. Nitrendipine in Secondary
        Prevention. See MOSES trial
MOSES trial
    baseline characteristics of patients, 217
        antihypertensive pretreatment, 218
    design, 216–217
    details of, 101
    results, 218
Multicenter Isradapine Diuretic Atherosclerosis
        Study. See MIDAS trial
Multiple regression analysis
    association between hypertension prevalence,
        demographic factors and BMI, 26
Mutagenesis, BYSTOLIC™, 334

N
National Health and Nutritional Examination
        Survey. See NHANES
National Institute for Health and Clinical
        Excellence. See NICE
National Intervention Cooperative Study in
        Elderly Hypertensives. See NICS-EH
        trial
Natural antihypertensive compounds, 69–70
Nebivolol. See BYSTOLIC™
NHANES, 22
NHANES III
    cardiovascular disease trends, 22
    high blood pressure in US adults, 21
    renal disease and, 240–241
NHANES IV
    key findings of hypertension, 22
NICE, 30
NICS-EH trial
    details of, 101
Nifedipine
    in ACTION trial. See ACTION trial
    in INSIGHT trial. See INSIGHT trial
    in PRESERVE trial, 181
    in STONE trial. See STONE trial
Nitrendipine
    in MOSES trial. See MOSES trial
    in SYST-EUR trial, 142, 144–145
    vs. placebo, 113
Nonpharmacologic treatment, 61–62
Nordic Diltiazem Study. See NORDIL trial
NORDIL trial, 151
    details of, 101
    results, 152

Normotensive hypertension, 57
    vascular changes and CV risk factors in
        borderline hypertension vs, 56
Nursing mothers
    BYSTOLIC™ for, 335
Nutraceutical supplements
    hypertension prevention and treatment trials,
        63–71
Nutritional supplements
    hypertension prevention and treatment trials,
        63–71

O
Obesity, 80
Omapatrilat in Persons with Enhanced Risk of
        Atherosclerotic Events. See OPERA
        trial
OPERA trial
    details of, 101
Oxidative stress
    to blood vessels, 14

P
Paleolithic diet, 63
PART-2 trial
    details of, 101
    results of, 205
PATE trial, 158
    details of, 101
PEACE trial
    details of, 101
    results of, 206
Pediatrics
    use of BYSTOLIC™, 335
Perindopril Protection Against Recurrent Stroke
        Study. See PROGRESS trial
Perindopril Regression of Vascular Thickening
        European Community Trial. See
        PROTECT trial
Peripheral vascular disease
    BYSTOLIC™ to patient with, 333
PHYLLIS trial
    details of, 101
    results of, 195
Physiological dysfunction, endothelium, 13
PIH. See Pregnancy-induced hypertension
Plaque Hypertension Lipid-Lowering Italian
        Study. See PHYLLIS trial
Postganglionic neuronal inhibitors, 317–319
Potassium, dietary supplement, 65
Practitioners Trial on the efficacy of
        Antihypertensive Treatment in the
        Elderly hypertension. See PATE trial
Preeclampsia, 291–292

Printed and bound by CPI Group (UK) Ltd, Croydon, CR0 4YY

Printed and bound by CPI Group (UK) Ltd, Croydon, CR0 4YY

16/04/2025

14658827-0001